# Clinical Examination

JOHN MACLEOD
Consultant Physician, Western General Hospital, Edinburgh
Consultant Physician, Royal Edinburgh Hospital
Consultant Physician, Clinic for Rheumatic Diseases,
Royal Infirmary Edinburgh
Head of University Department of Medicine,
Western General Hospital, Edinburgh

# Clinical Examination

A Textbook for Students and Doctors by Teachers
of the Edinburgh Medical School

*Editor*

JOHN MACLEOD

*Foreword by*

SIR STANLEY DAVIDSON

FOURTH EDITION

CHURCHILL LIVINGSTONE

EDINBURGH LONDON AND NEW YORK 1976

CHURCHILL LIVINGSTONE

Medical Division of Longman Group Limited

Distributed in the United States of America by
Longman Inc., 19 West 44th Street,
New York, N.Y. 10036 and by associated
companies, branches and representatives throughout
the world.

First Edition 1964
Second Edition 1967
Reprinted 1968
Reprinted 1970
Third Edition 1973
Reprinted 1974
Fourth Edition 1976
Reprinted 1977

ISBN 0 443 01437 X


**Library of Congress Cataloging in Publication Data**

Edinburgh, University. Faculty of Medicine. Clinical examination.

Includes index.
1. Diagnosis. I. Macleod, John George. II. Title [DNLM: 1. Diagnosis. 2. Physical
examination. WB200 U58c].
RC71.E33 1976 616.07'5 75-35601

Printed in Great Britain by
Butler & Tanner Ltd, Frome and London

# Foreword

A sound basis for treatment and a guide to prognosis can be provided only if the correct diagnosis is established. This in turn depends on a properly conducted clinical examination, supplemented where necessary by certain specialised procedures. This book is concerned with the taking of the history, the making of the physical examination and the evaluation of the information obtained.

Written in clear and concise language and in a style which holds the reader's interest, its aim is to provide the clinician with an up-to-date account of those methods of clinical examination which have proved to be of value. That this desirable objective has been fully attained is indeed not surprising because the book is written by a team of eight men in the prime of life who are close friends and who have had many years' experience of teaching undergraduate and postgraduate students. They are colleagues on the staffs of the Western and Northern General Hospitals, institutions which have played a notable part in maintaining and enhancing the reputation of the Edinburgh Medical School since their establishment as centres of teaching and research in 1946.

I can recommend this book unreservedly to medical students and general practitioners, and I also believe that many physicians working in hospitals would obtain from it both benefit and enjoyment.

STANLEY DAVIDSON.

1964.

'My first point is therefore this, that in any branch of university education, including medical education, we should aim at using the methods of education rather than instruction. We must teach the student how to collect the facts, to verify them, to assign a value to them, and how to draw conclusions from them and test those conclusions; in short, how to form a judgement. As Karl Pearson said, "the true aim of the teacher should be to impart an appreciation of method rather than a knowledge of facts," for method is remembered when facts have been forgotten, and method can be used in a new situation where there are no, or too few, facts. The student learns how to learn and can go on acquiring knowledge for the rest of his life.'

SIR GEORGE PICKERING
Medicine's Challenge to the Educator.
*British Medical Journal*, 1958.
Vol. 2, p. 1117.

# Preface to the Fourth Edition

Publication of a Fourth Edition within 12 years of the First has been prompted not by a need for fundamental changes but by a desire to ensure that the description of the clinical methods and their interpretation is in step with advances in the practice of medicine. The text has therefore been carefully revised once more. Constructive criticisms by colleagues and students from all over the world continue to give us an additional stimulus.

The aim of the book is to provide an account of the procedures carried out by a doctor examining a patient in the consulting room or at the bedside. We have sought to identify the principles on which these techniques are based and to analyse the information obtained in this way. Each chapter conforms to a general plan; starting with the history the reader learns how to elicit and evaluate symptoms; the methods of physical examination are then described and the significance of the findings is discussed. Finally an indication is given of the type of investigation which may be required as a logical extension of the clinical examination.

The contents are presented in the same order as in the Third Edition. An introductory chapter on the history and the general principles governing the physical examination is followed by an account of the assessment of the psychological state which must form at least part of the evaluation of every patient. The third chapter illustrates the analysis of symptoms and signs while the fourth stresses the importance of the observation of the patient and also describes those aspects of the clinical examination which cannot be assigned to any single system. Thereafter the examination of the cardio-vascular, respiratory, alimentary, genito-urinary, nervous and locomotor systems is described. Particular attention has been devoted to the anatomical and physiological background of the neurological examination and to the interpretation of the findings. After the accounts of the major systems the special problems concerned in the examination of the infant and child are described. Separate chapters are devoted to the use of the ophthalmoscope and to simple laboratory tests which constitute an integral part of the clinical assessment and which should be within the competence of any doctor. The appendices contain detailed information about anthropomorphic measurement at all ages and about traditional systems of case recording as well as the newer problem orientated medical records.

The book is intended primarily for undergraduates but we hope it will be of value to general practitioners and to the potential specialist. As the very junior medical student may feel overwhelmed at first by the range and detail of the methods involved, we have also produced a small pocket-book 'An Introduction to Clinical Examination' designed to be of service in the initial weeks of clinical training by selecting out and describing very simply the fundamental techniques of clinical examination. The Fourth Edition of *Clinical Examination* is also closely integrated with the Eleventh Edition of *Davidson's Principles and Practice of Medicine* in which most of the contributors and the editor participate.

The contributors are teachers of undergraduate and postgraduate medical students in University centres and include general physicians and a surgeon, a cardiologist, a respiratory physician, an endocrinologist, a neurologist, an orthopaedic surgeon, psychiatrists and a paediatrician. Although most sections have largely been the responsibility of one person, each contributor has been supported by uninhibited comment from his colleagues.

Throughout the book emphasis has been placed on the need to obtain valid evidence by reliable methods and for thinking in terms of clinical science. If we have succeeded in creating an urge to comprehend, as well as an ability to collect accurate data, we shall feel amply rewarded.

JOHN MACLEOD.

# Acknowledgements

We are indebted to the Medical Photography Unit and to the Department of Medical Illustration, University of Edinburgh, for assistance in the preparation of the plates and some of the diagrams, and also to Professor P. J. Hare and Professor I. C. Michaelson for permission to reproduce colour plates. We found some of our quotations in *Doctors by Themselves* compiled by E. F. Griffith, *The Quiet Art* compiled by Robert Coope and *The Medical Works of Hippocrates* translated by J. Chadwick and W. N. Mann. We are much obliged to these authors and their publishers for giving us permission to make use of their work.

We are indebted to Dr J. F. Munro who made many helpful suggestions about the book as a whole and to Dr N. C. Allan who revised the section on examination of the blood.

It is a special pleasure to acknowledge all the help we have had from our publishers in the preparation of the manuscript.

# Contributors

Carstairs, G. M., M.D., F.R.C.P.Edin., D.P.M. Vice-Chancellor, University of York. Formerly Professor of Psychological Medicine, University of Edinburgh.
*The Examination of the Psychological State.*

Forfar, J. O., M.C., B.SC., M.D. St. And., F.R.C.P.Edin., F.R.C.P.Lond., D.C.H., F.R.S.Edin. Professor of Child Life and Health, University of Edinburgh.
*The Infant and Child.*

Fraser, Sir James D., B.T., M.B., CH.B., F.R.C.S.Edin. Professor of Surgery, University of Southampton.
*The Examination of the Breasts, the Acute Abdomen Etc.*

French, E. B., B.A., M.B., B.CHIR.CANTAB., F.R.C.P.Edin., F.R.C.P.Lond. Reader, University Department of Medicine, Western General Hospital, Edinburgh.
*The Alimentary and Genito-Urinary Systems.*
*The Use of the Ophthalmoscope.*

Grant, I. W. B., M.B., CH.B., F.R.C.P.Edin. Consultant Physician, Respiratory Diseases Unit, Northern General Hospital, Edinburgh.
*The Respiratory System.*

Macleod, J. G., M.B., CH.B., F.R.C.P.Edin. Head of University Department of Medicine, Western General Hospital, Edinburgh.
*The History and the General Principles Governing the Physical Examination.*

Matthews, M. B., M.A., M.D.CANTAB., F.R.C.P.Edin., F.R.C.P.Lond. Consultant Cardiologist, Western General Hospital, Edinburgh.
*The Cardiovascular System.*

Mawdsley, C., M.D.Manch., F.R.C.P.Edin., F.R.C.P.Lond. Head of University Department of Neurology, Edinburgh.
*The Nervous System.*

Robson, J. S., M.D., F.R.C.P.Edin. Reader, University Department of

Medicine, Royal Infirmary, Edinburgh.
*The Examination of Urine, Blood, Vomit, Faeces and Cerebrospinal Fluid.*

Scott, J. H. S., M.B., CH.B., F.R.C.S.Edin. Consultant Orthopaedic Surgeon, Western General Hospital and Princess Margaret Rose Orthopaedic Hospital, Edinburgh.
*The Locomotor System.*

Strong, J. A., M.B.E., M.A., M.D.Dubl., F.R.C.P.Edin., F.R.C.P.Lond., F.R.S.Edin. Professor of Medicine, University Department of Medicine, Western General Hospital, Edinburgh.
*The General Examination and the Common External Features of Disease.*

Walton, H. J., PH.D., M.D., F.R.C.P.Edin., D.P.M. Professor of Psychiatry, University of Edinburgh.
*The Examination of the Psychological State.*

# Contents

# CHAPTER 1

# The History and the General Principles Governing the Physical Examination

'And I place the interrogation of the patient himself first, since in this way you can learn how far his mind is healthy or otherwise; also his physical strength and weakness, and you can get some idea of the disease and the part affected.'

RUFUS OF EPHESUS (c. A.D. 100)

The clinical study of disease is founded on two essential processes, the history of the patient's disability, and the doctor's physical examination. The term 'clinical examination' comprises both these components. Although in practice the two may be intermingled, an adequate clinical examination is based on a methodical and comprehensive routine to which the student should closely adhere, particularly throughout his apprenticeship. Flexibility will come with experience. This chapter gives an account of the sequence which should normally be followed by the doctor in the consulting-room or at the bedside.

## THE HISTORY

As Rufus of Ephesus pointed out almost 2000 years ago, the history is usually the most valuable part of the clinical examination in leading to a diagnosis. Every medical student is, rightly, taught this—and then spends the remainder of his life in practice relearning the lesson. The doctor's first task is to listen and observe, not only to obtain information about the current problem but also to understand the patient as a person and the life situation in which he finds himself.

The art of obtaining an accurate history expeditiously can be acquired and developed with practice, provided it is founded on certain fundamentals, the first of which must be a satisfactory approach to the patient. Secondly, ample opportunity must be given to the patient to tell his story. Thirdly, a competent interrogation must be made by the doctor to clarify the patient's account and, when indicated, to extract information regarding previous health, family and social and personal matters. The same sequence is followed with almost every patient, the emphasis changing in accordance with the current problem. When the basic technique has been acquired, skill will improve with experience until an efficient routine is at the doctor's command, flexible enough to deal with the manifold vagaries of clinical practice. Impatience is the commonest cause of failure.

## The Approach to the Patient

The individual who is ill and who is possibly apprehensive when confronted by a doctor is readily disturbed if first impressions are bad, for example, if the doctor appears indifferent or unsympathetic; an emotional barrier to effective communication is then erected. It is, therefore, essential that the patient is put at ease by being given a friendly greeting, and made to feel that he is the centre of interest. In the surgery or in the outpatient department it is easy to acquire the bad habit of completing notes about the previous case at the crucial moment when the newcomer should be welcomed. Rather it should become second nature for the doctor to have all his senses alert, particularly at the outset; the clinical examination begins from the moment of first contact with the doctor who must not miss the revealing, fleeting gesture or other non-verbal forms of communication.

The patient may be embarrassed by not knowing to whom he is speaking, and accordingly appropriate introductions should be made, for example by medical students. At the outset the doctor should do the talking while the patient adapts himself to the situation. Initial remarks should be about impersonal matters; a minute or so can be spent with profit in this way to help eliminate any preliminary diffidence. Any impression of hurry on the doctor's part must be avoided. One can then proceed to obtain particulars about name, address and occupation, and conversation can readily be built round the last while confidence accrues. Addressing the patient by his or her name is good for the individual's self-esteem and for establishing a less impersonal relationship—a discreet glance at the notes may be necessary to prevent an embarrassing mistake. It is also wise to be sure whether it is 'Miss', 'Mrs.' or 'Ms'. A satisfactory initial relationship has been achieved when the patient and the doctor have begun to get to know each other. Conditions should then be favourable for the patient to express himself.

## The Patient's Account of the Current Illness

The patient is now given an opportunity to tell his story in his own way, and in order to encourage him to do so the initial question must be of a general nature, e.g. 'Now please tell me about your trouble'. If he has difficulty in starting, ask 'What was the first thing you felt wrong?', followed by 'What happened next?'. As the history proceeds, the doctor should learn much about the symptomatology, the patient's intellectual capacity and his emotional reaction to his troubles. Premature interruption must be avoided; learning to listen comes with experience and patience and is particularly important when dealing with a psychological problem (p. 17). Further action depends on the initial assessment of the personality of the patient. While the possibilities are innumerable, certain situations commonly recur;

for example, there is the intelligent person who gives a clear unemotional account, the 'good witness'. This kind of description often points straight to the diagnosis with little further help from the doctor. The inarticulate person will require patient handling and help by the posing of very simple questions, whereas the verbose individual, giving irrelevant details, will need guidance to direct his attention to essentials; even so, there is still a danger of premature interruption by the doctor. The quasi-knowledgeable individual, in relation to medical matters, tends to give his own diagnosis rather than an account of his symptoms and speaks in terms of 'flu', 'gastritis', 'rheumatism'. 'migraine', etc. It is important not to accept such statements without reviewing their basis. The emotionally disturbed patient, worried by his illness or frightened in a doctor's presence, must be handled with sympathy, but the doctor must remain alert to detect sources of psychological stress which may require elucidation later. Elderly patients are liable to give the keen young doctor the answer they think will please him, deafness or early dementia may add to the misunderstanding, particularly if the doctor has failed to appreciate that the patient's mental functions are impaired. Timidity, guilt or fear of disease may lead to information being suppressed. In contrast, symptoms may be exaggerated in an attempt to ensure attention. Wilful deceit is rare except by alcoholics and drug addicts; the latter are often expert at faking symptoms, as are patients with Munchausen's disease whose motive is to gain admission to one hospital after another on the basis of a convincing but mendacious tale of illness. Other examples of personality disorder and sociopathy are described on page 26. In Trousseau's words, *'Il n'y a pas de maladies; il n'y a que des malades.'*

### Interrogation by the Doctor

**1. The Current Illness.** It is first necessary to clarify the patient's account to ensure that all the symptoms have been elicited and to evaluate them. The art of cross-examination, like the preceding technique, is also one which develops with practice, provided certain principles are observed. Questions should be formulated simply and clearly. When a satisfactory answer has been obtained, the same question should not be repeated, thoughtlessly, later. This usually results from inattention and gives a poor impression of the efficiency of the examiner. However, it may sometimes be necessary deliberately to pose the question again, possibly in a different way to obtain a more illuminating account, or if the subsequent interrogation throws doubt on the accuracy of the original answer. Many individuals are very open to suggestion and unintentionally provide erroneous information if a certain answer would appear to be expected. Biased and premature questions in conjunction with a perplexed patient open to suggestion and anxious to help the doctor, may result in a very distorted history. It is therefore important, particularly while the basic facts are being elicited, not to ask leading questions which may act as guides to the answers desired by the doctor. Later in the proceedings, however, it may be necessary to use such questions to elucidate the patient's account provided the fallacies involved are kept in mind.

The principal symptoms must be thoroughly analysed. Examples of this process are given in Chapter 3, but basically the doctor must satisfy himself that he has accurate information regarding the time and mode of onset of any important symptom, the circumstances in which it occurred, its duration and the existence of any ameliorating or aggravating factors. The relationship to other symptoms must be defined and a chronological account obtained of the development of the illness from the first symptom to the date of interview. If possible, exact dates should be recorded rather than imprecise statements such as 'last Saturday' or 'a few weeks ago'. It may be helpful to reproduce the symptoms and observe what happens, for example the patient who complains of breathlessness on exertion may be studied as he goes upstairs. If there is difficulty in describing a recurrent symptom of varying severity, the position may be clarified by asking for an account of the first or of the most severe attack. It is often necessary to record negative findings, e.g. cough but no sputum, or breathlessness but no cough.

*Systemic Enquiry. Drugs? Allergy?* When a clear record has been obtained of the current complaint it is advisable to make specific enquiries about the presence or absence of cardinal symptoms suggestive of involvement of various systems, such as cough, breathlessness, indigestion (the imprecise word is deliberately used to broaden the scope), bowel, urinary or menstrual troubles, pain, insomnia or change in weight. It is essential to know about any *drugs* taken on medical advice or otherwise and if the patient is *allergic* to any substance (p. 15). These questions can be asked very quickly and a comprehensive view of the patient's health thus obtained.

*Information from a Third Party.* It is necessary to obtain information from a relative or friend when the patient is unable to supply it because of immaturity, illness, senility or mental disturbance. Corroboration is often helpful when the patient is a poor historian. Every effort should be made to obtain an account from an eye-witness in the case of a person who has been unconscious or who may be suffering from epilepsy or from other conditions in which knowledge of the patient's behaviour or appearance may be useful. The description from an onlooker of the circumstances in which an injury occurred may be helpful, but in obtaining this evidence from a third party the doctor must be careful not to give to unauthorised persons information which may be confidential or have medico-legal repercussions. Important information is often obtained from relatives also by the nursing staff and by social workers, particularly in psychiatric problems.

**2. Previous Illness and State of Health.** Information should be obtained about previous illnesses, operations and accidents as indicated by the individual problem and preferably in chronological order. The patient may have forgotten about past illness and his memory may be stirred by being asked if he has ever been in hospital or been confined to bed at home. It must be remembered that the diagnosis supplied by the patient may not be correct, either because of misapprehension, misdiagnosis, or because, in the patient's interests, it had been judged advisable to give him a less harsh explanation; a gastric carcinoma may have been described as an 'ulcer'. If medical records are not available, the examiner may have to decide about past episodes on the patient's description of symptoms and circumstances at the time, but it is salutary to realise that what may now be obvious because of the progress of the disease may have been impossible to diagnose even in the recent past. Frequently patients incriminate an accident as being responsible for subsequent troubles; any claim of this kind must be considered critically. A history of venereal disease may be suppressed, because of a feeling of guilt, and when it is suspected on clinical grounds the individual must be asked, not only about venereal infection, but also about the occurrence of any extra-marital sexual inter-course, as the initial disease may have been unnoticed by the patient or suppressed by an antibiotic.

*Residence or travel abroad* and any illness which occurred may be relevant; a puzzling fever may prove to be due to malaria or amoebiasis contracted outside Britain. Air transport enables vast distances to be covered within the shortest of incubation periods so that almost any infection may be transmitted to an area where it is not normally encountered. Patients will not necessarily mention their journeyings unless specifically asked if they have been abroad. The onus is on the doctor to make the necessary enquiry.

*Previous Health.* Just as knowledge of previous illness may be necessary in assessing a clinical problem, so also may information about past health. A medical examination for insurance or employment purposes would give a good basis for comparison with the present findings. In all cases it is most helpful to know the date and result of any previous radiological examination, especially of the chest. The films should be reviewed if there is any doubt about the result.

**3. Family History.** Information regarding the age and health, or cause of the death of the patient's relatives is often valuable. The knowledge that there is a family history of diabetes, ischaemic heart disease, hypertension, gout or an infectious disease such as tuberculosis, should increase the doctor's awareness of the possible presence of such a condition in the patient. The symbols used in the construction of a family tree or pedigree chart are illustrated in Figure 1.

Often there is unwarranted anxiety on the patient's part lest like a parent he may be in the process of developing some potentially crippling disease such as rheumatoid arthritis. Considerable tact may have to be deployed when asking a new patient about features such as alcoholism or mental disorder in a close relative. Overall, however, a display of interest in the welfare of the family usually helps to secure rapport.

At this stage it is usually possible to obtain at least an impression of the individual's personal relationships but enquiry about more intimate matters, if deemed necessary, is best postponed until after the physical examination when a good measure of confidence should have been established. However, if the patient wishes to unburden himself about emotional disturbances at any phase of the proceedings he should be allowed to do so as the opportunity may not occur again. Sexual problems, a broken marriage, difficulties with elderly relatives living in the same house, problem children or adolescents, or an unhappy childhood are all very potent influences on an individual's well-being. On the other hand, the family may constitute a united group able to give substantial support to any member in difficulty.

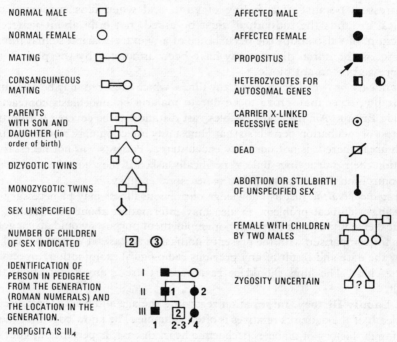

FIG. 1    Symbols used in pedigree charts.

Drawing up a family tree begins with the affected person first found to have the trait (*propositus* if male, *proposita* if female). Thereafter relevant information regarding siblings and all maternal and paternal relatives is included. From *Elements of Medical Genetics*, by A. E. H. Emery. Churchill Livingstone. 1974.

**4. Social History.** An individual's adaptation to his occupational and social environment may, like family influences, have profound repercussions on his health. Illness may ensue directly as in the case of silicosis or indirectly as in malnutrition; social problems may arise as a result of illness. The doctor working in hospital sees the patient in an artificial setting and it is important for him to have some knowledge of the individual's normal background, not only in relation to diagnosis, but also in the planning of rehabilitation.

A description ('profile') of how the patient spends an average day may be helpful in determining realistic therapeutic goals. The patient's functional capacity must be assessed and related to his employment, for example in cases of heart or lung disease, return to heavy work or to a polluted atmosphere may be contraindicated. Enquiry should, therefore, be made about home, occupation, personal interests and habits.

As regards the *home*, it may be necessary to know about the number of rooms and their occupants, the sanitary arrangements, the state of repair of the house and the financial obligations of the residents. Neighbours may create problems or may be very helpful in times of stress. A social worker can often obtain invaluable information by reporting on home conditions.

It is desirable to know not only the mere fact of the patient's *occupation* but what it involves. It is good practice to encourage conversation about this at appropriate times during the physical examination. Useful information is obtained, the anxious patient is diverted and the doctor's interest is usually appreciated. Attention should be paid to the congeniality or tedium of the employment, to any occupational hazards, and to stresses imposed by others or by the individual's own ambitions. Frequent change of employment may indicate an inadequate personality. Many married women have a part-time occupation, because of real necessity, because of the need to maintain hire-purchase commitments, or because of boredom at home. The type of work and the reason for undertaking it should be known. It is necessary to have at least some appreciation of the overall economic situation of the patient and his family.

The doctor should also be aware of the patient's *personal interests*, such as his leisure pursuits, the amount of physical exercise undertaken, and his educational background. *Habits* as regards food, tobacco and alcohol may have important implications in relation to nutritional problems, lung disease and psychological instability respectively. A dietetic history should be obtained if there is an obvious nutritional abnormality. In most instances an approximate assessment by the doctor of the patient's food and vitamin intake will suffice but he should not accept the corpulent woman's claim that she eats nothing or the statement by the girl with anorexia nervosa that she eats everything. Deficiencies of substances such as folate or vitamins C or D occur in elderly patients whose accounts of their eating habits may not be corroborated by a neighbour or by evidence obtained from a brief inspection of the larder. Occasionally a precise evaluation by a trained dietician is required.

Gradually a picture should emerge of the individual as a whole in relation to his background and with discrimination the details can be elaborated as demanded by the current problem.

**5. The Psychological History.** In all illness it is necessary to evaluate the part played by psychological factors. The account of the history and the manner in which it is delivered usually reveal much about the patient's personality. The reaction of the individual to distressing situations in the past is also significant, as similar patterns of behaviour tend to recur. Frequently this information, supplemented by negative findings on physical examination, will direct attention to the need for a more detailed psychological assessment by the examining doctor. In the earlier stages of the interview the doctor should have recognised any traumatising life events, such as bereavement, separation or rejection in the patient's experience and these should now be further explored. It is usually possible to start the patient talking about emotionally disturbing topics by such remarks as, 'You had begun to tell me about a disagreement with——', or 'Tell me more about your mother who died last year'. If no obvious opening presents, a more direct approach is necessary; the patient should be asked if anything is worrying him and thereafter any factor of possible significance must be further explored. Often specific questions must be posed about the existence of anxieties regarding financial, occupational, domestic, sexual or religious matters. Frequently fear of disease, such as cancer, is a potent source of stress, and the same fear may inhibit disclosure of what is in the individual's mind unless specific questions are asked. Many individuals have good insight into their own personality and it may be profitable to know about their evaluation of themselves, with reservations about the opinion offered. The patient should be encouraged to talk freely about his problems, and about current difficulties in his association with people important to him, as self-disclosure to an understanding listener is of value from the therapeutic as well as from the diagnostic aspect. When this is done, it often becomes apparent to the doctor and to the patient that the presenting symptom, apparently physical in origin, is in fact a manifestation of a psychological difficulty. Frank, unhurried discussion in privacy can be time-consuming but there is no doubt that the experienced doctor finds that it is time well spent, as many emotional problems are resolved when they are brought to the surface and ventilated in a neutral environment. When emotional distress persists or when significant abnormalities are apparent or suspected in the patient's personality or in his mental processes, a formal assessment of the patient's psychological state is required. The interview employed for this purpose is described in Chapter 2.

*The Doctor–patient Relationship.* In addition to the patient's response to his problem, the interactions between the patient and the doctor have also to be considered. This relationship is very complex as a result of the interplay between different personalities in potentially unstable situations and anything from harmony to antagonism can ensue.

The patient will 'transfer' to the doctor his habitual modes of behaviour, some of these deeply ingrained and learned from his parents. Thus an aggressive attitude to the doctor may represent the patient's habitual reaction to people regarded as uncompliant, in this case a doctor who does not speedily relieve painful or frustrating symptoms. The patient with hysterical symptoms characteristically masks his distress by a show of 'smiling unconcern'.

When the doctor points out to the patient his apparent need to present himself as jovial or indifferent, this form of defensiveness is often replaced by more appropriate anxiety. Other defence mechanisms include the repression of unpleasant matters, the projection of faults on to others, rationalisation and over-compensation.

Noxious intensifications of, the patient's relationship to the physician can occur. Erotic transference is the best known of these extremely troublesome developments. The patient comes to believe she loves the doctor and by gesture or statement conveys this to him. Occasionally, and disastrously, a clinician reacts by responding to this supposed sexual invitation. Erotic transference however is really indicative of a longing to be accepted without at the same time being exploited. The clinician is not called on to react to the overtly seductive statements but rather to the basically childlike behaviour of the patient. Thus, far from responding either on a similar level, or by rejection of the patient, the doctor can properly view the declaration of love as an aspect to be assessed as methodically and calmly as any other highly emotional communication.

The clinician should not depart from his professional position as a neutral non-judgemental observer and react to troublesome patients with criticism, anger, dislike, disapproval or dismissal. In contrast, some patients strive to manipulate him by flattery or other manoeuvres and the doctor may go to excessive lengths to meet their demands. Yet other patients cause the doctor to feel helpless and inadequate. By observation of his own feelings—i.e. the effect the patient has on him—the clinician can often gain a much clearer perception of what the patient is trying to achieve. The doctor can improve his management of a situation when the feelings aroused by the patient are carefully assessed, but not acted upon.

The adaptation of the medical student to his patient will be facilitated if he systematically gives consideration to interpersonal factors of this kind. Poise will come with understanding, self-awareness and self-control. In these circumstances it is seldom that the doctor loses control of the situation in his conscious efforts to create an effective relationship with his patient.

## The Taking of Notes

The human memory is far from reliable and its efficiency deteriorates with ageing and with the passage of time. It is, therefore, essential that a record be made of the findings without delay. The history should be written down as it is given; with practice this can be done quickly with little or no interruption of the patient's narrative. Some doctors develop a form of shorthand which may serve their own purposes, but it is obviously essential that notes should be legible and comprehensible if others have to use them. It will clearly not be necessary to write down all that is said as much may be irrelevant, but the recording of the patient's own words is particularly valuable in psychiatric illness (p. 18).

However, note taking may have an inhibitory effect when highly personal matters are being discussed; it may then be advisable to lay the pen aside and later record an appropriate account. A nervous patient often hurriedly jumps from one topic to another and then it is best to jot down headings and elucidate the sequence and details later. In some circumstances, for example if the history is very complicated, it may be good policy to make rough notes at the time and later elaborate these into an orderly account. This should commence by stating the presenting symptoms and their duration and be followed by a description of the development of the illness. Students will inevitably make mistakes at first, but with practice they will learn to sift the evidence, select the facts which merit prominence and record them in a coherent form.

### Conclusions on Completion of History

When the history has been obtained to the doctor's satisfaction the first step has been taken towards diagnosis. The information must be appraised, taking into account the reliability of the patient as a witness. The relevant facts must be separated from the irrelevant and evaluated objectively. The logical analysis and interpretation of the evidence may then lead either to a provisional diagnosis, to a differential diagnosis or to no conclusion. While the planning of the physical examination will be influenced accordingly, the doctor should remain unbiased and proceed to attempt to elicit further objective evidence which may confirm or refute the interpretation of the history or which may point in a wholly different direction.

## THE PHYSICAL EXAMINATION

During any clinical examination attention is frequently concentrated on one or more systems. However, a review of a patient's complaints too closely restricted to a single system can lead to errors in diagnosis as important disease elsewhere may be missed. It is not always possible to make a single diagnosis to embrace all the clinical features of disease encountered particularly in the elderly in whom multiple pathological lesions, not necessarily related and each requiring consideration, are commonly present.

The doctor carrying out a clinical examination must work on the assumption that he is entirely and solely responsible for seeking out the features of disease at all times rather than expect them to present or depend on the patient to draw attention to something that perhaps has been taken for granted. Occasionally and for a variety of motives, patients will not reveal what they regard as stigmata of disease, but as a rule failure to recognise these signs is due to careless or inadequate examination. Shortage of time may be a contributing cause. More commonly, however, the additional factor is the natural human failing either to recognise the obvious or to remain sufficiently alert when performing repetitive tasks.

For most purposes it would not be practicable for even the most obsessional of doctors to carry out all the minutiae of examination in every patient encountered, and some degree of compromise must be accepted. The undergraduate, however, must not hurry or attempt any short-cuts, but in all cases methodically follow a careful routine until he is thoroughly familiar with the procedure. Discrimination comes with practice and experience allied to a logical approach to the individual problem.

### Environment and Equipment

Before discussing a method of physical examination, consideration has to be given to the conditions under which it is conducted and to the equipment required.

Privacy is essential and this usually constitutes no problem in the home or in the consulting-room. In some families relatives may feel it is their duty to be present in numbers which may embarrass the patient and the doctor. The tactful dismissal of all, or all but one, is desirable. In a hospital ward, screens must be drawn round the bed before the examination begins. Steps should be provided for easy access to a high couch in the consulting-room. Comfort is necessary and encourages adequate relaxation. The examination couch should have an adjustable back-rest as it is easier for the patient in the semi-reclining position to converse, whereas he may feel at a disadvantage if lying supine at the outset. A back support is essential for the patient with heart failure who becomes breathless when lying flat. Illumination must be good. Exposure of the area to be examined must be adequate but not to an extent that might unnecessarily embarrass or chill the patient. Both patient and the doctor should be warm; auscultation of the chest of a shivering subject and palpation of the abdomen with cold hands are common faults, for apart from the discomfort, the consequent muscle sounds and the resistance of the abdominal wall impair the efficiency of the examination. Patients have, with good reason, perennially complained about such practices since the first century, when Martial wrote:

> I'm ill. I send for Symmachus; he's here,
> An hundred pupils following in the rear;
> All feel my pulse, with hands as cold as snow;
> I had no fever then—I have it now.

It is imperative that the handling of any painful area is gentle. Exhaustion, as a result of a prolonged examination, must be avoided; the risk of this is greatest in the frail or elderly. The needs of female patients require special consideration. While privacy is important, the presence of a relative or nurse is often desirable when dealing with a sensitive, frightened or hysterical woman and is essential when a rectal or vaginal examination is performed.

It is convenient for the doctor to carry on his person a stethoscope, a torch, a measuring tape, a pin and cotton-wool, and he should have ready access to a sphygmomanometer, an ophthalmoscope with auriscope attachment, a tendon hammer, a clinical thermometer, disposable wooden tongue-depressors, finger stalls, lubricant and a proctoscope. A weighing machine and a height scale should be available in the consulting-room and also facilities for procedures such as the testing of the urine described in Chapter 12.

## A Method of Examination

While the doctor must think about and record his findings in terms of systems, the actual sequence of examination should be conducted primarily with the comfort of the patient in mind. After a general inspection, the hands, upper limbs, head, neck, chest, abdomen and lower limbs are usually dealt with in turn. Thus information about the heart, lungs, breasts, axillary lymph nodes and spine is generally obtained at one time while dealing with the thorax, whereas facts relating to the nervous system are usually acquired piecemeal. This compromise presents difficulties to the student. At the outset of his training he should concentrate on the individual systems in turn and, later, learn to integrate his techniques. Practice may be obtained, at an early stage, by examining, and being examined by a student colleague. This will help to attain proficiency and will also give some insight into the patient's point of view. A routine is gradually acquired which should be both methodical and flexible. The experienced doctor varies the emphasis as a result of information obtained from the history. In some cases a comprehensive examination of all systems is imperative, while in other instances one system may require special attention and the remainder need only a very brief review. A word of explanation to the patient may be advisable if the examination commences at a point remote from the site of his complaint. Procedure will vary with individuals and circumstances and the method which is outlined here is intended to provide only a provisional working basis; it should be adapted as the occasion demands.

1. General inspection of the patient (demeanour, colour, physique, etc.) and his surroundings, e.g. the temperature chart in hospital.
2. Feel pulse and examine hands and arms.
3. Examine head and neck.
4. Proceed now either to area mainly affected or to anterior chest (heart, lungs, breasts and axillae) and then to back (lungs and spine).
5. Examine abdomen, groins and external genitalia.
6. Examine lower limbs.
7. Record blood pressure either now or later if the patient is still not relaxed.
8. Ophthalmoscopic examination.
9. Rectal or vaginal examination if indicated.
10. The temperature, weight and height can be recorded and a specimen of urine obtained either at the outset or at the end of the examination.

If unexpected abnormalities are elicited, a further change in emphasis in the examination may be required and it may be advisable to reassess some of the earlier findings considered then to be negative. Errors may be made by misinterpreting normal findings, for example regarding haemangiomata as indicative of purpura. It must also be remembered that the normal range of biological measurements such as the blood, like those of height and weight, is very wide.

Even the most unbiased and alert doctor must be constantly critical of his clinical abilities. The scientific training of the preclinical years should have engendered an objective attitude of mind in the medical student but even so the human failing of evolving preconceived ideas about one's findings is ever present. This is illustrated in Figure 2. When the diagrams have been studied

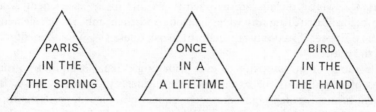

FIG. 2   The Three Triangles.

it will be found that most observers have interpreted the legends incorrectly as 'Paris in the spring' 'Once in a lifetime', and 'Bird in the hand'. We also tend to pay attention to findings which we consider significant and to ignore those which we judge unimportant. We are not aware of making this judgment and if it is faulty, errors arise. The verdict may be influenced unduly by other information and as a result varying interpretations of the same material are possible. This has been demonstrated by the differing reports given by experienced physicians when confronted by the same clinical problem, such as the site of the apex beat, the state of nutrition of a child or when interpreting a radiograph or an electrocardiogram; furthermore, when the same evidence is reviewed at a later date by the same individuals the second reports often differ significantly from the first. The range of observer variation and error is thus very wide. The junior clinician must be even more fallible, but mistakes should be fewer when there is a constant awareness of one's limitations, and a testing of one's conclusions against other objective findings. Errors can be put to profit if the reasons for them are critically analysed.

## FURTHER INVESTIGATION

At the conclusion of the clinical examination it may be possible to offer either a final or a provisional diagnosis. In the latter event consideration should be given to the further investigations which may be indicated. The scope and use of these should be regarded as logical extensions of the clinical examination. The number of investigations carried out varies extensively between one doctor and another depending upon knowledge, experience or philosophy. Some are insufficiently critical of the deficiencies of clinical methods, whereas others employ a large number of routine tests and also innumerable investigations, many of which may be only remotely connected with the problem under consideration. This latter practice has become possible in Britain where the National Health Service involves no increase in expense to the individual patient. However, even the simplest test costs money in time and materials; laboratories are apt to be so swamped with work that inaccuracies tend to occur; the patient may suffer unnecessary discomfort, and the doctor's clinical acumen does not develop in proportion to increasing experience. Many pitfalls are avoided if a full clinical assessment is always made before instituting any investigation, and then only those selected for a specific purpose. If in doubt it is helpful to ask oneself—'What benefit will this be to the patient?'.

The range of investigation is ever widening. Visual examination may, by means of instruments, be extended to the inner eye, the ear, nose, larynx, trachea, bronchi, oesophagus, stomach, duodenum, pleura, peritoneum, lower gut, urinary bladder and vagina. Biopsies may be obtained directly from many sites and also by aspiration methods, blindly, from the stomach, small intestine, pleura, lymph nodes, liver, spleen, kidney and other organs. Information may be obtained by recording electrical activity in the body by electrocardiography, electroencephalography and electromyography. Much help comes from the radiologist and in the laboratory area from the biochemist, microbiologist, pathologist, physicist and the pharmacologist and discussion of the problem by the clinician with other workers is often rewarding. However, all tests are prone to errors of measurement and interpretation and it should be the doctor in charge of the patient who finally weighs up all the evidence before deciding on diagnosis and prescribing treatment.

## CASE RECORDING

It is essential, whatever sequence may have been followed in the course of the physical examination, that the findings are recorded in a systematic form. When acquiring clinical experience, the undergraduate should take every opportunity of examining his patients in detail and of making a comprehensive written report of his findings. Later he will learn how the account may be adapted to meet the needs of the individual patient; in many circumstances quite brief notes will suffice. With most hospital patients, however, a detailed systematic report is usually essential. Records of normal or negative findings often prove very helpful when comparison has to be made at a later date. Problem orientated case records are discussed on page 469.

Case notes should be precise and free from any irrelevant or facetious comment which might cause embarrassment in more formal circumstances elsewhere. It is as well to remember that courts of law are empowered to demand a view of official records. The value of adequate notes, accurately and promptly recorded at the time of the illness or injury, has repeatedly been emphasised by Medical Defence Societies.

The record must be legible and easily understood. Incomprehensible abbreviations and symbols must be avoided, but simple diagrams are often useful adjuncts in demonstrating the site and extent of certain findings such as swellings (Fig. 4, p. 49). The abdomen in particular lends itself to the graphic illustration of abnormalities such as tenderness, guarding, palpable masses and enlargements of the viscera or lymph nodes (Figs. 39, p. 212; 42, p. 215). Diagrams are also helpful in illustrating neurological abnormalities (Fig. 90, p. 334) and the effects of trauma (Fig. 91, p. 335).

### Danger Signals

Many highly effective modern drugs have dangerous as well as beneficial potentialities. Interactions between drugs can also occur with adverse effects. It is therefore essential nowadays to find out about recent medication and know how this may influence the clinical features or indeed may be the cause of disease. When treatment entails a known risk it should be recorded prominently on the front of the case notes and it may be advisable for the patient to carry a card. Such warnings are particularly necessary when there is an idiosyncrasy to a drug, when overdosage is hazardous and when the therapy has profound effects on the metabolism of the recipient. Thus a careful history often reveals that an individual is hypersensitive to a substance in common use. Serious repercussions and even fatalities may be prevented if, for example, **penicillin allergy** is clearly noted. Long-term treatment is easily overlooked in an emergency and the danger of haemorrhage forgotten if a reminder is not readily available that the patient is having **anticoagulant therapy.** An even more important example is the hazard of acute adrenal failure in persons receiving **treatment with corticosteroids** and who are exposed to the stress of an acute infection or an operation. This risk may persist for many months after a preparation such as prednisolone has been withdrawn. It is fatally easy to forget about the danger involved unless the doctor is alerted by a conspicuous entry in the case notes.

### A System of Case Recording

This is given on page 466. It also outlines the main features dealt with in this and later chapters.

# THE METHODS IN PRACTICE

Diagnosis is an intellectual process requiring the integration of information derived from many sources. The medical student must learn first how to collect the facts and then, by analysing them, how to reach a diagnosis. With increasing experience it becomes possible at an early stage in the clinical encounter to decide on a provisional explanation. This is an hypothesis which is formulated to account for the symptoms and signs. This hypothesis is then tested systematically by a flexible and progressively more specific interrogation, by further physical examination and by special investigation; these lead to the confirmation or adjustment of the hypothesis or sometimes to its total replacement. In the last event alternative hypotheses are selected and analysed in turn as further data are collected until the presenting problem is solved. The student, trained in scientific method, will recognise that this attitude conforms to the current scientific approach in studying a biological phenomenon whereby explanatory hypotheses are tested and are given up when refuted by new evidence.

Some clinical problems must be explored in detail before they are solved; others are less obscure and a more direct pathway can be taken to the diagnostic destination. In either event a series of decisions is involved, the effective taking of which characterises the thinking of the competent doctor whose knowledge is well organised.

Making and testing diagnostic judgments constitutes a strict but rewarding discipline of continuous educational value; but, in addition to the intellectual approach required to reach a diagnosis, decisions made by scientific methods must then be applied effectively to meet the needs of the individual human being.

# CHAPTER 2
# The Examination of the Psychological State

'The most important practical skill which a student has to learn during his clinical instruction in psychiatry is the use of the interview as a technique of enquiry.'

(Royal Commission on Medical Education 1965-1968)

Examination of the psychological state consists of four parts:
1. The psychiatric history.
2. Examination of the mental state.
3. Evaluation of the personality.
4. The diagnostic formulation.

The interview is the method involved. While this is essentially history taking, the process is less formal than that involved in dealing with a purely physical problem and also differs in that therapy is involved at an earlier stage, if only by the fact that the patient is encouraged to talk to an understanding listener. A series of interviews may be necessary before the clinician acquires all the information needed to comprehend both the genesis and the course of the psychiatric illness. In the first interview the goal is at least a preliminary overall history; in the course of this, prominent abnormalities of the mental state will be detected; moreover, a tentative assessment of the patient's personality will be obtained and a working diagnosis should be possible. A diagnosis is a hypothesis about the nature of the illness and about its main aetiological factors. It is derived by the clinician from an informed synthesis of the facts elicited. Because diagnosis comes before therapy and because the clinician may wish to begin treatment in the course of the first interview, he aims to reach his preliminary diagnosis as soon as possible. The initial interview takes an experienced practitioner about half an hour. Subsequent interviews may be briefer and can be arranged as required to obtain further information and to extend the psychiatric examination.

While a theoretical knowledge of interviewing procedure is essential and while this process is a practical skill which can be acquired only through direct experience with patients, students can learn from studying practised interviewers at work. Furthermore, regular supervision is needed if technical errors are to be identified and corrected. An invaluable aid is provided by the use of videotape; the trainee interviewer has his psychiatric examination of the patient recorded, and when it is subsequently played back, he and his instructor have the actual clinical data before them for review.

When conducting the psychiatric examination, the clinician inevitably makes use of his own personality: he relies on his own capacity for communication. He would like to have an objective view of the extent to which he succeeds in expressing himself as he intends. His instructor and such aids as tape recording and television help to show him whether he is accurate in his impression about the way he affects people.

## THE CLINICIAN'S APPROACH

In the conduct of a psychiatric examination the clinician and his patient should sit in chairs placed more or less at right angles. They are then free to look at one another when they wish, without imposing any requirement for fixed stares as would be inevitable if the two participants were directly facing each other. A directorial station behind the office desk is of course altogether inappropriate. The room should be quiet and interruptions minimal.

A question and answer technique is not appropriate. The psychiatric history should flow smoothly from one topic to a related one in a sequence meaningful to the patient. The clinician acts as a catalyst. His primary function is to assist the patient to relate a clinically useful account of personal experience. The clinician writes steadily, to obtain an accurate, factual and full record of the interaction. Any questions he asks are also noted so that the verbal stimuli offered to the patient are recorded. A good history is neither nebulous nor abstract. When the patient mentions somebody, that person should be named; for example, 'I was going with a man friend at that time'. The clinician asks 'What was his first name?'. This is then recorded; if this person again enters the patient's account, in the present or a later examination, he can be rapidly identified and related to the earlier information.

The competent clinician does not take the patient firmly in a dull routine through each step in the historical sequence of events. He leaves the patient relatively free to reflect, to overcome hesitations, to go back and amplify, and to alter earlier statements as confidence is established. The clinician gently guides the patient, advises him when inconsequential detail threatens to crowd out important events and indicates quite frankly when he thinks the patient is following a blind alley. The clinician's task is to gain possession of the necessary facts in each of the crucial areas.

This apparent discursiveness is easier to permit the more experienced the clinician becomes. It is appropriate for him to indicate quite plainly to evasive patients that he must have the necessary information. He does not need to encourage the patient with phrases of approval or expressions of sympathy. It goes without saying that he should never convey moral censure or disapproval, although unwittingly clinicians sometimes do. He has no call to become autobiographical himself, and tell the patient about his own trying experiences, child rearing practices, or opinions and attitudes.

In the course of the examination the matters about which people are sensitive can be dealt with sensibly and directly as technical data. Behaviour usually regarded as wrong or unusual can be broached without equivocation, no hint of moral evaluation entering, e.g. 'Have you thought of ending your life?' Such an enquiry may be welcomed by a depressed patient as a much needed opportunity to disclose painful impulses towards suicide; the very process of speaking about these intentions may effectively serve to deter the patient from making a suicide attempt. Sexual experience is discussed in terms which the patient is sure to understand, checking where necessary the patient's term for a part of the body or a sexual activity. The contemporary patient will almost certainly know what 'masturbation' means, but not always; the clinician will often perceive that more explicit explanations or simpler words are needed to obtain the information he seeks.

While the patient is not constrained to give a formal, chronological and precisely sequential account, the clinician examining the psychiatric patient has a technical task to complete, a schedule of operations to be performed. This he aims to perform as methodically as he would examine any other clinical sector, the neurological system for example. Thus if he has not examined the ocular fundus, he will be aware of this omission, and if he neglects to test the plantar responses, the trained clinician likewise knows that his examination is incomplete. Similarly with the psychiatric assessment; if, for example, the clinician has not found out about the patient's family relationships, his understanding of the patient's personality is the poorer; if the patient's job record has been neglected, the history is also incomplete. The psychiatric examination is a technical skill, within the competence of all clinicians. One can know about a person's mind with more or less certainty according to one's ability to carry out the relevant clinical procedures.

## 1. THE PSYCHIATRIC HISTORY

**A. The Description of the Patient.** The patient's name, age, occupation, marital status, sometimes his religious affiliation and finally the method of his referral are facts the clinician will want to record. Eliciting such relatively neutral information may be a useful way of starting the history-taking; as he replies, the patient is able to settle in his chair as comfortably as possible, and to assess the situation in which he finds himself. The patient needs an opportunity to size up the clinician as the examination begins.

**B. The Reasons for the Consultation.** The clinician then ascertains why the patient has come, and what the patient requires of him. The patient's reason for the interview may on occasion be straightforward or at times bizarre. He may come on account of his own distress. The police may send a patient for examination, as occurs when a psychiatrist is asked to examine a woman who has harmed her children physically and has then attempted to kill herself. It may be a relative who brings the patient, as occurs when a mother tells the clinician she has been worried recently about her small son, and describes mannerisms which alarm her. The presenting reason for the referral of course may be merely the introductory gambit, to be extended when the clinician has gained the patient's confidence: a man complaining initially of indigestion may later disclose that he has actually come on account of impotence.

**C. The Present Illness.** Having established why the patient has requested to be seen, the clinician then obtains a detailed account of the patient's symptoms. Each complaint should be recorded scrupulously, in terms close to the patient's own. If the patient mentions a pain in the heart, that is to be noted as his symptom; it should not be translated into clinical jargon, such as 'praecordial pain'. If the clinician rephrases the patient's actual self-description into medical terminology, he impairs his own grasp of the patient's experience of illness. An adequate description of the illness has been reached when the clinician has traced chronologically each manifestation of the disorder.

**D. The Family History.** This consists of a verbal sketch by the patient of both his parents and of all his brothers and sisters. 'You mentioned your father—what sort of person is he?'. The question causes some patients to pause in perplexity, until after hesitation they describe the father as one of the best, or portray him as strict but perfectly fair, or as a mean man who terrorised the family when drunk at weekends. The clinician can usually determine whether the father was perceived positively, in a neutral light, or negatively. The importance of this information is that it conveys the role which a parent took in the formation of a patient's personality; a concept of each parent is incorporated during growing-up, forming an aspect of the patient's self.

The mother has also to be characterised and this can usually be done with less trouble. A patient may say of her that she was kind and gentle, or two-faced, or a virago who started her persecution before the patient's birth by striving to abort herself. Again, in describing his mother the patient is disclosing a significant relationship which contributed to his personality structure.

His position in the sibship may be important. If he was an only child, alone with his mother until 5 years of age when his father was demobilised from the army, then to have a baby sister arrive on the scene, the patient may proceed to describe a rivalry which agitated his childhood and coloured his subsequent social relationships in adult life with envy and competitiveness. The size of the sibship is obviously relevant. The clinician's perception of the parental family is filled out when the patient is asked to comment on the general atmosphere which existed in the home. Finally, the patient is asked to give details of any psychiatric illness suffered by his first and second degree relatives.

**E. The Personal History.** This can follow naturally from the account of the parental family. The clinician finds out if the patient thought he was a wanted child, whether he acquired control of his sphincters at the usual age, whether he bit his nails, and at what age he stopped using temper tantrums as a means of attempted mastery of the household—but these crucial facts are seldom elicited by blunt questions. To grasp in addition whether the patient separated from his mother without difficulty and managed to start his school attendance without anxiety, whether he had an early conduct disorder like stealing, or an early neurotic illness such as a childhood obsessional state, calls for an ability on the part of the clinician to empathise with the patient, so that the patient realises how accurately he is being understood.

One then discovers from the patient about the onset of puberty, the development of his sexual awareness and information, and the form of his erotic imagery. He tells whether he had a chum, a first close friendship. His progress at school is studied. The course of his adolescence discloses whether he was able to separate off gradually as an independent individual from his parents, and whether this social growth—if it occurred—was relatively untroubled, or took the form of a disruptive rebellion. Identity-formation proceeds rapidly from the middle teens, and if arrested the youngster does not arrive at an understanding of his personal potentiality, nor a decision about the work he is fit for, nor a definition of the values he wants to advance. He may be greatly troubled about sexual aspects of this stage of maturation, with prolonged or recurrent fears about homosexuality or masculine inferiority. The girl may reject aspects of feminity. In the later teens the capacity for close relation with another person begins to develop if personal maturation is proceeding smoothly, the individual finding greater purpose when deeply fond of somebody else.

The clinician then inquires about courtship, marriage and the patient's own children. The patient may tend at first to deny any sexual or personal difficulties in his marriage, revealing these only later, when he has gained confidence in his doctor. The account of the personal history is completed by following the jobs the patient has had during the course of his working life and noting the quality of the patient's relationships with his employers, his workmates and acquaintances beyond his family circle.

**F. Previous Illnesses.** These are then studied; physical disorders are described more readily by the patient and can be rapidly surveyed. They can of course have emotional consequences, especially if they occurred early in life or left a disability which interfered with the patient's social participation.

Previous psychological disorders are sometimes more difficult to track down. They are often revealed if careful questioning is directed to the major stressful epochs· in the biography; the start of schooling, puberty, later adolescence, courtship, marriage and the onset of middle life with the realisation of advancing years. Any previous psychiatric disorders and the way they were managed are recorded in order of occurrence.

**G. The Previous Personality.** This is especially relevant in understanding the patient's illness. The onset of serious disease or psychosis may constitute a break with the patient's former self. Suddenly unheralded the delusion took form; the cheerful, busy man altered to become anxiously preoccupied and troubled by convictions that he suffered from cancer.

The previous personality is important not only to define the time of onset of

B

illness. It is also important because from his understanding of it the clinician can identify special strengths—perhaps obscured by the symptoms of illness—which the patient will be able to call on when recuperating; values and habits of mind, initiative, friendships and other social relationships, membership of groups, clubs and organisations, and special interests may be useful assets at this time.

As the patient speaks, the clinician writes. His transcript of the interview may not be orderly, but when he recasts material in systematic form, he will have obtained data in each of the important sectors of the patient's biography.

## 2. THE MENTAL STATE

Many of the clinical signs characterising the mental state of the patient will have become apparent during history taking. The clinician then has the opportunity to study any aspect of the psychological state which calls for special further evaluation.

**A. General appearance and behaviour.** The patient is described tersely but vividly, to provide a record which will suffice to call him to mind as he looked when in the examination room in terms of his posture, his expression, his clothes, his mannerisms, his reactions to the clinician, and his mode of presenting himself. In the case of a mute or stuporous patient this aspect of the mental state may be among the most revealing.

**B. Thought processes.** Talk is externalised thought; thus the clinician notes how ideas are handled and the manner in which the patient arranges and expresses his concepts. The major abnormality may be in this psychological sector. It may be disclosed in disordered syntax, as when a schizophrenic patient juxtaposes apparently unrelated references to a portion of his body and the river he lived close to as a child: 'This is my arm and the Thames is in England'.

SAMPLE OF TALK. A segment of conversation is written down, in the patient's own words, to convey in precise context his major preoccupation, and his way of expressing himself.

**C. Mood.** The clinician has probably already obtained much evidence about the prevailing affect before he asks the patient, 'How do you feel in yourself?' or 'What is your mood like?'. The patient may then state in dispirited tones that nothing that takes place means anything any more—'It's all flat'. In some instances sadness is not mentioned directly; instead the patient talks of a dead sensation in his chest or a heaving in his head, or the deeply pessimistic patient describes the surrounding world as grim and hopeless. In contrast, the hypomanic patient feels elated, full of energy, 'on top of the world'.

**D. Delusions.** The patient may disclose that he has developed false beliefs, misinterpreting everyday events as specially significant or attributing unwarranted intentions to people with whom he comes into contact. They are seen as intensely concerned with him, pestering him or maligning him or scorning him. He may not arraign particular people, but may consider himself under the control of outside influences: 'I know from the way I've been feeling that there is some evil force that is directed onto me by supernatural powers'.

**E. Hallucinations.** When a patient perceives sensations—visual, auditory, tactile, and so on—in the absence of any actual external stimulus, he may conceal the mental experiences which he himself has found startling, or may readily tell the examiner about them:

'During the morning of the 10th of March I was de-frosting my refrigerator when I distinctly heard my husband in his office, which is completely away from our house in an entirely different street. I heard him having consultations with three different people and then dictating letters to his secretary. During the early afternoon I was most disturbed to hear a strange male voice which was loud and clear. I got absolutely no peace from this voice which was accompanied by music and a mixed choir.'

This patient had alcoholic hallucinosis. In schizophrenia hallucinations also occur in a setting of clear consciousness, whereas in delirium they are accompanied by altered awareness.

**F. Obsessions.** These are thoughts—ideas or images—which the patient regards as foreign or silly and tries to dispel, but which nevertheless persist:

'The idea keeps coming back that I may be pregnant. I can't be quite certain. I've never had intercourse, and my periods never stopped, so with my logical mind I know it's impossible. I think over and over again that I may be having a child. I've sent away to an agency for a pregnancy test, and I saved up for an abortion.'

Compulsions are repetitive actions, the motor counterpart of obsessions in overt behaviour.

**G. Evidence of Intellectual Defect.** When there is either acute or chronic brain impairment, leading respectively to temporary or permanent intellectual defect, disorders of the following functions may be detected:

(a) ORIENTATION. An estimation of the patient's capacity to orient himself in time and space emerges as the history is taken and more accurate assessment is gained by testing the patient. The following five questions can be used, a score of one point being awarded for each correct answer: What year is this? What month is this? What day of the month is this? What is the place you are in now? In what town is it?

(b) MEMORY. This is tested by assessing the patient's ability to recall remote and recent events. The clinician may already have noted gaps or inconsistencies in the patient's account of himself. An unimaginative but effective question is to ask what he had for breakfast.

(c) ATTENTION AND CONCENTRATION. These are attributes of a normal person whose sensorium is intact. In delirium, in contrast, alertness and attentiveness are clearly deficient. Less obvious impairment may be revealed by the patient's inability to calculate an arithmetical sum correctly. The 'serial sevens' is a classical test. The patient is asked to subtract seven from 100 and to continue to take seven from what remains as rapidly and as accurately as he can. Most people will complete this task within one minute and will make no more than two mistakes.

(d) GENERAL INFORMATION. This is tested by asking the patient questions such as: Who is on the throne? Who ruled before? Who is the Prime Minister?

(e) INTELLIGENCE. This is assessed from the detail and subtlety of the patient's account of himself, his capacity to reason, the extent of his knowledge, and the level of his occupational attainment. Accurate measurement is made by use of standardised intelligence tests. These can be carried out by the clinician himself, or by a clinical psychologist and are expressed as the patient's Intelligence Quotient (I.Q.), the normal range of which is 80–120.

**H. Insight and Judgment.** This is the final sector in the examination, and deals with the extent of the patient's recognition that he is ill, his grasp of the nature of the disorder, and the realism of his judgment about his future.

## 3. EVALUATION OF THE PERSONALITY

The personality may be defined as the sum total of a person's actions and reactions—the individual as he appears to others, by reason of those persistent behaviour patterns which distinguish him from his fellows, and which form the basis of predictions about how he can be expected to act. Abnormalities of personality are expressed particularly in the individual's relationships with other people and these are unusual, in specific ways, when the personality is disordered.

The clinician diagnoses the personality by two clinical techniques. The first is applied during the history-taking. At the same time as he gathers facts about the illness, he takes note of the characteristic and repetitive behaviours which the patient describes—e.g. a man may give repeated instances of gross and passive dependence, first on his mother and later on a teacher, an employer, his wife, etc. The patient may ask for special tonics, may indulge in special pleading for another appointment in the very near future, may comment on the extent of his reliance on the doctor to take good care of him, etc. The clinician registers mentally, as he notes down these specimens of the patient's social responses, that a morbid pattern of clinging passivity appears to be emerging.

The second procedure depends on the use by the clinician of his own personality as an instrument in the clinical interaction. The clinician knows—or should know if adequately trained in interviewing—what effect he has on people—i.e. what behaviour he evokes from them. He knows from experience what reactions to him are exceptional, as when a patient becomes unduly aggressive or when excessive demands are being made of him. A patient with abnormal passivity may convey by his general demeanour that he will become a burden to the doctor, a 'dead weight'. The tentative personality diagnosis which may have been suggested by the patient's own account will then have been supported by his dependent mode of relating to the doctor, a characteristic which impairs the patient's social adaption. The doctor has observed his own responses to the patient, and made use of these as clinical information.

A third possible step to confirm these two sources of clinical information about the personality structure is to request formal personality testing, to be carried out by a clinical psychologist. Tests commonly used evaluate neuroticism (anxiety proneness), extroversion-introversion, hysterical and obsessional traits, and the level of aggression.

## 4. THE DIAGNOSTIC FORMULATION

The fourth part of the psychiatric examination is a technical decision-making procedure. The doctor coordinates all the data he has derived from the patient, decides on the relative weighting he will give to the different elements in the case and arrives at a diagnosis. In psychiatry this consists of two parts:

**A. The naming of the disorder** (or nosological diagnosis). The term to be applied to the illness depends on the most prominent symptoms and signs in the case, constituting one of the syndromes or disease patterns which can be found described in standard psychiatric texts, e.g. depressed mood, suicidal impulses, loss of appetite, retardation of thinking, physical apathy, self reproach and early wakening point to endogenous depressive psychosis.

**B. The psychodynamic formulation.** The second part of a psychiatric diagnosis lists, in a coherent sequence, the pattern of factors which the clinician considers to have contributed to bring about the illness, e.g. 'The patient, the submissive member of an identical twin pair, is less attractive than her sister; during childhood her mother discriminated against her, and the patient is now resentful and hostile. She tried to suppress these impulses in order to win affection from those to whom she forms overdependent attachments (e.g. twin sister, husband). Her illness began when she found evidence in her husband's wallet that he was associating with another woman.'

Because in successive examinations the patient may communicate fresh biographical material, the psychodynamic formulation becomes gradually fuller as confirmation is obtained for particular dynamic factors in the patient's adaptive pattern. The nosological diagnosis may also in some cases have to be revised. The formulation of the illness can well be tested—in many cases—by communicating it to other members of the medical team, who have also had contact with the patient. The value of concensus also enters for example, when the formulation is discussed with a general practitioner who has close knowledge about the patient and his environment.

## THE METHODS IN PRACTICE

### 1. The Recognition of Abnormal Personality

This example has been chosen because it is important that the clinician should be aware of the clinical presentation of the main types of abnormal personality. Such deviations can be identified from the information obtained by the application of the method set out in Section 3. Two degrees of severity can be recognised, the lesser being the personality disorders and the more severe being known as sociopathy.

#### A. PERSONALITY DISORDERS

There are three types of personality disorder:

(a) **Obsessional personality.** The obsessional person is rigid, over-attentive to details, and prefers to have everything predictable and orderly. He is over-careful, methodical, concerned with neatness and orderliness. He is meticulous, punctual, and over-organised, and becomes upset if his routines are disturbed. He may work compulsively and be unable to use opportunities for relaxation.

(b) **Schizoid personality.** The schizoid person is solitary, aloof and detached from other people. He may be pre-occupied with some impersonal activity in such realms as electronics, physics, mathematics or engineering. The personality deviation is recognised from the person's quietness and shyness, his disinclination to mix socially and his preference for solitary pursuits.

(c) **Hysterical personality.** Such people crave attention and appear insincere. They are characterised by excessive displays of emotion. The clinician diagnoses the disorder from the patient's showiness, histrionic manner and dress, and need to be appreciated. Speech is superficial, with ample exaggeration. The hysterical man cannot form any enduring attachment to one woman. The hysterical woman is often frigid sexually.

#### B. SOCIOPATHY

This is the more severe degree of abnormality of personality. The sociopath has a serious defect in his capacity for feeling. He has a severely defective conscience, and is often described as affectionless. He cannot form satisfactory relationships and major failures repeatedly occur in his marriage, his work and his social life. He is seen as indifferent, loveless and destructive. He comes into conflict with the customs and laws of the community. He does not learn from his failures, nor are his social transgressions corrected by punishment. His social ineptitude causes him to be persistently in trouble. Many sociopaths are superficially likeable and charming, and initially mislead well-meaning people, whom they subsequently disappoint and distress. A characteristic of sociopathic behaviour is impulsiveness. Uncontrolled emotional outbursts occur in the absence of sufficient provocation.

The sociopath may be punished repeatedly for the same unacceptable behaviour, continuing his antisocial behaviour pattern despite the harm it does him. He disregards possible consequences of his actions, and gives scant consideration to the welfare of those on whom he depends. There are two types of sociopathy:

(a) **Aggressive sociopathy.** Persons of this type make hostile attacks on other people, cause damage to property and often come to legal attention because of thefts or fraud.

(b) **Passive sociopathy.** A person of this type is seriously inadequate and chronically dependent and passive. Some are placid and responsive while others are cold, withdrawn and apathetic. They may adapt at so poor a level as to exist as aimless drifters to be found in places where hobos congregate. However, if the family is accepting and supportive, the inadequate sociopath may manage a sheltered existence under the protection of his relatives.

## 2. The Recognition of Psychiatric Illness

Analysis of the various forms of abnormal personality just described does not call for the detection of any signs or symptoms, but for the recognition of certain traits, qualities present in normal people also. These traits are found in excess in abnormal individuals, e.g. too much aggressiveness, or too high a degree of dependency.

To diagnose psychiatric illness, in contrast, the clinician requires the presence of symptoms or signs, i.e. new manifestations which are not present in normal people, such as those set out in Section 2, The Mental State. For example, the patient is psychiatrically ill when he has obsessions, suffers from a delusion or is hallucinated.

**Psychosis.** This is the first category of psychiatric illness to be sought clinically. By this is meant what the layman calls madness, and what used to be termed insanity. The patient's whole personality is affected by the illness. It has often come out of the blue, not being precipitated by some personal setback. Contact with reality is grossly impaired. The patient himself considers that he is drastically changed; a break has happened in his life, so that the person he is differs clinically from the individual he had formerly been.

Psychoses are either organic or functional. The former, when acute, is termed *delirium,* or a toxic confusional state. In the United States this is referred to as the acute brain syndrome. The person is hallucinated, deluded, seriously restless, his sensorium is impaired by some blunting of consciousness. The last feature is often diagnostic but may be so subtle as to be evident only to trained observers. Deliria run short courses lasting only a few days.

*Dementia* is the chronic organic psychosis. It is characterised by impairment of memory, chiefly recent memory. The patient has no difficulty recalling remote events, and may accept with relief a question about his youth rather than about news in the morning paper or the name of the present Prime Minister. In addition to amnesia, the patient with intellectual deterioration will have some disorientation for person and place, will show blunting of finer sensibilities so that the personality in time becomes a caricature of its former self, and will deteriorate to inability to give any accurate account of his present condition or of the surrounding realities. Dementia is progressive and irreversible.

The functional psychoses are not subdivided according to whether they are acute or chronic, but according to the prominent symptoms and signs. *Manic-depressive psychosis* is characterised, in the depressive phase, by a lowering of mood, so that the person is morbidly sorrowful, to the extent of depressing the clinician also. He believes all is hopeless, the future black; he is self-reproachful and often suicidal. In the manic phase such patients are unduly elated, with hyperactivity, unwarranted optimism, high physical drive and conspicuous lack of insight.

The second great category of functional psychosis is the *schizophrenias*. In these disorders the chief symptoms and signs are in the sector of thought. The patient's disordered thought may show a lack of expected connections between phrases, so that a sense of fog is generated in the clinician. The bizarre impression may be enhanced by blunting of feeling. In addition to thought disorder and affective blunting, the patient is autistic (detached from reality). These symptoms are not confused with organic psychosis, because the state of consciousness is absolutely clear.

**Psychoneuroses.** These are the minor psychiatric illnesses. Here only part of the personality is involved, so that only rarely is hospitalisation necessary. The housewife can manage many of her duties and the man his job. Insight is not impaired, as is the case with the psychoses. The illness follows a special psychological stress; this setback is not always stated plainly but becomes evident to the clinician, and often to the patient also, only after detailed exploration. The essential clinical feature is the presence of a psychoneurotic syndrome, i.e. a characteristic constellation of symptoms and signs typical of each type of psychoneurosis. Depending on the symptoms and signs which are most prominent the neurotic illness diagnostically may be one of the following: anxiety neurosis; hysterical neurosis, either conversion or dissociative type, depending on whether the symptoms are somatic or, in the latter type, consist of altered awareness such as occurs in psychogenic amnesia; phobic neurosis; reactive depressive illness; obsessional psychoneurosis.

As indicated in the description of the method for examining the mental state, the clinician may find the psychoneurotic patient is helped considerably by the mere communication of distressing experiences during the course of the interview.

# CHAPTER 3
# The Analysis of Symptoms and Signs

'If there is a fault in us bred of familiarity it is, I believe, the old fault
of omitting to probe sufficiently deeply into causes; the fault of accepting
the fact of common symptoms without trying to explain them.'

JOHN A. RYLE (1948).
*The Natural History of Disease*. London: Oxford University Press.

A comprehensive account leading to a complete understanding of all symptoms is not only outside the scope of this textbook, but is beyond the limits of
the present state of knowledge. The object of this chapter is to demonstrate by
a few examples how to obtain in full and to analyse in detail the information
which may be derived from a symptom or sign. Three symptoms have been
selected because they are common and important, because they illustrate
different but fundamental points, and because they are not within the
province of any single system subsequently described. *Pain* is a purely
subjective complaint. *'Blackouts'* show among other things the importance of
the interrogation of eyewitnesses. *Breathlessness* is often associated with
objective findings and can, if necessary, be reproduced.

Two signs have been chosen; *swellings* because they require systematic examination and because they may be encountered in almost any part of the
body; *oedema* because it provides a simple example of the clinical application
of physiological and pathological knowledge.

The junior student may find that the understanding of this chapter will be
facilitated after reading about the examination of the major systems.

## PAIN

**General Considerations.** The importance of pain in diagnosis cannot be
overestimated. Its subjective nature is such that it is only through personal
experience of pain that a doctor can have insight into the meaning of the
descriptions given by patients. Further understanding may be acquired by
careful enquiry and by observation. Sudden or severe pain may be accompanied by objective signs such as the withdrawal of a limb when the skin is
pricked or the muscle spasm which accompanies deep pain. Examples of the
latter are the sudden fixation of the lumbar spine in flexion at the onset of
lumbago, the catching of the breath due to pleurisy or the rigidity of the
abdominal wall in the presence of peritoneal inflammation. Other signs may
include pallor, sweating, vomiting or fainting, an involuntary shout evoked by
pain of abrupt onset, screaming attacks due to intestinal colic in children, and

groaning or crying due to protracted pain. Relief may be sought by characteristic actions such as the adoption of specific postures, the application of heat to the affected area or the use of appropriate medicines such as aspirin or alkalies. Pain as a symptom is poorly suited to investigation by animal experiments. Much of our knowledge has been gained by clinical observation and extended by experiment in human beings.

The distribution of pain resulting from the injection of hypertonic solutions at various sites has been studied. In addition many observations, particularly those made upon the raw bases of artificial blisters, have led to the identification of certain pain-producing substances. Among these, in concentrations which may be achieved in pathological circumstances, are hydrogen ions, potassium ions, acetyl-choline, histamine, 5-hydroxytryptamine and various polypeptides such as bradykinin. It is of interest that many of these substances are present in combination in the stings of nettles, wasps, hornets and other insects.

It is assumed here that the student is conversant with the anatomical and physiological facts about sensation. The nervous pathways for the conduction of pain are described on page 290. Briefly it may be recalled that while several sensations arise from the skin, pain is the main conscious feeling originating in the deep structures. In the skin, pricking, cutting, pinching and extremes of heat and cold cause pain, whereas considerable stretching fails to do so. In the viscera spasm of smooth muscle or distension may cause pain, but the other stimuli mentioned above do not produce any sensation. Ischaemia induces pain in all types of muscle, while the parenchyma of several structures including liver, spleen, kidneys and brain is completely insensitive. Rapid stretching of the capsules of these organs may cause pain such as that which arises from the liver in acute congestive cardiac failure.

The solution of a clinical problem demands that every aspect of a pain is elicited from the history. There will be many occasions when the cause of a pain is obvious without entering into details, but even then it is good practice, when time permits, to make a full enquiry. The experience gained through the variations which are encountered will improve diagnostic accuracy in difficult cases.

### The Analysis of a Pain

Information should be obtained by a system of analysis of pain based upon questions about the undernoted 10 features:

| | | | |
|---|---|---|---|
| 1. | Main site | 6. | Frequency and periodicity |
| 2. | Radiation | 7. | Special times of occurrence |
| 3. | Character | 8. | Aggravating factors |
| 4. | Severity | 9. | Relieving factors |
| 5. | Duration | 10. | Associated phenomena |

**1. Main Site of Pain.** With the eyes shut, it is possible to point precisely to the site of a pinprick on a finger-tip, yet on the skin of the back a spot several centimetres away from the point pricked may be indicated. Similarly two pinpoints can be distinguished from one when they are separated by about 3 mm over the finger-tip, yet the distance required between them may be as much as 50 mm on the leg or back. Localisation is proportionately less accurate in structures from which sensory stimuli rarely reach consciousness. For example, pain arising low in the thoracic spine may be felt in the hypogastrium, whereas a kick on the shin bone is correctly localised. Misinterpretation of the source of pain in the muscles of the trunk can be demonstrated by injecting hypertonic saline into the erector spinae on one side. This will cause an immediate pain in the back, poorly localised by pointing. The pain soon radiates through anteriorly on the same side. Muscle spasm and localised tenderness may then appear in front, signs which in other circumstances might lead to the erroneous supposition that an inflammatory lesion lies somewhere immediately beneath the examining finger.

By contrast with skin, normal viscera rarely give rise to conscious sensation, and localisation is poor. The oesophagus is, however, sensitive to extremes of temperature, and the bladder and rectum arouse characteristic sensations when they are full. To some extent therefore we are trained in the knowledge of the position of these organs, and for this reason pain arising in them tends to be correctly orientated. Localisation of pain originating in other viscera is far less accurate or specific. Thus pain in the epigastrium may arise from the stomach, duodenum, biliary tract, liver or pancreas. Unpaired structures such as the heart, pericardium, alimentary tract, liver, biliary system, pancreas, bladder and uterus tend to give pain deep in the midline anteriorly. Such mal-localisation could well be called referred pain, but the term is more conveniently reserved for spread beyond the main site. Paired structures such as muscles, bones and joints, eye, pleura and renal tract cause unilateral pain on the affected side. The localisation of pain in limb joints is usually accurate, presumably owing to training through sense of position, but a notable exception is the frequency with which pain from a disorder of the hip is referred to the knee, through mutual innervation by the obturator nerve.

While studying the main site of any pain it is often profitable to find out whether it is localised or diffuse, and at the same time to note any gesture made by the patient. For example, the pain of myocardial ischaemia is usually retrosternal and is often indicated by the flat of the hand laid upon the centre of the chest, by both hands outstretched over the pectoral regions or by a clenched fist pressed upon the centre of the sternum. The epigastric pain of peptic ulcer, on the other hand, is often indicated by three fingers or just one finger localising the affected area. The palm of the hand rubbed diffusely over the epigastrium may be used to indicate the pain of biliary colic or acute hepatitis.

The common sites of pain arising from the various organs and structures of the body are mentioned in the appropriate chapters.

**2. Radiation of Pain.** Two main aspects of the radiation of pain from the site of the initial lesion must be considered, namely referred pain and spread of pain due to extension of disease.

REFERRED PAIN. In contrast to pain arising in the skin, deep pain may sometimes be felt in or may spread to areas remote from the main site or point of origin, and the distribution of such a referred pain may be highly characteristic. Diaphragmatic pleurisy, for example, or involvement of the undersurface of the diaphragm by acute peritonitis may be referred, through the phrenic nerve, to an area of skin over the shoulder-tip. Even so, it must be pointed out that pain over the shoulder does not invariably indicate involvement of the diaphragm. Local lesions of the skin or of the fourth cervical root may give pain in a similar distribution, while in a few patients with biliary colic or acute cholecystitis pain may similarly be referred to the tip of the right shoulder through involvement of some twigs of the phrenic nerve supplying the gall-bladder.

The distribution of referred pain may be more complicated and less readily explained than in the examples already given. Thus the pain of myocardial ischaemia may spread beyond the main retrosternal site to any or all of the following areas: the left pectoral region; down the left arm to the finger-tips (often mostly felt in the elbow and the wrist); the throat; up the left side of the neck to the lower jaw and the tongue; through to the back; sometimes down the right arm and up the neck to the right side of the jaw. The pain may even radiate symmetrically to both arms, or to the right arm only. Sometimes referred pain may be felt without the main pain, and diagnosis then depends on other features. Thus pain in the left forearm could be due to cervical spondylosis, the carpal tunnel syndrome or perhaps even a hiatus hernia, but regular induction by exercise and relief by rest would point to myocardial ischaemia as the cause.

Pain due to pressure upon a nerve root or to sensory nerve involvement by a disease (e.g. herpes zoster) is referred to the corresponding dermatome. For example, compression of the fifth lumbar nerve root by a prolapsed intervertebral disc may cause pain in the ipsilateral buttock, the posterolateral aspect of the thigh, the anterolateral aspect of the leg and the dorsum of the foot. However, the pain may be felt only in the buttock, leg or ankle, or there may be a pain-free gap. In fact, nerve root pains may be indistinguishable from pains originating in the viscera or other deep structures.

SPREAD OF PAIN DUE TO EXTENSION OF DISEASE. Appendicitis is most readily diagnosed when pain, first felt in the umbilical area, moves after some hours to the right iliac fossa, where it is accompanied by tenderness and muscle guarding. Extension of the inflammation to the serous surface of the appendix with involvement of the overlying parietal peritoneum accounts for this change in the site of pain. Less frequently pain and tenderness due to extension of the inflammation may occur elsewhere, according to the position of the appendix.

Pain due to extension may be the first indication of a latent disease. For instance, peptic ulceration may occur without causing pain. Hence the condition may remain symptomless until pain from penetration into surrounding structures develops. Diagnostic difficulties and errors will result unless such a possibility is borne in mind.

**3. Character of Pain.** As the result of carefully controlled studies in man it has been shown that all pain arising in the skin has a pricking quality if brief or has a burning quality if protracted. However, it is common experience that pains due to a pinprick, burn, cut, pinch or wasp sting can be distinguished, mostly by the context in which they occur, but also by the intensity, duration and distribution of the pain, and by various associated sensations such as heat or traction.

Deep pain is a diffuse aching sensation such as that reproduced by squeezing the tendo achillis; yet its site and duration lead to variations which are described in comparable terms by different patients. Sometimes these descriptions are highly imaginative, and such expressions as 'like being in a vice', or 'like an iron band round the chest' not infrequently replace the common terms 'tight', 'heavy', 'crushing', 'pressing', or 'like a weight' which are used for the retrosternal pain of myocardial ischaemia. It is remarkable how seldom such a pain is described in any other terms. Yet when myocardial pain is felt in areas of reference elsewhere it does not have this special quality. It appears to be the retrosternal site which determines the character of this pain. A similar crushing pain may be due to pericarditis, dissecting aneurysm of the aorta, collapsed thoracic vertebra, fractured sternum, peptic ulcer or hiatus hernia. The retrosternal pain of pulmonary embolism is probably due to myocardial ischaemia.

The epigastric pain of peptic ulcer on the other hand is never described in these terms, but is usually said to have a gnawing, aching or dull quality. Pain across the epigastrium which is described as burning should lead to suspicion of a psychogenic disorder.

As a final example, headaches of organic origin are described in terms of pain which is intermittent, felt mostly over the frontal, occipital or occasionally temporal regions and usually relieved by suitable analgesics. By contrast, psychogenic headaches are indicated by the flat of the hand pressed down on top of the head; they are described in terms of a pressure or perhaps a tightness or lightness, they are continuous and the patient may frequently resort to aspirin in spite of the experience that it has no effect upon the headache.

**4. Severity of Pain.** In some diseases pain is characteristically severe, while in others it is mild or may vary in severity. Thus in most cases of perforated peptic ulcer, acute pancreatitis, biliary and renal colic, and dissecting aneurysm of the aorta, the pain is usually so bad that it is unusual to obtain a description of quality. Pain due to trigeminal neuralgia, glaucoma, toothache, earache, pleurisy and myocardial infarction is often severe.

However, individuals vary so much in their tolerance to pain that a mere statement of severity is insufficient; it is the doctor's responsibility to form a reasoned judgment on the evidence available. In doing so it must be remembered that the intensity of a pain depends greatly upon the patient's state of mind. Thus a remarkable indifference to pain may be observed in states of mania, religious fervour and hypnosis or after prefrontal leucotomy. Pain suffered on the football field is apt to be borne much more easily than that due to an injury of similar severity inflicted in the home. On the other hand, mental depression, anxiety and introspection tend to aggravate the severity of pain. Such facts must already be familiar to the reader, but it may not have been realised that similar influences affect the appreciation of all subjective symptoms. For example, the tick of an alarm clock may irritate some people to the extent of interfering with sleep, yet others may not hear either the tick or the alarm bell at the bedside. Similarly the incessant sounds (tinnitus) which may accompany disorders of the cochlea and its connections may make life miserable for some patients, yet others can be persuaded to ignore these noises so successfully that they no longer hear them without a conscious effort to do so.

When all these factors are taken into account, an assessment of the severity of a pain, though sometimes misleading, is usually of considerable diagnostic value. The behaviour of the patient while pain is present may be of great help. In biliary and renal colic, patients are usually restless and, having unsuccessfully sought relief by lying down in all sorts of positions, they try sitting, standing or walking. By contrast, the perforation of a peptic ulcer tends to make the patient lie still. Severe pain is commonly associated with pallor, sweating, vomiting, an increase in the pulse rate and blood pressure and a leucocytosis. Hysteria or acute anxiety may lead to restlessness and groaning, but many of the other features are absent and diversion by conversation may immediately calm the patient. With very little experience a reasonably accurate judgment of the true intensity of a pain may be made if the patient is seen during its occurrence. An account of the pain and details of the patient's behaviour, supplemented if possible by evidence from witnesses, may enable a retrospective assessment of severity to be made.

**5. Duration of Pain.** Estimations of time without actual measurement are often very inaccurate. Yet the duration of pains of various origins may range from less than a second to several days, so that even inaccurate guesses of time may be very helpful. Thus the lightning pain of the now rare tabes dorsalis, or the excruciating jabs of trigeminal neuralgia, last for less than a second at a time. Each of the griping pains of intestinal colic is felt for less than a minute. The pain of angina of effort ceases two or three minutes after resting, whereas that of a myocardial infarct may continue for hours. The head pain of migraine may be relieved in an hour or so, or it may persist for days.

**6. Frequency and Periodicity of Pain.** In some instances pains may occur at regular intervals every few minutes as in labour or intestinal colic. At

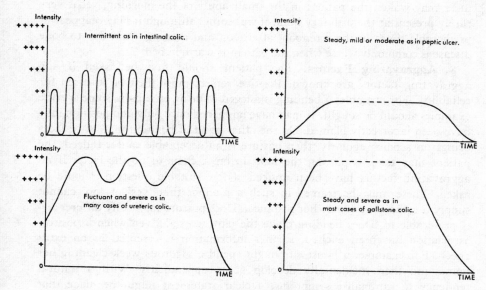

FIG. 3   PAIN    Examples of Time-Intensity Diagrams.

the other extreme the recurrence of pain may be unpredictable as in biliary colic, which may return more than once in a day, though an interval of days, weeks, months or even years may elapse between two attacks. On the other hand, the symptoms of peptic ulcer recur in attacks lasting for one to several weeks, interspersed with pain-free intervals of weeks or months. During an attack the pain usually appears at predictable times on more than one occasion during the 24 hours. A further example is trigeminal neuralgia, in which attacks of pain may be followed by intervals of remission.

The information about the severity, duration and frequency of a pain may be usefully summarised in the form of a time-intensity diagram (Fig. 3).

**7. Special Times of Occurrence.** Is is sound practice to ask if the pain recurs at any special times. Although these may not have been noticed it is remarkable how informative it may be to review an average day. Are symptoms present on wakening? Do they occur in the forenoon, afternoon, evening or night? The results of such interrogation may lead to the recognition of a rhythm which can then be related by the doctor to activity, meals, posture, etc.

Migraine, for example, may occur especially in the morning, or every weekend, or at the menses. Most other headaches are intermittent but some occur at special times such as that associated with arterial hypertension which is often present on wakening, or the 'eleven o'clock' headache of frontal sinusitis, so often at its peak a few hours after rising. The pain of duodenal ulcer may waken the patient in the small hours of the morning, yet is very rarely present at the ordinary hour of wakening, although it may reappear at predictable times in the forenoon, afternoon and evening. Pain due to bone disease is commonly worse when the patient is warm in bed.

**8. Aggravating Factors.** The patient should first be asked if any aggravating factors are known. Positive replies must then be assessed for reliability. For example, if bending is alleged to bring on a pain, some specific examples should be sought. It may have happened once only and position may have been incorrectly blamed. On the other hand, if bending to tie shoe-laces brings on a pain regularly, then posture is an acceptable cause. Indeed, the patient may take to putting the foot up on a chair to tie the laces. If no aggravating factors have been noticed, a few suitable questions should be asked. These must be framed in such a manner that 'yes' or 'no' cannot supply a complete answer. For instance, 'Does posture make any difference?' is preferable to 'Does bending make the pain worse?' Even when a positive association has been elicited, further information is essential as an extra check. For example, a housewife might spend a vigorous week cleaning her home and then incidentally develop acute appendicitis. With a natural tendency to rationalise symptoms, a clear statement might be made that unusual exercise involving repeated bending had been the cause of the pain. Such false deductions can be eliminated only by enquiry into the precise time relationships.

**9. Relieving Factors.** Similar caution must be exercised before accepting patients' statements about relieving factors. Many pains subside spontaneously, and the evidence upon which the patient's belief is based must be obtained in detail and carefully considered. For example, epigastric pain due to peptic ulcer is relieved by alkali in 5 to 15 minutes, but never immediately nor in an hour or more, and even half an hour is a suspiciously long time. Yet the patient may deduce that alkali has helped a pain if there is slight relief after a week's treatment or complete relief after two hours, but in either case the doctor can assume that this deduction is incorrect. A combination of faith and gratitude may convince a patient that his condition has improved as a result of treatment which has in fact had no real effect.

**10. Associated Phenomena.** Some pains may be accompanied by other manifestations which are of diagnostic value. Migraine, for example, is often preceded by visual disturbances and accompanied by vomiting, thus giving rise to the lay terms 'blinding headache' or 'bilious attack'. Rarely, premonitory symptoms such as hunger, an unusual sense of well-being or depression, may precede the attack by a day or so. Added to these characteristics there are usually other members of the family who suffer from recurrent headaches. Further examples are the rigors and pyuria of acute pyelonephritis, the haematuria which may accompany renal colic, or the brown urine, pale stools and yellow sclerae which may follow gall-stone colic.

## Conclusion

Almost any pain can be analysed in relation to these 10 features. An example is given of the application of the method in the assessment of chest pain (p. 105). When these principles are employed the examiner will not only progress a long way towards a diagnosis of the individual problem, but will often increase his own store of knowledge.

# BLACKOUTS

The complaint of blackouts is common, and presents a fascinating diagnostic exercise since the causes range from the trivial to the serious. In the clinical approach it is first essential to understand what the patient means. Although the term 'blackout' is most frequently used to describe some form of lapse of consciousness, it is also sometimes employed to denote attacks of vertigo, of weakness and of psychiatric disturbances such as fugue-like states.

The nature of episodes wherein consciousness is lost is best diagnosed by a trained observer who has witnessed such an attack. However this is not often possible and the interpretation has to be inferred from the patient's accounts of the events which precede and succeed the attack, supplemented whenever possible by interrogation of a witness of the incident.

The most fruitful technique in the elucidation of the history is to direct the patient's mind back to the time and place of the attack, and to encourage him to relive his experiences in his own words. He should then be questioned about any circumstances which immediately preceded the episodes and about any precipitants or consistent time relationships of such attacks. Of equal importance is the patient's account of his sensations during the period immediately after he has recovered some awareness of his surroundings.

A detailed history along these lines should enable the clinician to decide whether the sudden episodes of unconsciousness are due to reduction in the flow of blood to the brain (syncope) or to an alteration in electrical activity of the brain (epilepsy). Further evidence may be provided by the physical examination which should in addition help to determine the underlying cause of the syncopal or epileptic attack. There are also less easily classifiable conditions such as hysteria and narcolepsy which may present with a complaint of blackouts.

## 1. REDUCTION OF BLOOD FLOW TO THE BRAIN

Disturbance of consciousness may be due to a temporary decrease in the flow of blood to the brain as a result of a number of mechanisms. There may be an inadequate venous return to the heart as when vasomotor control is impaired and blood is pooled in the peripheral circulation. This is the process which underlies faints. Venous return may also be impaired because of raised intrathoracic pressure occasioned by coughing or by straining during micturition. Inadequate venous return leads to diminished cardiac output, which may be more directly due to dysfunction of the heart caused by arrhythmias, myocardial damage or valvular lesions. The cerebral circulation may be interrupted by narrowing or occlusion of arteries supplying the brain.

*Simple faints* (vasovagal attacks) are the commonest form of syncope and occur most frequently in adolescent females. There are often precipitating factors such as pain, fright, anxiety or a hot crowded environment. Simple faints most often occur when the patient is standing, are uncommon in the sitting position and are rare when the patient is lying down or during exercise. There is usually a prodromal period which often lasts for several minutes before loss of consciousness and when the patient may complain of weakness, nausea, sensations of heat or of coldness, sweating, light headedness, buzzing in the ears or blurring of vision.

The sufferer rarely falls precipitately, but rather sinks to the ground. During the attack she is usually described as limp and pale. The period of unconsciousness is brief, rarely lasting longer than a minute. Occasionally, if the faint is prolonged, and particularly so if the patient is maintained in an upright posture by the pressure of a crowd, the sufferer may manifest the features of a grand mal fit (p. 39).

*Syncope on standing up* (postural syncope) is a feature of impairment of the vasomotor reflexes (p. 118) and is particularly common when arterial hypertension is over-treated. Postural hypotension occurs in the elderly, and in diabetic patients, but it is usually overlooked unless the blood pressure is measured with the patient standing as well as lying flat. Those who are liable to this symptom suffer more severely after being confined to bed; indeed it is a fairly common complaint at any age, on rising from bed after prolonged illness.

*Syncope following movements of the head* suggests either a hypersensitive carotid sinus reflex or inadequacy of the vertebral arterial supply. In the former, confirmation should be obtained by observing whether pressure on one or other carotid sinus (p. 118) causes extreme bradycardia. The pressure should be released once the response has been estimated for if it is too firm and too protracted cardiac arrest may occur. Lapses of consciousness due to insufficient blood flow in the vertebral arteries are often attended by other features of brain stem ischaemia such as double vision or vertigo.

*Cough syncope* refers to a transient loss of consciousness at the end of a purple-faced paroxysm of coughing in some patients with chronic bronchitis and is particularly liable to occur in over-weight, thick-set men, addicted to tobacco and alcohol.

*Micturition syncope* is rare and occurs in the male who leaves a warm bed at night; the upright position and straining are contributory factors.

Some schoolboys learn the trick of performing the so called *'fainting lark'* by which they contrive to reduce the blood flow to the brain to the point of syncope. It consists of a series of manoeuvres, the first of which is to squat, which traps blood in the legs. Simultaneously the subject over-breathes; hyperventilation is known to produce peripheral systemic vasodilatation and cerebral vasoconstriction. Standing erect and performing a Valsalva manoeuvre, i.e. forceful expiration against resistance (p. 118), reduces the cardiac output to such an extent that syncope follows. Those who wish to try it for themselves should take precautions against injury!

*Syncope on exertion* is found in some patients with extreme limitation of cardiac output due to severe obstruction at the aortic or pulmonary valve, the signs of which would usually be evident; it may also occur in patients under treatment with drugs which block the sympathetic nervous system.

*Erratic syncope* may be due to Adams-Stokes attacks, which usually occur in old age and at the most there is only a very brief warning. During the attack the patient appears to be dead and recovery is accompanied by an obvious facial flush in many cases. This physical sign is so characteristic that a description of it by an observer may enable a precise diagnosis to be made even in those few patients who have a normal pulse and electrocardiogram between attacks. The onset of paroxysmal tachycardia or atrial fibrillation with a rapid ventricular rate may lead to syncope, but usually only when significant disease of the heart muscle or valves is also present. If the paroxysm is brief, diagnosis is difficult or impossible without information about the pulse during the attack.

## 2. Epileptic Attacks

An epileptic fit is a transient disturbance (not necessarily a loss) of consciousness due to a brief, excessive electrical discharge of cerebral neurones. The abnormal electrical discharge may remain localised to a small area of the brain, or it may become generalised.

Characteristically an epileptic fit is of abrupt onset. Fits may occur at any time and in any situation. Sometimes, however, in an individual they run to a pattern; some epileptics have fits only during sleep, or when they are pyrexial or during menstruation. A minority of patients develop seizures in response to specific stimuli such as flashing lights or noise. It is important to explore these relationships and precipitants during the taking of the history.

The features of a *grand mal* fit with its tonic phase ushered in by a cry or groan followed by the jerking movements of the clonic phase, are so distinctive that most lay observers can diagnose such an attack. In the absence of an observer the patient's history will often be indicative as the fall may cause the patient to injure himself and there is frequently incontinence of urine, or tongue biting during the attack.

The very short lived 'absences' of *petit mal* when clearly described by an observer present an easily recognisable pattern. The sufferer, almost always a child, is described as looking vacant or blank for a few seconds. Petit mal seizures are usually very frequent; scores of attacks may occur daily.

In some varieties of *focal epilepsy* consciousness is not entirely lost and the clinical features may be unusual or bizarre. Seizures which originate in the temporal lobe (the commonest type of focal epilepsy) may give rise to diverse manifestations, depending on the site of the initial electrical abnormality and the extent to which it spreads. In the most characteristic variety the onset is associated with a hallucination of smell which is almost always unpleasant. On occasion the prodromal features of a temporal lobe fit are manifest by the patient developing an intense feeling of familiarity with his surroundings—the '*déjà vu' phenomenon*. Visual *hallucinations* of a specific organised nature occur; miniscule men or animals may be seen in one part of the patient's visual field. Less commonly the patient may describe auditory hallucinations; voices or music may be heard.

These and allied phenomena will be accompanied by variable loss of consciousness and commonly attacks will go on to complete loss of consciousness. When consciousness is retained to some extent the patient may carry out motor acts of a bizarre or even antisocial nature. He may appear to the outside observer to be in control of his actions, but the patient afterwards has no memory of his behaviour. Sometimes too this form of *automatism* occurs after the major events of a fit are over.

In *Jacksonian attacks* also the patient can retain contact with his environment. He may be able to describe involuntary movements beginning in one part of the musculature and spreading to contiguous areas. The fit may then cease or he may lose consciousness and the features of a grand mal seizure supervene. Occasionally after a Jacksonian fit the affected parts of the body exhibit a temporary paresis, rarely lasting for more than one or two hours.

**The Underlying Cause.** The recognition that a patient's blackouts are of epileptic nature is the first stage in the diagnostic process. The underlying cause of the fits must then be determined. Epilepsy may be due to genetically determined factors of unknown nature, to any intracranial injury or disease, or to a variety of systemic illnesses or metabolic disturbances. Close attention should, therefore, be paid to the age of onset of the fits, the family history, the previous medical history, associated symptoms and the results of neurological as well as the general systematic examination. In practice one is particularly concerned to define the group of epileptics whose fits arise from a potentially curable cause.

A history of generalised fits which began in childhood and which have been present for many years in a patient who knows of relatives similarly affected, strongly suggests that there is no underlying structural lesion. Fits of recent onset and focal nature, developing for the first time in an adult raise the possibility of a primary cause such as an intracranial tumour. Associated features such as headache or focal neurological signs would reinforce this suspicion. Fits which occur only in the early morning before breakfast or after prolonged fasting should evoke consideration of an insulin-secreting tumour resulting in periodic hypoglycaemic fits. Clinical features of renal or hepatic failure may point to the underlying cause of epilepsy.

It is becoming increasingly important always to explore the possibility that fits may be drug induced. Some drugs, such as L.S.D., are epileptogenic. The sudden withdrawal of many hypnotic drugs, including alcohol, after their long continued and regular ingestion may result in convulsions.

### 3. Miscellaneous Causes of Blackouts

Narcolepsy and cataplexy may sometimes mimic epileptic attacks. *Narcolepsy* is characterised by attacks wherein the patient has an irresistible desire to sleep. These episodes often occur in situations which normally produce drowsiness, such as sitting in front of a fire, watching television, or sitting for long periods in a lecture theatre. But they occur too in most inappropriate circumstances as when eating a meal, or driving a motor car. Sometimes narcolepsy may be accompanied by *cataplexy* wherein the patient suddenly becomes intensely weak and may fall to the ground but throughout remains fully conscious.

*Hysterical attacks* are often bizarre in their manifestations and are rarely accompanied by the stigmata of tongue biting and incontinence of urine. Cross examination of an eye witness would reveal none of the features of deviation of the eyes, or cyanosis which are observed in epileptic attacks. Hysterical seizures usually take place in the presence of others, and create maximal disturbance. Movements of the limbs often occur in hysterical episodes but these are coordinated and may be aggressively directed towards other people.

### Conclusion

The approach to blackouts exemplifies how a clinical problem may be clarified by the analysis of a single symptom in meticulous detail, seeking evidence from diverse sources, notably in this instance from the cross examination of eye witnesses.

## BREATHLESSNESS

A complaint of shortness of breath (dyspnoea) implies that the act of breathing has become a conscious effort. Although many dyspnoeic patients breathe rapidly, there is no direct correlation between the observed rate of breathing and the subjective sensation of dyspnoea. Patients with acute pneumonia, especially children, may take as many as 60 breaths per minute without experiencing respiratory discomfort, while in other conditions, such as respiratory paralysis, a feeling of shortness of breath may not be accompanied by any increase in the rate of breathing. There is also considerable variation in what might be called the 'dyspnoea threshold'. Some patients with objective evidence of gravely impaired respiratory function may complain of relatively mild dyspnoea, while others with only slight disturbance of function may experience quite severe respiratory distress.

## Factors contributing to the Production of Dyspnoea

While *hypoxia* and dyspnoea frequently co-exist, hypoxia *per se,* unless it is severe, plays a relatively minor part in the production of dyspnoea. Many patients with severe dyspnoea are not hypoxic, while in hypoxic patients dyspnoea is not invariably a conspicuous symptom. There is a similar lack of direct correlation between dyspnoea and *hypercapnia.* Although a rise in the carbon dioxide tension of arterial blood causes hyperventilation and dyspnoea in normal subjects, it may not do so in patients with chronic ventilatory inadequacy in whom the respiratory centre may have become unresponsive to carbon dioxide.

The disturbances of respiratory function which may contribute to the production of dyspnoea are now well recognised. The most important of these are an increase in the work of breathing, increased pulmonary ventilation, and weakness of the respiratory muscles. Each of these disturbances has a variety of causes, and there are thus many factors which may operate, singly or in combination, to produce dyspnoea in an individual case.

### 1. DYSPNOEA ASSOCIATED WITH AN INCREASE IN THE WORK OF BREATHING

Airways obstruction, decreased pulmonary compliance ('stiff lungs') and restricted chest expansion all increase the work of breathing.

*Airways obstruction* is the main cause of dyspnoea in patients with obstructive lesions of the larynx, trachea and main bronchi, bronchial asthma, chronic bronchitis and emphysema. Those conditions in which *decreased pulmonary compliance* may contribute to the production of dyspnoea include all forms of diffuse interstitial lung disease, including interstitial pulmonary oedema, which is probably the main cause of cardiac dyspnoea. Pneumothorax, pleural effusion and pleural thickening may also restrict pulmonary expansion and produce disturbances in respiratory function similar to those caused by decreased pulmonary compliance. Dyspnoea due to *restricted chest expansion* may occur in patients with severe pleural pain, kyphoscoliosis, ankylosing spondylitis and extreme obesity.

### 2. DYSPNOEA ASSOCIATED WITH INCREASED PULMONARY VENTILATION

An increase in the respiratory dead space, severe hypoxia, metabolic acidosis, hyperthyroidism and severe anaemia may all be responsible for an increase in pulmonary ventilation. Hyperventilation may also be a manifestation of hysteria.

An *increase in the volume of the physiological dead space* occurs in certain forms of emphysema, when numbers of alveoli are under-perfused but adequately ventilated. In these patients there is an inordinate rise in pulmonary ventilation in response to exercise, although the resting level may be normal. In massive pulmonary embolism a drastic reduction in pulmonary blood flow produces a very large increase in dead space. Patients who survive a massive embolism for a few hours may exhibit a striking degree of hyperventilation ('air hunger'), but this is usually overshadowed by the clinical features of a sudden severe reduction of cardiac output, such as low blood pressure, thready pulse and syncope.

*Severe hypoxia,* in conditions such as pneumonia, pulmonary oedema and interstitial lung disease, increases pulmonary ventilation by reflex stimulation of the respiratory centre via the aortic and carotid chemoreceptors.

In *metabolic acidosis,* caused for example by diabetic keto-acidosis or renal failure, the respiratory centre is stimulated by the increased hydrogen ion concentration in the blood, and the resultant hyperventilation may produce the sensation of dyspnoea.

*Hysterical hyperventilation* is also accompanied by a sensation of breathlessness. Breathing is often irregular, and may be sighing. If the hyperventilation is sufficiently severe and prolonged, it may lead to tetany, or even to an epileptic fit.

### 3. Dyspnoea associated with Weakness of the Muscles of Respiration

Neuromuscular lesions, such as high spinal cord injuries, poliomyelitis, polyneuritis and myasthenia gravis, may cause partial or complete paralysis of the muscles of respiration, with the result that the patient is no longer able to meet his ventilatory requirements.

### 4. Dyspnoea associated with Multiple Factors

In some cases a single factor may be chiefly or even entirely responsible for the dyspnoea, as for example in patients with airways obstruction or with respiratory paralysis. In most conditions, however, the mechanisms responsible for the production of dyspnoea are much more complex. Two examples are given below:

(a) In *pneumonia* the restriction of chest expansion by pleural pain is probably the chief cause of dyspnoea in the early stages of the illness; later, if the lungs become extensively consolidated, dyspnoea is mainly due to a combination of decreased pulmonary compliance and increased pulmonary ventilation caused by hypoxia.

(b) *Pulmonary oedema* of cardiac origin begins in the alveolar walls and causes dyspnoea by reducing pulmonary compliance and increasing the work of breathing. At a later stage, oedema within the alveoli aggravates the dyspnoea, at first by increasing pulmonary ventilation in response to hypoxia, and finally by producing airways obstruction.

### Clinical Forms of Dyspnoea

The sensation of dyspnoea is apparently the same, whatever its cause, but its mode of presentation varies considerably. There are, however, two main patterns, which may occur either independently or together, namely *paroxysmal dyspnoea* and *exertional dyspnoea*.

**Paroxysmal Dyspnoea.** This usually develops when the patient is at rest, but in some conditions is precipitated by exertion. It is by definition acute in onset and may be intense and alarming. An acute attack of dyspnoea is usually due to the rapid development either of airways obstruction or of a restrictive lesion of lungs or pleura. Rarely, as in massive pulmonary embolism, it may be associated with a sudden increase in the volume of the physiological dead space. The differential diagnosis therefore includes the following conditions:

1. Obstruction of the larynx, trachea or main bronchi by exudate or vomitus, or by an inhaled foreign body.
2. Retention of secretions in the air passages of a patient with chronic bronchitis and emphysema or with respiratory paralysis.
3. Bronchial asthma.
4. Left-sided heart failure.
5. Massive pulmonary embolism.
6. Spontaneous pneumothorax.
7. A rapidly accumulating pleural effusion.

HISTORY. A carefully taken history is often of great help in identifying the cause of an acute attack of dyspnoea. In children the possibility of a *foreign body* in the larynx or of membranous exudate obstructing the air passages should not be forgotten. In adults unable to cough effectively because of advanced chronic pulmonary disease or weakness of the respiratory muscles, the *retention of secretions* may produce acute dyspnoea.

An attack of *bronchial asthma* is in most cases readily recognised. As airways obstruction in this condition is maximal during expiration, the latter is slow and laboured while inspiration is relatively rapid and impeded only by the fact that the lungs may already be almost fully inflated. Wheeze and rhonchi are almost invariably present and are predominantly expiratory. If, as is often the case, there have been previous episodes, these will probably have responded promptly to a bronchodilator drug. It is more difficult to recognise from the history alone a patient's first attack of asthma. This is particularly a problem in the child, as anxious parents are often unable to give an accurate account of the episode. The diagnosis usually becomes obvious, however, when a subsequent attack is witnessed by a trained observer.

Attacks of dyspnoea occurring during the night (*paroxysmal nocturnal dyspnoea*) may be due to bronchial asthma, but in middle-aged and elderly patients *left heart failure* is the most likely cause. Although the term 'cardiac asthma', often used to describe paroxysmal dyspnoea of cardiac origin accompanied by wheeze, has now fallen into disrepute, it serves to emphasise the difficulty which may occasionally arise in distinguishing this condition from bronchial asthma. In most cases, however, a previous history of exertional dyspnoea can be elicited and the patient will often state that he sleeps more comfortably in the upright position, supported by several pillows. The attack usually develops in the early hours of the morning as he slides into the recumbent position during deep sleep. He then wakens with intense breathlessness, which often produces feelings of suffocation and panic. His usual reaction is to sit bolt upright with his feet over the side of the bed, and his hands clutching the back of a chair if he can find one. He may even struggle to an open window in the hope that cool fresh air will ease his breathing.

In most cases the attack subsides spontaneously in about half an hour, but there is always a danger that acute pulmonary oedema (p. 147) will extend from the interstitial tissues into the alveoli and the bronchial tree. In some instances the picture may be less dramatic and heart disease may not at first be suspected, particularly if the patient is already known to have chronic bronchitis or bronchial asthma. In these cases it is inadvisable to attempt to make a diagnosis from the history unless it is supported by objective evidence clearly incriminating the heart or the bronchi.

Paroxysmal nocturnal dyspnoea is seen most frequently in left ventricular failure secondary to hypertension, ischaemic heart disease or aortic valvular lesions. It is uncommon in mitral stenosis except during pregnancy or as a result of a change in cardiac rhythm. In the later stages of left heart failure paroxyms of dyspnoea may develop whenever the patient lies down. Such intolerance of the recumbent position is known as *orthopnoea*. Some patients with severe emphysema are also orthopnoeic, but for a different reason. In left heart failure the recumbent position is avoided, possibly because it is liable to induce pulmonary oedema. In emphysema, on the other hand, the upright position is more comfortable because it improves pulmonary ventilation by facilitating the range of movement of the thoracic cage.

Paroxysmal dyspnoea may also be experienced during the phase of hyperpnoea in *Cheyne-Stokes breathing* (p. 174).

The dyspnoea which follows *massive pulmonary embolism* produces a sensation of suffocation in which the patient feels desperately short of air, although he may, in fact, be breathing deeply ('air hunger'). It is invariably accompanied by profound circulatory collapse caused by a fall in left ventricular output, and often, if the patient survives for an hour or two, by evidence of pulmonary hypertension and right ventricular failure. The differential diagnosis from cardiac infarction may be very difficult or even impossible by clinical methods, particularly in the elderly who may experience pain of a similar character in the two conditions, but if the dyspnoea is of the character described above and no crepitations are heard on auscultation of the lungs, pulmonary embolism is the probable diagnosis.

Dyspnoea caused by *spontaneous pneumothorax* usually develops suddenly, not infrequently in the morning when the patient wakens or shortly after he gets out of bed. In other cases the dyspnoea is slight at first but becomes more severe when the patient exerts himself or if he has a bout of coughing. Unilateral chest pain or 'tightness' typically precedes or accompanies the onset of dyspnoea.

*Fluid in the pleural space* produces acute dyspnoea only if it accumulates very rapidly. Massive intrapleural haemorrhage is probably the only condition in which this occurs and can usually be recognised without difficulty, as the dyspnoea is accompanied by symptoms of acute blood loss.

PHYSICAL EXAMINATION. The following findings are of particular value in the differential diagnosis of acute dyspnoea. These are described in detail in Chapters 5 and 6 but are summarised here for convenience.

1. Clinical features indicating a possible cause for left heart failure, e.g. mitral stenosis, aortic valvular disease, diastolic hypertension, myocardial infarction.

2. An increase in jugular venous pressure (p. 122) which is often, but not invariably, raised in acute dyspnoea of cardiac origin and in massive pulmonary embolism.

3. Cyanosis. Central cyanosis (p. 110) is a relatively late feature in acute dyspnoea of cardiac origin but develops at an early stage in severe airways obstruction of all types. In massive pulmonary embolism cyanosis is chiefly of the peripheral type (p. 110) which, in combination with intense cutaneous vasoconstriction, imparts a slate-grey colour to the lips and cheeks.

4. Hypotension, which occurs in massive pulmonary embolism and also in extensive cardiac infarction, and may be associated with acute dyspnoea in both conditions.

5. Physical signs indicating either a primary abnormality in bronchi, lungs or pleura, or a pulmonary abnormality secondary to a cardiac lesion:

(*a*) Expiratory rhonchi which, if the sole clinical abnormality, strongly suggest a diagnosis of bronchial asthma.

(*b*) Markedly diminished or absent breath sounds on one side of the chest, accompanied by hyperresonance on percussion in spontaneous pneumothorax and by stony dullness in massive pleural effusion or haemorrhage. When sufficiently gross to cause severe dyspnoea, both these conditions are easily recognised from the physical signs. Failure to discover a spontaneous pneumothorax in such circumstances is usually the result of inadequate examination of the chest in the stress of the emergency.

(*c*) Basal crepitations which, produced by pulmonary oedema, are often present in association with acute dyspnoea of cardiac origin.

When the cause of acute dyspnoea cannot be clearly identified from the history and clinical examination, a portable chest radiograph and an electrocardiograph may provide information which will enable a precise diagnosis to be made.

**Exertional Dyspnoea.** The significance of breathlessness on exertion can be assessed only by reference to the level of physical activity at which it is induced. A series of standard questions make it possible to grade the severity of dyspnoea as follows:

GRADE 1. The patient can walk at a normal pace on level ground and can walk up mild inclines and stairs without feeling short of breath.

GRADE 2. The patient can walk at a normal pace on level ground but becomes short of breath on walking up mild inclines or stairs.

GRADE 3. The patient cannot walk at a normal pace because of shortness of breath but can walk on level ground for a distance of a mile or more at a slow pace.

GRADE 4. The patient cannot walk for a distance of more than 100 yards without having to stop to regain his breath.

GRADE 5. The patient becomes short of breath on taking a few steps and while washing or dressing.

HISTORY. Once the existence of an abnormal degree of exertional dyspnoea has been established and an estimate made of its severity, the next step in history-taking is to determine the duration of the symptom and to find out whether it is sustained at a uniform level or whether it varies from day to day or even from hour to hour. Patients with sustained exertional dyspnoea should be asked whether it is increasing in severity, stationary or improving, and an attempt should be made to estimate the rate at which any change is taking place. When dyspnoea is intermittent or varies in degree, the circumstances under which these changes occur should be carefully noted. It may be important to discover whether it is worse at any particular time, and if it is aggravated by sudden alterations in atmospheric temperature, by exposure to smoke, dust or pollens or by sudden variations in the level of pulmonary ventilation caused, for example, by coughing, laughing or emotional disturbance. An enquiry into the symptoms accompanying exertional dyspnoea often yields useful information, and should always be made. Symptoms of particular importance in this respect are cough, wheeze, chest pain, palpitations, and swelling of the ankles. It should also be remembered that dyspnoea may occur in disorders other than those of the cardiovascular and respiratory systems, such as obesity, hyperthyroidism, severe anaemia, psychoneurosis and neurological conditions involving the brain stem and the neural pathways to the respiratory muscles.

PHYSICAL EXAMINATION. The clinical investigation of exertional dyspnoea calls, in particular, for a detailed examination of the cardiovascular and respiratory systems. Amongst the abnormalities which should be looked for with special care are, in the cardiovascular system, the physical signs of congestive cardiac failure, cardiac enlargement, left ventricular hypertrophy, cardiac arrhythmias, valvular lesions and hypertension, and in the respiratory system, severe chest deformities, the stigmata of emphysema and the physical signs of airways obstruction, pulmonary oedema, interstitial lung disease, pleural effusion and pneumothorax. In many cases, however, clinical examination fails to elucidate the cause of exertional dyspnoea and it is necessary to submit the patient to a series of special investigations, including radiological examination of the heart and lungs, electrocardiography, and respiratory function tests (including arterial blood gas studies) in order to reach an exact diagnosis.

### Conclusion

Breathlessness may be the presenting complaint in a large number of important cardiovascular and respiratory diseases. A correct assessment of its significance requires a clear understanding of the disturbances in physiology with which it is associated, and of the pathological processes by which these disturbances are created. By means of a carefully taken history the possible causes of dyspnoea in an individual patient can usually be narrowed down to two or three conditions, and a final diagnosis can often be made from the physical signs. In some cases, however, special investigations, such as radiological examination of the chest or tests of respiratory function, may be required.

Breathlessness illustrates how an important symptom is analysed. Other complaints may be interpreted in a similar way by correlating their physiological and pathological basis with the clinical findings.

## THE EXAMINATION OF SWELLINGS

A swelling is a common presenting feature. The patient may find a lump in the neck, in a breast or elsewhere, or a mass may first be noted during a physical examination. By systematic attention to detail it should be possible to determine the origin of the swelling if the examiner is acquainted with the anatomy of the region. The local findings should also give at least some indication of the pathological nature of the swelling—whether this is due to trauma, inflammation or neoplasm.

In the first place, inspection may show the position, the approximate size and shape, and any unusual colour of the mass. By palpation, further information should be obtained about the position, size, and shape of the mass, tenderness may be elicited, the mobility, consistency, surface texture, and type of edge of the mass may be determined, and any enlargement of the regional lymph nodes can be detected. Other methods of examination, such as auscultation, are usually much less informative.

### Inspection and Palpation

**Position.** The anatomical situation of a mass must be defined as accurately as possible. Frequently this will present little or no difficulty, as in the case of a swelling in the breast, in the thyroid, or in the parotid gland. Elsewhere, however, the precision with which a lump can be located will vary in spite of the most careful palpation, especially with some masses in the abdomen. In these circumstances, other features, such as the shape or movement of the mass, will help to identify its anatomical origin.

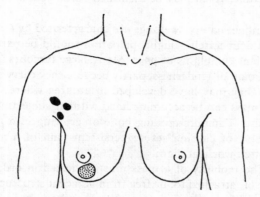

FIG. 4    THE USE OF DIAGRAMS IN CASE RECORDING.
Lump in right breast and axillary lymphadenopathy in patient with carcinoma of the breast.

**Size.** The size of a swelling should always be measured. A diagram, indicating the dimensions, position and shape of the swelling should be recorded and dated (Fig. 4). In this way, significant changes, which may occur later, can be recognised. In contrast, vague statements about size, such as large, medium or small, or comparisons with fruit, eggs or vegetables, are inaccurate and misleading.

**Shape.** Many swellings have characteristic shapes, as, for example, diffuse enlargement of the thyroid gland with its two lobes linked by the isthmus. The swollen parotid gland of mumps fills in the hollow between the posterior border of the mandible and the mastoid process, and often lifts up the ear and extends forward on to the cheek below the zygoma as the accessory parotid gland. The characteristic outline of a mass in the appropriate position should simplify the recognition of an enlarged spleen or liver, a distended bladder, or the fundus of the uterus in the later months of pregnancy. Even with these familiar examples, however, errors can arise, and some additional evidence may be required, such as the disappearance after catheterisation of a swelling when this was due to a full bladder.

**Colour and Temperature.** The skin over acute inflammatory lesions near the surface is usually red and this may be accompanied by a rise in temperature due to an increase in blood flow. A vascular skin tumour may range in colour from red to blue or purple according to the proportions of reduced haemoglobin present and the depth of the layer of skin through which it is seen. Other colour changes over swellings may occur, for example in haematomas the pigment from extravasated blood may produce the range of colours caused by various breakdown products of haemoglobin so familiar in a bruise. Melanin deposition may be responsible for brown pigmentation in the skin over swellings when there is any undue pressure from clothing and other causes. A brown or black colour is common in melanomas, though some are not pigmented. A xanthoma is a small skin nodule which may be identified by its yellow colour due to the lipids it contains.

**Tenderness.** Inflammatory swellings are characterised by tenderness. While this sign must be deliberately sought, palpation should be particularly gentle whenever the patient complains of pain. Many large tumours, in contrast, are entirely free from pain or tenderness, partly because they carry no nerve supply and also because they may have developed in an area where tissue tension is low and where a mass can be accommodated without subjecting any structure to undue stretching. Tumours eroding bone or growing into nerve roots and plexuses are capable of causing severe persistent pain of a most intractable type, and this is often worse at night.

**Movement.** The mobility of a mass must be tested in order to determine whether it is part of, attached to, or free from adjacent structures, such as skin or bone. So far as the skin is concerned, this may be tested by attempting to pick up a fold of skin over the swelling and comparing this with the mobility of the skin over other structures in the vicinity. Fixation of the skin may be associated with a fine dimpling at the opening of the hair follicles resembling 'pigskin' or 'orange skin' when there is lymphatic obstruction. Such a change is most commonly due to malignant disease.

Fixation to deeper structures such as bone or muscle will be recognised by attempting to move the swelling in different planes relative to the surrounding tissues. For example, with a tumour in the breast, the patient is asked to press the hand firmly on the hip of the affected side. The mobility of the mass may then be tested in relation to the contracted and immobilised pectoral muscle. Again it may be difficult to decide whether a mass is situated in the abdominal wall or within the abdominal cavity. This distinction is made by noting the effect of contraction of the rectus and other muscles on the accessibility of the swelling, as described on page 213. In the case of the thyroid, movement of the gland relative to the larynx or trachea will be very slight, but most goitres will move up and down on swallowing because the pretracheal fascia which envelops the thyroid gland is attached to the larynx.

Adherence to adjacent structures such as a blood vessel, a nerve or a viscus, may cause pulsation, paralysis, pain or obstructive symptoms. Pulsation of a lump will readily be appreciated if the palpating hand is kept still for a few moments. It is then necessary to determine whether this is the expansile pulsation of an aneurysm or a vascular tumour, or whether the movement is transmitted from an artery nearby.

An impulse on coughing is characteristically felt in certain swellings within which a rise in pressure may occur because their contents communicate with the thoracic or abdominal cavity. The commonest example is an inguinal hernia.

**Consistency.** The consistency of a swelling may vary from soft and fluctuant through increasing degrees of firmness until this may be so striking as to merit the term 'stony hard'. Very hard swellings are usually malignant or calcified, or consist largely of dense fibrous tissue.

Fluctuation indicates a fluid-containing swelling, such as an abscess or a cyst. Soft tumours such as lipomas may also show some degree of fluctuation. The sign is elicited by detecting with one finger the bulge created by compressing the swelling suddenly with another finger placed at a distance. Fluctuation should be detectable in two planes before the sign is regarded as positive.

**Surface Texture.** The surface of a swelling may vary widely from the uniform smooth to the grossly irregular, as is commonly illustrated in enlargements of the thyroid gland and the liver. The surface of a simple goitre and of some primary toxic goitres is usually uniformly smooth, whereas other goitres, especially those of long standing, may be so irregular in outline that they are described as nodular. A similar variety of texture may be noted on palpation of the liver, ranging from the smooth surface usually found in congestive cardiac failure, through the irregularity of portal cirrhosis, to the gross degree of nodular change in some cases of metastatic tumour. However, a thick abdominal wall may make it impossible to appreciate these variations with confidence.

**Margin.** The edge or margin may be well or ill-defined, regular or irregular, sharp or rounded. The margins of enlarged organs such as the thyroid gland, liver, spleen or kidney can usually be defined more clearly than those of inflammatory or malignant masses. The indefinite margin of a mass is sometimes a valuable indication of an infiltrating malignant growth as opposed to the clearly defined edge of a localised benign tumour.

**Associated Swellings.** The nature of a lump can sometimes be inferred by identifying others with similar characteristics. Conditions in which multiple swellings occur include neurofibromatosis (Plate IV), lipomatosis, metastases in the skin, lymph nodes in reticuloses, and nodules in the breast in chronic mastitis. The suspicion that a tumour is malignant should invariably lead to a thorough examination for evidence of involvement of the lymph nodes draining the area concerned.

### Additional Methods of Examination

**Percussion.** This technique is of very limited value in the examination of a swelling, although occasionally it may be helpful in defining an abdominal mass (p. 218).

**Auscultation.** *Vascular Sounds.* If the blood supply through a tumour is very large, a systolic murmur (bruit) may be audible over the swelling. A murmur is commonly present over vascular goitres and, if it is sufficiently marked, a thrill may also be palpable. Systolic murmurs may also be heard over arterial aneurysms, while over the very rare swellings due to arteriovenous aneurysms there is a continuous murmur, often accompanied by a thrill, similar to the bruit of a patent ductus arteriosus (p. 139).

*Foetal Heart Sounds.* These may be audible over the pregnant uterus after the 30th week.

*Bowel Sounds.* (p. 220). These may be heard over a hernia which contains intestine.

*Friction.* This may sometimes be heard over an enlarged spleen or liver when fibrinous perisplenitis or perihepatitis is present.

**Transillumination.** This is occasionally a useful test in distinguishing between a swelling composed of solid tissue and one consisting of transparent or semi-transparent liquid which may be under such tension that fluctuation cannot be elicited. The sign is sought in darkened surroundings by pressing the lighted end of an electric torch into one side of the tumour. A cystic swelling will light up like a lantern if the fluid within it is translucent provided that the covering tissues are not too thick. The sign is useful in helping to distinguish a hydrocele from a solid tumour of the testis, though it must be borne in mind that a testicular tumour may lie within the hydrocele.

**Further Investigation.** *Radiographs* may define a mass either directly or by the use of various contrast media.

*Biopsy* is often required and must be carried out if there is any suspicion of malignancy.

### Conclusion

The examination of a swelling illustrates the value of a strictly methodical approach, making particular use of two of the basic procedures in physical examination, namely, inspection and palpation. The same principles are applied in defining the physical characteristics and in deducing the nature of any mass wherever it may be situated.

## OEDEMA

Oedema means swelling of the tissues due to an increase in interstitial fluid. It may be generalised due to a disorder of the heart, kidneys, liver or gut, or it may be local from venous or lymphatic obstruction, allergy or inflammation. Sometimes, as is explained later, oedema may be postural and relatively unimportant. An appreciation of the physiological and pathological background is required in order to understand the significance of oedema.

### Clinical Manifestations of Oedema

The doctor may be consulted because of swelling of the ankles, face or abdomen, breathlessness or a rapid gain of weight. When oedema is due to generalised fluid retention, for whatever reason, its distribution is determined by gravity. Thus it is usually observed in the legs, back of the thighs and the lumbosacral area as in cardiac failure in the semi-recumbent patient. If a patient can lie flat quite comfortably, it may readily be seen in the face and hands as in many children with acute glomerulonephritis. Regional rises in venous pressure also determine the distribution of oedema fluid as exemplified by pulmonary oedema in left heart failure or by ascites when there is portal hypertension.

The cardinal sign of subcutaneous oedema is the indentation or pitting made in the skin by firm pressure maintained for a few seconds by the examiner's fingers or thumb. The pitting may persist for several minutes until it is obliterated by the slow reaccumulation of the fluid which had been displaced. However, pitting on pressure may not be demonstrable until an increase in body weight of as much as 10 or 15 per cent has occurred; day to day alterations in weight usually provide much the most reliable index of progress or response to treatment.

Myxoedema in contrast to oedema is characterised by swelling which does not pit on pressure and which is due to infiltration of the tissues by a firm mucopolysaccharide. Chronic lymphoedema may also fail to pit on pressure for reasons that will be described later.

### The Genesis of Oedema

Generalised oedema is bound to occur if, after allowing for water loss through the skin, the breath, the stools or discharges, the fluid intake exceeds the renal excretory capacity. The latter may be reduced by disease of the kidneys, or renal function may be altered by extrarenal factors. For example,

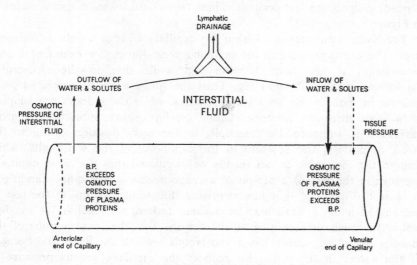

FIG. 5   The Formation and Disposal of the Interstitial Fluid.

C

a fall in renal blood flow leads to a reduction in glomerular filtration rate and an increase in obligatory water absorption by the proximal tubule as in the early stages of cardiac failure. Renal tubular reabsorption of water may be greater when a rise in circulating aldosterone enhances the reabsorption of sodium as occurs in some patients with hepatic cirrhosis, the nephrotic syndrome or cardiac failure. The retained fluid dilutes the plasma and so causes a drop in the osmotic pressure of the proteins and consequent oedema (Fig. 5). However, many instances of generalised oedema and all forms of local oedema are due to alterations in the factors which control the formation and disposal of interstitial fluid at capillary level. In some types of oedema, such as that due to advanced cardiac failure, the genesis is multifactorial.

### THE FORMATION AND DISPOSAL OF INTERSTITIAL FLUID

Interstitial fluid is formed as the result of filtration through the capillary walls, and it is removed partly by reabsorption into the capillaries and partly by drainage along the lymphatic channels. It is convenient to regard the capillary wall as a semi-permeable membrane although the full explanation of the transport of water and solutes across it is much more complicated. The main force causing filtration is the hydrostatic pressure within the vessels; in addition, there is the osmotic pressure of the proteins in the interstitial fluid. The latter is normally very low as albumin in a concentration of not more than 20 mg per cent escapes through the intact capillary. In inflammatory, allergic and lymphatic oedema, on the other hand, there is a high concentration of protein which retains tissue fluid by its osmotic effect. Reabsorption of the fluid is determined by the osmotic pressure of the plasma proteins (oncotic pressure) with an additional effect from tissue pressure depending upon site and position. These factors are shown diagrammatically in Figure 5.

The hydrostatic pressure within the capillaries varies widely at different sites. The mean pressure in the pulmonary capillaries, for example, during recumbency is less than 10 mm Hg, while that in the glomerular capillaries is about 75 mm Hg. Thus the lungs are well protected from oedema in spite of the low tissue pressures, while the kidneys are adapted to a high filtration pressure. Other capillaries are subjected to gross variations in pressure. For example, in the erect posture, owing to the effect of gravity, the pressure in the capillaries of the scalp falls, while that in the feet rises. It can readily be calculated that the mean capillary pressure in the feet of a person of average height during quiet standing is at least 110 mm Hg. It is not surprising that some swelling of the feet at the end of a day's work may be normal. Indeed, the swelling of the feet would be much greater were it not for the fact that contractions of the muscles pump the venous blood and lymph towards the heart and because of the valves in the veins this reduces the capillary venous pressure to some 20 mm Hg. Similarly, some puffiness under the eyes for a short time after rising in the morning is an unflattering sight familiar to many. This is due to the rise in capillary pressure during recumbency in areas where the tissue is lax and the pressure is lower than elsewhere.

### The Types and Causes of Oedema

Oedema may be generalised or localised and it results from factors disturbing the physiological control of body fluid.

#### GENERALISED OEDEMA

The causes of generalised oedema (anasarca) may conveniently be considered under three headings, namely, hypoproteinaemia, cardiac failure and renal causes. As will be seen, several factors may contribute to the production of the swelling in some instances.

**1. Hypoproteinaemia.** The oncotic pressure is mostly due to the serum albumin so that a fall in the concentration of this protein in particular predisposes to oedema. One or more of five mechanisms may lead to hypoproteinaemia:

(a) *Inadequate intake* of protein may be responsible as in kwashiorkor, the most important and widespread nutritional disorder in the world. Famine conditions, the diet of food faddists, or pyloric obstruction with vomiting, may also impair the protein intake.

(b) *Failure of digestion* of dietary protein results from impairment of the exocrine secretion of the pancreas, as in chronic pancreatitis.

(c) *Failure of absorption* of the products of digestion may occur after resection of considerable lengths of small intestine or in diseases such as gluten induced enteropathy.

(d) *Reduced synthesis* of albumin is found in diseases of the liver, such as cirrhosis. When the portal venous pressure is high, ascites is a more prominent feature than dependent oedema.

(e) *Excessive loss* of protein may occur, especially in the urine in the nephrotic syndrome, and less commonly in the stools from a protein-losing enteropathy, or in exudates or discharges through fistulae. The repeated removal of ascitic fluid by paracentesis may also cause depletion of protein.

**2. Cardiac Failure.** The causes of oedema in cardiac failure are multiple and are not fully understood. Significant factors are:

(a) *Impairment of Renal Blood Flow.* In cardiac failure a 'rationing system' gives priority to the maintenance of the coronary and cerebral circulations at the expense of other organs. The renal blood flow is reduced and the fall in glomerular filtration rate promotes excessive reabsorption of water and salt by the renal tubules.

(b) *Increased Venous Pressure.* In cardiac failure there is a rise in venous pressure proximal to the failing chamber. Thus in right-sided failure the increase in venous pressure can be measured by inspection of the neck (p. 121). In left-sided failure, pulmonary venous congestion is inferred from the symptoms of dyspnoea and cough and from the auscultatory findings of crepitations in the lungs. It is possible to measure the rise in pressure by a catheter wedged in a branch of the pulmonary artery. However, the heights of these rises in venous pressures do not correlate with the degrees of oedema and it is clear that the hydrostatic effect does not account for the major part of the fluid retention.

(c) *The Effect of Aldosterone.* In some cases of cardiac failure secondary hyperaldosteronism occurs. The sodium retention, which is part of this process, contributes to the oedema.

(d) *Antidiuretic Hormone.* There is evidence of an increase in antidiuretic substances in the urine of some patients with cardiac failure.

(e) *Lymphatic Factors.* Lymphangiectasis, incompetent valves, and poor lymph drainage have been demonstrated in cardiac failure.

(f) *Oncotic Pressures.* A combination of chronic passive congestion of the liver reducing albumin synthesis, a poor appetite, and loss of protein into the oedema fluid and the urine may account for a significant drop in the concentration of the serum albumin in some cases.

Acting in the opposite direction is an increase in the protein content of the interstitial fluid. In cardiac failure, this may rise to as much as 1 g per cent compared with only 0·02 g per cent in normal interstitial fluid. This change has sometimes been interpreted as evidence for an increase in capillary permeability supposedly due to ischaemia, but it is likely to be mainly due to lymphatic failure.

(g) *Vasodilatation.* In wet beriberi (vitamin $B_1$ deficiency) the extremities are characteristically hot and oedematous. An abnormal accumulation of carbohydrate metabolites causes peripheral vasodilatation, and high output cardiac failure often ensues. The vasodilatation leads to a rise in capillary pressure which contributes to oedema formation just as very hot weather induces swelling of the feet in unacclimatised persons.

**3. Renal Causes.** The oedema of the nephrotic syndrome has been discussed under hypoproteinaemia. In acute glomerulonephritis inflammatory swelling of the glomeruli leads to a fall in the glomerular filtration rate, a relative increase in tubular reabsorption and consequent reduction in urinary volume. Should normal fluid intake be maintained, oedema results. This also applies to any condition in which urine production is diminished (oliguria) or negligible (anuria).

## LOCALISED OEDEMA

This may be due to venous, lymphatic, inflammatory, or allergic causes.

**1. Venous Causes.** External pressure upon a vein, venous thrombosis or incompetence of the venous valves due to varicose veins may each contribute to a rise in capillary pressure in the areas of drainage. A common example is thrombosis in a leg vein complicating an operation, pregnancy, or an illness which confines a patient to bed. Venous return will also be impaired if the normal pumping action of the muscles is diminished or absent, and accordingly oedema may occur in an immobile bedridden patient, in a paralysed limb, or even in a normal person sitting still for long periods as, for example, during air travel.

**2. Lymphatic Causes.** The small quantity of albumin filtered at the capillary is normally removed through the lymphatics. In the presence of lymphatic obstruction, the water and solutes are reabsorbed into the capillaries as the tissue pressure rises, but the protein remains until its concentration approaches that in the blood. Ultimately, fibrous tissue proliferates in the interstitial spaces and the whole part becomes hard and no longer pits on pressure.

Lymphatic oedema is common in some tropical countries due to obstruction by filarial worms. One or both legs, the female breast, or the external genitalia in either sex, are the parts most frequently involved. The skin of the affected area eventually becomes very thick and rough—elephantiasis. Lymphatic oedema is comparatively rare in Britain. It is the cause of the peau d'orange appearance (p. 50) in some instances of mammary carcinoma. It may be due to congenital lymphangiectasis or hypoplasia of the lymph vessels of the legs (Milroy's disease) and may affect an arm after radical mastectomy and irradiation for carcinoma of the breast.

**3. Inflammatory Causes.** As a result of damage to tissues by injury, infection, ischaemia, or chemicals such as uric acid, there is liberation of histamine, bradykinin, and other factors which cause vasodilatation and an increase of capillary permeability; the inflammatory exudate, therefore, has a high protein content which upsets the normal balance of forces. The resulting oedema is accompanied by the classical signs of inflammation, namely, redness, heat and pain. Testing for pitting on pressure in inflammatory oedema causes pain and should be avoided.

**4. Allergic Causes.** Increased capillary permeability also occurs in allergic conditions but, in contrast to inflammation, there is no pain, there is less redness, and eosinophil cells rather than polymorphs and red cells make their way into the exudate, which has a high protein content. Angio-oedema is a specific example of allergic oedema; it is particularly prone to affect the face and lips. The swelling develops rapidly, and it is pale or faintly pink in colour. The condition may constitute a serious threat to life by suffocation if the tongue and glottis are affected.

## Conclusion

In analysing the pathogenesis of oedema, it is desirable to think particularly in terms of disturbance at the capillary level, where the fluid exchanges are taking place. Thereafter, further evidence should be sought from the associated clinical features in order to determine the primary cause. Physiological principles can be applied along similar lines to the interpretation of many other clinical situations.

# CHAPTER 4

# The General Examination
# and the
# External Features of Disease

'The trouble with doctors is not that they don't know enough, but that they don't see enough.'

CORRIGAN (1853)

The object of this chapter is to describe those aspects of clinical examination which it would be inappropriate to assign to any single system. These include the observations made on first meeting the patient, while the history is being taken. Several other important elements of a general clinical examination are also described, for example the hands, the head and neck, the lymphatic system, the breasts and the skin.

The general examination begins as soon as the patient enters the consulting-room or the doctor approaches the bedside. Early impressions will certainly be formed while taking the patient's history and all the doctor's faculties should be on the alert from the outset. The aphorism which heads this chapter serves to emphasise the importance of inspection and this will be evident, not only throughout this chapter, but also particularly in the chapter devoted to the examination of the infant and child. At the start of the formal examination an analysis is made of the patient's demeanour, complexion, physique and the other features which together constitute his appearance. Thereafter the hands, head and neck are examined in turn. With constant practice this part of the examination can be dealt with expeditiously. At first the student must be prepared to take his time and develop a methodical routine. With increasing familiarity and experience, he will gradually acquire facility and speed as well as the ability to discriminate between the details of examination that are vital in one case and superfluous in another. To compromise too early in this respect is to invite disaster.

## GENERAL OBSERVATIONS

### Demeanour

Early impressions of the patient's condition are compounded from many factors. Much may be learned simply by noting how he stands or dresses, from his greeting and from his handshake. His gait may indicate the presence of a neurological or locomotor disturbance (pp. 243, 322). In bed the posture of the patient can be most revealing. Is he able to adjust his position independently or has he to be helped to do so? Does he sit up or lift his head spontaneously when addressed, or has he to be supported or propped up on several pillows? Does he tend to lapse helplessly into some awkward position and seem to disregard the attendant discomfort?

Facial expression may serve as an initial guide to physical or mental disorder. A look of pain, fear, excitement, anxiety or grief does not require a medical training for its recognition. More subtle, however, is the appreciation of such features as the agitation of hyperthyroidism or hypomania, the apathy of hypothyroidism and of some types of depression and the poverty of facial movement in Parkinsonism. However, without in any way intending to deceive, the more intelligent patient will often manage to conceal his apprehension, or he may cloak his feelings in an air of feigned cheerfulness. He may occasionally make light of his symptoms or signs, or deal facetiously with features about which he feels the most anxiety; the doctor should avoid adopting the patient's light-hearted attitude, but on the other hand should not be too ponderous. The inexperienced doctor will do well to behave naturally and so eliminate risks of misunderstanding.

## Complexion

Everyday experience leads to familiarity with the wide variety of the physical characteristics of the face. Among these, abnormalities of complexion may be the first to be noticed by patients or by their friends or relations. When these simple observations are reinforced by medical training, complexion may become a remarkably sensitive index of disease. It must be remembered, however, that lighting conditions affect the appreciation of colour. This is well enough known to shoppers when choosing materials and cosmetics, but the effect of light on the complexion is not so widely appreciated. For instance, jaundice deep enough to be obvious to anyone in daylight, may be undetectable in artificial light.

The colour of the face depends upon variations in oxyhaemoglobin, reduced haemoglobin, melanin and, to a lesser extent, carotene. Unusual colours, excluding those which have been applied externally, are due also to abnormal pigments such as sulphaemoglobin and methaemoglobin (bluish tinge), carboxyhaemoglobin in carbon monoxide poisoning (pink), jaundice (yellow or greenish), and uraemia (sallow with a brownish tinge).

**Haemoglobin.** The contribution of haemoglobin to the normal complexion is largely determined by the amount which is present in the subpapillary venous plexus and the proportion which is oxygenated or reduced. Abnormal pallor may be due to vasoconstriction as in fright, to draining of blood from the face as is seen when the upright subject faints, or may be due to anaemia. It is common knowledge that a sallow face is not necessarily an indication of anaemia, but it is not so widely recognised that vasodilation may cause a deceptively pink complexion in spite of a severe degree of anaemia. An unduly plethoric complexion may be seen in some chronic alcoholics, in Cushing's syndrome or in polycythaemia. Cyanosis is discussed on pages 110 and 166.

**Melanin.** This pigment is normally formed in the deepest layer of the epidermis and colours the skin in varying shades of brown or even black according to the amount present. The colour is largely determined by hereditary influences but may be modified by a number of factors mentioned below. The pigment diminishes or increases in amount with withdrawal from or exposure to ultra-violet light. Absence of melanin from the skin may occur in patches, described as vitiligo; these depigmented areas are often associated with autoimmune disease. Total absence of pigmentation occurs in albinism as a result of a genetically determined failure to form tyrosinase in the melanocytes, and this may occur in any race. An acquired form of failure to synthesise pigment is largely responsible for the pallor which is so characteristic a feature of hypopituitarism in the white races. By contrast, in Addison's disease reduction in the output of adrenocortical hormones is associated with excessive production of melanocyte-stimulating hormone by the pituitary, and this in turn is usually accompanied by the development of brown pigmentation of the skin, particularly in creases, in scars, overlying prominent bones and on areas exposed to pressure from belts, braces and tight clothing. Melanin may also be formed in the mucous membranes of the lips and of the mouth. In both Addison's disease and hypopituitarism vasoconstriction occurs in the skin, so that pigmentation and pallor respectively are accentuated by the absence of the normal red background. Pregnancy is also commonly associated with a blotchy pigmentation of the face, the so-called pregnancy mask—chloasma gravidarum—and melanin is also formed in the areolae, the linea alba and around the genitalia. Increased melanin formation can be induced by heavy metals deposited in the skin, as for example, iron in haemochromatosis. Local over-production of melanin is responsible for freckles and for the pigmentation of moles.

**Carotene.** This yellow pigment is unevenly distributed and is seen particularly in the face, palms and soles but not in the sclerae. A distinct yellow colour of the face may appear in hypothyroidism because of impaired metabolism of carotene in the liver, but it must be borne in mind that hypothyroidism sometimes occurs coincidentally with pernicious anaemia and in this condition the yellow colour may be due to bilirubin. Carotenaemia occasionally occurs in vegetarians or in food faddists, particularly in those who elect to eat quantities of raw carrot.

**Bilirubin.** In haemolytic (acholuric) jaundice, the sclerae and the skin are a lemon-yellow colour. The stools are dark and the urine looks normal, but contains an excess of urobilinogen (p. 435). This form of jaundice is due to an increase in serum bilirubin attached to albumin which is not excreted in the urine.

In hepatocellular or obstructive jaundice bilirubin has been split from the albumin and conjugated with glucuronic acid by the liver. It is water soluble, readily passing through the renal glomerular filter (p. 434). The urine is brown like beer and the stools tend to be pale in colour like putty, because of the reduction in the amount of bile in the faeces. If the jaundice is deep and of long standing a distinct greenish colour becomes evident in the sclerae and in the skin due to the development of appreciable quantities of biliverdin. Scratch marks may be prominent on the skin as a result of the pruritus which occurs in obstructive jaundice from the retention of some unidentified factor normally excreted in the bile.

### Abnormal Movements

Involuntary movements may be due to organic disease of the central nervous system, particularly when the extrapyramidal system is involved (p. 279). Disorders of movement may also result from primary disease elsewhere. The 'flapping tremor' of encephalopathy due to hepatic failure is such an example and may not be apparent unless deliberately sought by inspecting the outstretched arms. The sign consists of jerky movements of the hands due to flexion and extension of the wrists in a manner somewhat resembling the action of a bird's wing, though less regular and rhythmical. Irregular twitching movements not unlike those seen in liver failure may occur in renal failure ('uraemic twitchings') and in respiratory failure with carbon dioxide retention. In thyrotoxicosis the tremor is more fine than in Parkinsonism, that is, its amplitude is less and frequency greater, and it is best seen in the hands. The patient is also often very restless or fidgety, a state of affairs sometimes described as hyperkinetic.

Anxiety is a common cause of tremor which will vary with the patient's emotional state. Senility and chronic alcoholism also may cause a fairly coarse rather irregular tremor.

### Abnormal Sounds

Sounds which are heard either by the doctor or the patient or another witness, may be of considerable value in diagnosis. Foremost amongst such is the information to be gained by attention to peculiarities of voice and speech.

The factors which contribute to the production of the voice include the ability to expel sufficient air from the lungs and the integrity of the mucosa, muscles and nerve supply of the larynx. Normal speech depends also upon the tongue, lips, palate and nose. The neurological abnormalities which cause disturbances of voice and speech are described on page 238. Many of the other causes can be recognised by examination of the mouth, nose and throat. Deformity, as for example a cleft palate, nasal obstruction, loose dentures, or a dry mouth (xerostomia) for any of several reasons, including apprehension, stomatitis or glossitis, should all be readily apparent. Hoarseness of the voice, again excluding neurological causes, may be due to laryngitis of inflammatory origin, or it may result simply from excessive smoking with or without a persistent accompanying cough. The chronic alcoholic is frequently hoarse, but in such cases there are probably several factors concerned, including that of smoking.

The voice in myxoedema may be so characteristic that the diagnosis can be made without even seeing the patient, perhaps over the telephone. The normal inflections of tone disappear, speech is low-pitched, slow and deliberate, and seems to require more effort than normal; it sounds 'thick', in that it flows less freely than normal, and the patient may stumble over individual syllables. Many of these changes in myxoedema are attributed to infiltration of the tissues concerned in voice production, but there are also changes in cerebral cortical function which probably contribute to the disability.

Several other types of sound may be heard, especially in connection with the respiratory system. Wheezing, stridor, rattling or crowing noises may help in the differentiation of paroxysmal dyspnoea. The character of a cough may be revealing (p. 156). Witnesses may give an account of a whoop suggestive of pertussis or the cry of an epileptic fit. Loud noises of cardiovascular origin and various sounds arising from the alimentary tract are described in the appropriate chapters.

### Abnormal Odours

Though the olfactory sense is poorly developed in man, there are occasions when the smell of a patient is so offensive that it is tempting to give him a wide berth. Some odours are sufficiently characteristic as to be diagnostic, like the sickly 'foetor hepaticus' of liver failure, or the sweet smell of acetone in the breath in diabetic coma, which is so obvious to some but not appreciated at all by others. Apart from their value in diagnosis, bad smells may be a source of great embarrassment to patients. One of the major sources of malodour in any patient, apart from dirty clothing and general soiling, is the skin, particularly of the axillae, under the breasts, of the external genitalia and the feet. In most highly organised communities with access to the usual amenities, odour due to dirt should not occur, except in the very young, the elderly infirm who are incapable of looking after themselves and their toilet, and some of the mentally defective, for whom inadequate provision outside an institution may have been made. Nevertheless, from time to time one comes across patients who have access to the necessary facilities but who are too lazy or incompetent to take the trouble to keep themselves clean, and who show little if any embarrassment at what is sometimes the filthy state of their skin, and particularly of their feet.

*Halitosis* is an affliction which is less readily avoided. Malodorous breath often passes unrecognised by the patient but may be particularly offensive to others. This condition may be associated with de-composing food wedged between the teeth, unclean or carious teeth, gingivitis, stomatitis, atrophic rhinitis, and tumours of the nasal passages, as well as pulmonary suppuration. Less acute disease such as bronchiectasis may be associated with offensive breath, and in some cases the patient may notice that expectorated sputum tastes foul. It is surprising that achalasia of the cardiac orifice of the stomach does not produce similar complaints, since foodstuffs which must undergo fermentation and putrefaction often appear to lie for long periods in considerable quantities in the dilated oesophagus. In patients with pyloric obstruction from scarring or associated with carcinoma of the stomach, foul-smelling eructations may occur, but probably the most offensive odour of this type is associated with a gastro-colic fistula, due to the faecal contents of the stomach. It should be noted that some individuals are afflicted with halitosis for which no adequate explanation can be found.

The smell of alcohol may prompt the doctor to ask appropriate questions about the patient's habits, but he should also remember that a comatose patient may have been given whisky or brandy as a remedy by a well-intentioned layman, and that alcohol may not be responsible for the patient's disability.

The source of other smells is usually only too easy to identify if the cause is excessive sweating of the feet, gangrene, chronic suppuration, necrotic tumours or some skin disorders.

## Anthropometry

A routine examination should include the measurement of *weight* and *height,* both for their immediate value and for future reference. Other measurements such as *span, sitting height* and *pubis to ground height* are made occasionally when a more precise evaluation of growth and development is required. The special measurements applicable to infants and young children are described on pages 384–385 and detailed on pages 459–463.

The *weight* of an adult patient taken in the outpatient department or consulting-room should include normal indoor clothing without shoes. Patients in hospital should be weighed in bed-clothing and dressing-gown, again without shoes. The *height* should be recorded with a suitable rigid arm sliding on a vertical scale, and with the patient standing on an even floor surface, so that his heels, calves, buttocks, shoulders and occiput can be aligned against the vertical plane.

*Giantism* as a feature of hyperpituitarism is very uncommon, but the appearance of some patients with hypogonadism and of patients with Marfan's syndrome may give the impression that they are disproportionately tall. In hypogonadism the limbs continue to grow for longer than is appropriate because of the absence of sex hormones, particularly oestrogens, which normally serve to close the epiphyses soon after puberty. Thus the sitting height of the patient (head, neck and trunk) will be considerably less than half the height of the patient measured standing. Alternatively, the height from the top of the symphysis pubis to the ground can be taken, and this as a measure of the length of the lower limbs will be found to exceed the sitting height very considerably. The span of the arms measured fully extended will be found to exceed the height standing or, more significantly, twice the sitting height, thus once more emphasising the disproportionate length of the limbs in contrast to the trunk.

In Marfan's syndrome the appearance of the patient is rather similar, that is to say, the limbs are much longer than is appropriate to the length of the trunk. As a rule there are additional features to distinguish the patient with Marfan's syndrome from the hypogonad patient, in particular long slender hands (arachnodactyly, Plate I) and narrow feet, dislocation of the lens or dilation of the aorta causing aortic regurgitation or an aneurysm.

*Dwarfism* may be due to many causes; from among these the most striking contrast to the conditions just described is provided by achondroplasia. Gross shortening of all four limbs with a normal trunk length is a constant and characteristic finding. The stunted growth of rickets is usually associated with some limb deformity, particularly genu valgum (knock knee) or varum (bow leg). If cretinism has remained untreated or has been inadequately treated for sufficiently long for growth to be restricted, there will usually be some other signs of persistent hypothyroidism, particularly impairment of mental development.

## Nutritional Status

The necessity for a proper relationship between height and weight cannot be over-emphasised if the complications of obesity are to be reduced or avoided. For this purpose a desirable weight for height should be recommended rather than an average weight, since this would include data derived from abnormal individuals. In Britain or America where many of the standard tables in common use were prepared from life insurance and similar figures, the individuals studied for these purposes belonged to social and occupational classes in which the average weights observed were usually in excess of the ideal. Tables of desirable weight in relation to height and frame (body build) will be found in the Appendix (p. 464).

A simple clinical method of estimating the amount of fat is to measure the skin fold thickness usually over the triceps or below the scapula by means of a special pair of callipers. Such a measurement, of course, includes two thicknesses of skin and subcutaneous fat.

Although the majority of adult patients in Britain requiring dietetic advice are suffering from the effects of overeating, some patients are encountered with disorders attributable to undereating (or starvation) or to specific deficiencies particularly of protein, of iron, or of vitamins in the diet. The last is especially liable to occur in elderly men living alone. A major proportion of nutritional deficiency disorders seen in Britain is due to malabsorption in disorders of the small intestine. The features of malnutrition are unlikely to be confined to those of a single factor. In addition to loss of weight and anaemia, signs of vitamin deficiency are occasionally seen, for example on examination of the skin and mouth.

**Abnormalities of Fat.** In the normal individual fat is stored mainly in the mesentery and in the subcutaneous tissues. In the *common type of obesity*, excess fat is widely but not always uniformly distributed. In more gross cases, the abdomen is predominantly affected and fat deposits may be so great as to make palpation of the abdomen uninformative. The hernial orifices may remain relatively accessible, since the tightness of the skin about the flexural folds, including the inguinal region, restricts the accumulation of fat in these areas. Next in order, the breasts, the buttocks, and the thighs will usually show signs of undue accumulation of fat. As a rule, the amount of fat deposited on limbs is greatest nearer the trunk and tapers towards the wrists and ankles, very little excess being deposited on the hands or feet. In some the excess of fat may extend uniformly to just above the wrist or ankle, where it ceases abruptly, producing on the legs an appearance like turkish trousers. The neck and face usually share in the accumulation of fat.

The distribution of fat in the body, particularly excess fat, may be abnormal in *Cushing's syndrome,* or in patients being treated for prolonged periods with moderate or large doses of *corticosteroids.* These hormones increase the appetite and may lead to a mixture of a simple form of obesity, together with the more striking changes due to excessive corticosteroid production or administration. Under the influence of these hormones fat deposition tends to be restricted to the trunk, neck and face, together with an increase of the normal pad of fat over the lower cervical and upper thoracic vertebrae. The limbs remain relatively thin or are actually wasted, the whole impression giving rise to the descriptive term of 'buffalo obesity'. The complexion often becomes florid, the face round and the neck thick. The so-called 'mooning of the face' is the earliest and sometimes the only change to appear (Plate VI). Osteoporosis causing collapse and wedging of the thoracic and lumbar vertebrae leads to shortening of the spine, increased protuberance of the abdomen, and further exaggeration of the abnormalities described. Cutaneous striae (p. 94) are often present in patients of this type.

*Localised deposits* of fat may occur, particularly in middle-aged or elderly females and large pads of fat, which are sometimes tender, may form on the limbs. Lipomas are commonly found around the trunk and are rather soft, circumscribed, lobulated swellings.

The term *progressive lipodystrophy* is used to describe a rare condition in which subcutaneous fat disappears sequentially from the face, neck, arms, chest and trunk. Fat remains or may even be deposited in excess on the lower trunk and thighs, the line of demarcation varying from case to case.

*Localised atrophy of subcutaneous fat* may occur occasionally in diabetics, in areas where insulin is habitually injected. The cause is usually obvious, though it may be puzzling to the observer if it is not realised that the patient is a diabetic, and if the punctures in the skin have disappeared, as they do when the site of injection is changed.

**The Significance of a Change in Weight.** A history of a recent change in weight must be regarded critically until it has been explained. *Loss of weight* may be due to inadequate intake, malabsorption or a metabolic disturbance. A coincident loss of appetite in a middle-aged person who has previously enjoyed his food should bring the possibility of gastric carcinoma to the doctor's mind.

Emaciation may occur in young women suffering from anorexia nervosa; these patients frequently take a great deal of trouble to conceal the fact that their diet is grossly inadequate. Anxiety at any age is a common cause of loss of appetite and weight.

Alimentary disease, with malabsorption as a feature, may be expected to cause some loss of weight, but in this condition, as in many others, the accumulation of latent or overt oedema may go far to counter the change in weight that might be anticipated when nutrition is unsatisfactory or inadequate.

Weight loss accompanied by a history of increased or unchanged appetite suggests the possibility of diabetes mellitus or hyperthyroidism. The former would usually be readily confirmed by examination of the urine for glucose. Thyrotoxicosis, likewise, of sufficient severity to lead to a complaint of loss of weight, would usually be confirmed by direct questioning and informed examination once the possibility has been suspected.

Radiological examination of the chest should invariably be carried out if weight loss is unexplained, since pulmonary tuberculosis does not always produce symptoms indicating chest disease. Furthermore, primary carcinoma of the lung or metastatic disease originating elsewhere may be recognised only in this way even at a time when it has progressed so far as to produce a loss of weight.

A *gain in weight* is frequently encountered in hypothyroidism, in patients treated with corticosteroids or as a result of the endocrine adjustments which occur during adolescence, following pregnancy or at the menopause. A very rapid increase over a period of days is often due to fluid retention, for example in patients with cardiac failure.

### The State of Hydration

The state of hydration should be assessed in all cases of fluid loss, notably from vomiting, diarrhoea, sweating and polyuria. Unless the possibility of dehydration is given special thought, its existence may be overlooked or its severity underestimated. A detailed history of the nature and quantity of fluid loss is of first importance. If the patient's usual weight is known, much the most satisfactory assessment is obtained by weighing. However, this may not be possible. A dry tongue is apt to be deceptive as it may be due to mouth breathing alone. In an adult, after 4 to 6 litres have been lost, the blood pressure may be low and the skin dry, loose and wrinkled. Loss of elasticity of the skin can be demonstrated by pinching up a fold which then remains as a ridge or subsides abnormally slowly. The eyeballs are soft, due to lowering of the intraocular tension.

All these methods, except weighing, are crude and inaccurate. If it is known that the patient was not anaemic before the episode of dehydration occurred, and has not lost blood, an estimation of the haemoglobin concentration or of the packed cell volume (p. 449) will be very informative, and serial readings will indicate when treatment of the dehydration has been adequate.

### Temperature, Pulse and Respiration

Examination of the pulse and respiration is discussed on pages 111 and 174 respectively. Body temperature is estimated by taking readings from the skin (axilla, groin, natal cleft), beneath the tongue or in the rectum. Rectal temperature is usually about 0·5°C higher than the mouth which in turn is 0·5°C higher than the skin. As a compromise between convenience and accuracy it is common practice to read sublingual temperatures, but precautions are required to prevent infection being spread by the thermometer. Clinical thermometers are classified as half-, one- or two-minute instruments; the time indicates how long they should be left in place before being read. Although these timings are underestimates, they are sufficiently accurate for most clinical purposes. Rectal readings are more reliable and should always be taken when there is any doubt about the authenticity of recordings from the mouth or axilla.

The normal oral temperature is 37°C. Diurnal variations of about 0·5°C occur, the lowest in the early morning. Fever is usually due to organic disease, though occasionally this is not the case. An otherwise inexplicable transient rise may be due to a recent hot drink or a hot bath. Malingerers sometimes falsify their temperatures by a variety of tricks, including the use of hot-water bottles, in order to feign illness.

The temperature of the skin as noted with the observer's hand provides a very unreliable indication of body temperature. The skin of a patient with a normal temperature may feel remarkably cold, and an apparently normal skin temperature does not exclude hypothermia. When hypothermia is present, it is commonly overlooked because the ordinary clinical thermometer reads only as low as 35°C and it is not always shaken below this level before a patient's temperature is measured. Clinical thermometers which record down to 30°C are readily available and should be used routinely. Rectal temperatures as low as 27°C are not uncommon in patients left exposed to cold after the onset of a cerebrovascular accident of sufficient severity to immobilise the patient and in patients with hypopituitarism or hypothyroidism. The deliberate reduction of body temperature to points approaching these figures is used in cardiac surgery.

# THE HANDS

After the history has been obtained and advantage has been taken of the opportunity that this provides for making an early general appraisal of the patient, the more formal physical examination usually commences with a scrutiny of the hands and pulse. Attention will have been paid to the strength of the patient's grip when shaking hands. Does it suggest a robust or an apathetic attitude? While the pulse is being examined and when appropriate, compared with that in the other arm, the *temperature of the hands* will be noted and contrasted. Whereas arterial insufficiency in the arms and hands is rare, Raynaud's disease (p. 141) is very common in some degree, particularly in women. In winter in Britain chilblains have a considerable nuisance value. They are usually seen as localised, red, raised, itchy areas about the dorsum of the fingers, hands and feet, associated with considerable swelling.

Unusually warm hands should raise the possibility of fever or of vasodilation for one of many other reasons, such as hyperthyroidism, chronic respiratory failure or pregnancy. The *colour of the hands* also calls for comment. Conclusions regarding pigmentation do not differ from those applying to the skin in general (p. 60). The brown staining of the fingers of the heavy or careless smoker should be reconciled with whatever history of smoking may have been given. Coal miners may have small blue tattoo marks on the skin of their hands, their arms, and in other sites where particles of carbon have been embedded in the scars of minor injuries.

The *size* of the hands as well as of the feet is notably increased in acromegaly. Radiological examination will make it clear that this enlargement is due mostly to increase in the bulk of the soft tissues.

*Tremor* of the hands should be noted and its characteristics defined (p. 61). Attention should also be paid to *deformities* due to trauma or disease.

**The Nails.** The fact that well-manicured nails are things of beauty and a social asset may account for disproportionate distress when an abnormality is present. It is important to study the nails because changes occur there which are useful diagnostic guides to systemic disease; this tends to affect all the nails to some extent as opposed to local influences which usually involve one or more nails only. While the form of the nails varies considerably between individuals it is not difficult to recognise what is abnormal.

A change in the shape of the nails may be a feature of general disorders. Koilonychia is the name given to finger-nails which are initially brittle and then flat or spoon-shaped (Plate I). They occur in long-standing iron deficiency anaemia. Poor quality nails are also a feature of impaired nutrition and if this is rapidly corrected, nail growth abruptly becomes normal, leaving a transverse furrow at the corresponding level in each finger. Longitudinal ridging by contrast is much less important. It tends to increase with advancing years, the ridges sometimes taking on a faintly beaded appearance. An increase in the normal longitudinal and lateral convexity of the nails is a feature of finger clubbing (p. 167).

Apart from alterations in shape, other changes in the nails may need to be considered. 'Splinter' haemorrhages in the nail bed are discussed on page 153. Leuconychia (white nails) may occur in chronic liver disease, but this is uncommon and should not be confused with the small isolated white patches often seen in the nails of normal persons.

Bitten nails suggest the need to take an element of neurosis into account in making the final assessment.

Primary disorders of the skin, such as dermatitis, frequently involve the

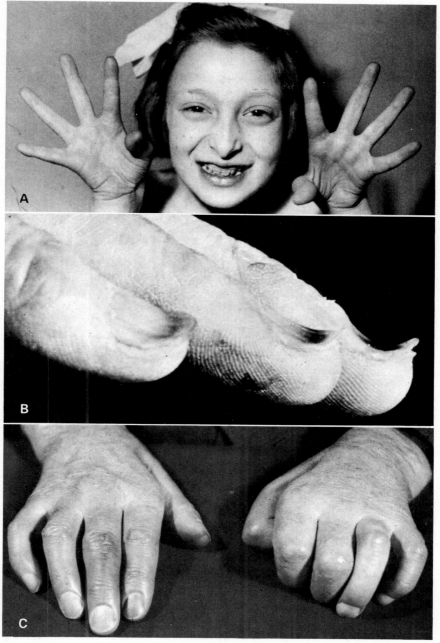

PLATE I.   THE HAND AS A DIAGNOSTIC AID

A, Arachnodactyly. This girl had other manifestations of Marfan's syndrome, including a congenital cardiac defect. (Photo by courtesy of Dr R. J. G. Sinclair.) B, Koilonychia. This is an unusually marked example. C, Syringomyelia. Note the wasting of the first dorsal interosseous muscles and the flexion deformity of the fingers. Trophic lesions were present on the finger-tips. (Photo by courtesy of Dr John Marshall.)

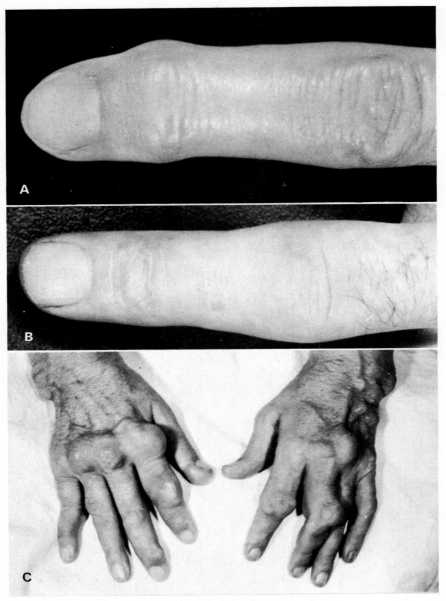

PLATE II. THE HAND AS A DIAGNOSTIC AID

A, Osteoarthrosis. Note the Heberden's nodes at the distal interphalangeal joint. B, Rheumatoid arthritis. Note the characteristic fusiform swelling of the proximal interphalangeal joint.
C, Gout. Note the irregular peri-articular swellings due to tophi. This is an unusually advanced
example.

nails which become irregularly malformed. Psoriasis may affect one or sometimes all the nails and its effects vary from a slight pitting to gross distortion and yellow discoloration; the most severe cases are invariably accompanied by obvious skin lesions. Fungal infection may lift the nail from the bed and form a heaped up dirty looking mass which gradually grows in towards the root of the nail.

Injury is by far the most common of purely local causes of changes in the nails and nail growth may be permanently impaired. Abnormalities of hereditary origin also occur; these may be a cause of embarrassment to the patient and a source of interest to the geneticist.

**Skin of the Hands.** Atrophy of the skin of the hands commonly occurs with advancing years. It is often particularly marked on the dorsum of the fingers and the metacarpus of the patient with rheumatoid arthritis, in osteoarthrosis and in patients with senile purpura. The skin may appear almost transparent, so that the tendons and their sheaths as well as the veins on the dorsum of the hands are conspicuous. In scleroderma changes in the skin covering the fingers may be striking. The collagen fibres in the dermis become swollen and then sclerotic. The skin has a shiny glazed appearance and is tightly stretched over the underlying tissues, limiting the movements of the fingers which are then held in a semi-flexed position.

The skin on the palms of the hands will show keratosis or hyperkeratosis according to the extent of heavy work undertaken by the patient involving gripping instruments, equipment or utensils. In patients with painful disabilities of the hands, this type of activity is avoided, and the skin of the palm and volar aspect of the fingers may become soft and smooth like that of an infant, just as may the skin of the soles of the feet in anybody immobilised for long periods and unable to bear weight. The hands of many people show signs of trauma; these are always worth investigating and sometimes lead to useful information with a bearing on the patient's presenting complaints or occupation.

The term 'palmar erythema' (liver palms) is used to describe the bright red colour often seen in the skin over the hypothenar eminence and sometimes on the thenar eminence and on the pulps of the fingers in patients with chronic liver failure. The intense cutaneous vasodilation responsible for this sign is not confined to patients with liver disease, but may also occur in normal people. Similarly Dupuytren's contracture may be seen in hepatic cirrhosis associated with alcoholism but also in normal persons. There is thickening and shortening of the palmar fascia and flexion deformities of the fifth, ring and middle fingers.

Dermatitis and other changes on the skin of the hands and elsewhere may be due to external irritants. The housewife adopting a new detergent or an unaccustomed soap powder may develop dermatitis, involving inflammatory changes in all the layers of the skin and of relatively uniform distribution in those parts exposed to the irritant, though frequently not confined to these areas.

**Muscles of the Hands.** Wasting of the muscles of the hands often accompanies rheumatoid arthritis and is attributable in part to disuse atrophy. A variety of neurological causes includes motor neurone disease, syringomyelia (Plate I), poliomyelitis, and lesions of the eighth cervical and first thoracic roots of the brachial plexus. Specific muscle groups are involved in ulnar and median nerve lesions (p. 334). In the first instance it is important to note that muscle wasting exists, and identification of the cause may need to be deferred until later when a systematic examination has been completed.

**Joints of the Hands.** Examination of the joints of the hand is described on page 335; two common varieties of disease are found. Rheumatoid arthritis (Plate II) affects the proximal interphalangeal, metacarpo-phalangeal and carpal joints, and causes pain, diffuse swelling, restriction of movement and ultimately sometimes gross disorganisation of the joints. Osteoarthrosis (Plate II ) affects mainly the terminal interphalangeal joints and usually causes little or no disability. In this condition the joint changes are characterised by Heberden's nodes, which are visible and palpable osteophytes projecting from the dorsal surface of the base of the terminal phalanges. If the terminal joints are affected by a diffuse swelling along with apparent rheumatoid changes in other joints, then psoriatic arthritis should be suspected and skin and nail lesions should be sought (p. 69). In gout there are acute episodes of pain, swelling, redness and tenderness in one or more joints and in severe cases, tophi may be found in the ears or around the affected joints (Plate II).

# THE HEAD

For purposes of convenience, the examination of the various components of the head is described in topographical sequence from above downwards—the cranium, hair, face, eyes, ears, nose and mouth. In practice the examination will probably commence with the structure mainly involved.

## The Cranium

The examination of the cranium in infancy and childhood can be most informative (p. 385). This is in striking contrast to the paucity of positive findings in the adult. In the latter, inspection may reveal generalised enlargement in Paget's disease or localised bony bossing overlying one of the intracranial venous sinuses as a reaction to a meningioma. In cranial arteritis the temporal arteries are often visibly and palpably enlarged and tender. On auscultation a bruit may occasionally be detected in the presence of an arteriovenous malformation (p. 139).

## The Hair

While the examination of the hair of the scalp and face is being described it is convenient to refer to abnormalities of the growth of hair in other sites.

**The Scalp.** Many of the characteristics of the hair on the scalp are too familiar to require a description here, but the distribution of this hair is sufficiently important to merit some discussion. In the normal adult male after puberty, the hair margin of the forehead tends to recede, or at least to become thin, particularly at either side; this is described as temporal recession, and when present in females, particularly if they show other evidence of virilisation, is to be regarded as of some importance. Loss of this hair in the male commonly occurs spontaneously, even in relative youth. The tendency to do so appears to be genetically determined in part. Loss of hair over the area of scalp approximately covering the frontal bone is an almost constant finding in dystrophia myotonica, and is then associated with other features such as cataract formation and wasting of muscles.

The most common local disease of the hair of the scalp is alopecia areata in which the hair becomes brittle and breaks off near the scalp. The broken hairs are found at the periphery of the bald area which is clean and smooth in contrast to fungus infection in which the whole area is bristly. Lice and nits of *Pediculus capitis* may also be found, particularly in women with long hair and living in poor social circumstances (p. 98).

**Facial and Body Hair.** Apart from examination of the hair of the scalp, useful information may be gathered from examination of the facial hair and of that upon the trunk and the limbs. Many of the features encountered are related to endocrine function, particularly of the gonads and adrenals, but it is still difficult or impossible to provide an adequate explanation for some of the abnormalities, especially in the female.

In any form of adrenocortical or gonadal dysfunction in the female associated with virilisation, the distribution of the hair usually undergoes changes in the direction of a masculine appearance. Associated with this, there will frequently be some abnormal growth of hair, at first particularly in the beard or moustache areas, and when this is dark in colour, it may cause serious embarrassment. In addition, the pubic hair may spread from its normal flat topped distribution up towards the umbilicus. Hair may also make its appearance on the limbs. At first this is most marked on the forearms and on the thighs, but later may become conspicuous on the legs as well, where in any case there is normally more to be found than in other situations on the limbs.

Secondary sexual hair on the face in the male, and in the axillae and on the pubis of both sexes, may fail to develop in hypogonadism; it may diminish in quantity in old age or be lost in hypopituitarism or as a result of hepatic cirrhosis. In severe hypopituitarism the loss is ultimately complete, including the hair follicles, so that the axillae and pubis return to the smooth appearance seen in childhood.

The amount of hair on the eyebrows varies very widely. This usually diminishes with age, and although the statement is frequently made that thinning of the outer third of the eyebrows is a feature of myxoedema, this is so common in normal people as to be of little value in diagnosis.

## The Face

Some facial appearances are pathognomonic of disease, for example the immobile stare of Parkinsonism, the startled appearance of hyperthyroidism in a young person, the pale, puffy face of nephritis, the coarse features of myxoedema or the eyes of the mongol. To the experienced observer the briefest glimpse of one of these patients will suffice. In addition, a patient's face, rather like his clothing, may serve to indicate some features of his personality. This perhaps applies with greater force to women, and the evidence of time, expense and care devoted to a person's appearance may be informative. In children, study of the facial appearance is particularly rewarding (Plates V and VI).

In most cases the characteristics which blend to form the facies must each be considered separately. While no attempt will be made to offer a complete compendium of facial characteristics, some examples of the more common and more significant findings will serve to illustrate the importance of this aspect of the examination of a patient.

## The Eyes and their Surroundings

It must be emphasised that in addition to numerous disorders confined to the eyes, there is scarcely a disease of other systems that may not have some possible manifestations in and around the eyes. Some aspects of this are described on pages 168, 253 and 388. The present section deals with features which are not considered in these more specialised fields.

During the period when the history is being taken, the patient's eyes will be under special observation. Allowing for normal variations, any asymmetry between the eyes is likely to have been noted. These differences may affect the whole or part of the globe and the eyelids and include squint, abnormalities of the conjunctiva, iris or pupil, exophthalmos or enophthalmos, lid retraction or ptosis and oedema or other affections of the lids.

**The Eyelids.** When the patient is alert, the eyelids are normally held in such a position that, with the individual looking directly ahead, both partly cover appropriate segments of the cornea. In bright light the orbital fissure narrows, while pain, particularly when this involves the eye or its environment, may cause spasm of the eyelids, *blepharospasm*, which can be so intense that retractors or the use of a local anaesthetic may occasionally be required before the eye can be properly examined. The term 'photophobia' is used to describe the reluctance to face the light, characteristic of patients with conditions such as meningitis and painful conditions of the eye.

*Retraction of the eyelids,* both upper and lower, is a common feature of hyperthyroidism. When asked to look at the examiner's finger, the eyelids of a patient with hyperthyroidism may separate appreciably, but after a moment or two they may come together again sufficiently to cover the upper and lower margins of the iris. The term 'lid retraction' implies that the sclera is visible above or below the iris while the patient is gazing straight ahead. In hyperthyroidism the upper lid may fail to follow the movement of the eyeball when the gaze is directed downwards, or may follow only after a delay—a useful confirmatory sign known as 'lid lag'.

*Swelling of the eyelids* occurs readily and is apt to be gross owing to the low tissue pressure under the skin of the lids and to looseness of the peri-orbital tissues. Swelling due to local traumatic and inflammatory lesions is sufficiently common to be familiar to the layman. Periorbital oedema is often due to drugs or to contact dermatitis (Plate III) from cosmetics or hair dyes. Among possible systemic causes of swelling of the eyelids may be included glomerulonephritis (Plate VI), hypothyroidism, angioneurotic oedema, infestation with Trichinella spiralis (trichinosis) and in South Americans or travellers from that continent, infestation with *Trypanosoma cruzi* (Chagas' disease). Swelling of the eyelids may be quite conspicuous in patients with right ventricular failure who are sufficiently free of dyspnoea as to be able to lie flat. The swelling may be greater on the side on which the patient has been lying.

Swelling of the eyelids is almost constant in hypothyroidism and in myxoedema, but in hyperthyroidism it may also be sufficiently marked to cause diagnostic confusion. In myxoedema the characteristic swelling is due to the accumulation of mucoprotein together with water and electrolytes. This material infiltrates between the cellular elements of the dermis and accumulates in the subcutaneous tissue. Failure to pit on pressure distinguishes myxoedema from oedema due to a simple increase in the amount of extracellular fluid, but frequently the two co-exist. Some pitting on pressure cannot therefore be taken to exclude suspected myxoedema.

A *meibomian cyst* is a painless swelling due to blockage of a tarsal gland on the internal surface of the lid. A persistently *watering eye* suggests that a nasolacrimal duct is blocked; the opening of the upper ends of these ducts can be seen at the medial end of each lid. The lacrimal glands lying in the upper and outer quadrant of the orbits are not normally visible.

Yellowish plaques consisting of deposits of lipoid material (*xanthelasma*) are frequently present in the skin at the medial ends of the lids and may be associated with hypercholesterolaemia. Xanthomatosis is described on page 99. The most common site of *rodent ulcers* (p. 100) is on or near the eyelids, particularly near the inner canthus.

**The Eyelashes.** Many common abnormalities of the eyelids result from disorders affecting the eyelashes. Thus a *stye* is due to staphylococcal infection of a hair follicle and *blepharitis* is the term applied to chronic infection of the edges of the lids; *ectropion* refers to eversion of the lids and *entropion* to inversion; in the latter condition the eyelashes tend to damage the cornea.

**The Conjunctiva.** The palpebral conjunctiva of the lower lid may readily be inspected if the lid is gently everted while the patient looks up. The colour gives a very approximate assessment of the patient's haemoglobin level. If there is any doubt, the haemoglobin must be estimated (p. 440) as significant and reasonable degrees of anaemia are easily overlooked, particularly in the elderly.

The upper lid may be everted by using the upper margin of the tarsal plate as a hinge. The patient looks down and the lashes and free margin are grasped between the index finger above and the thumb below. By a twisting movement the tarsal plate can be made suddenly to turn back to front (Fig. 6). The bulbar conjunctiva can be readily inspected at the same time. The two most common abnormalities are foreign bodies and conjunctivitis. The latter is commonly accompanied by photophobia, excessive lacrimation and adhesion of the lids by sticky purulent exudate on wakening. Purulent exudate does not accompany the painful, red subconjunctival injection of scleritis which otherwise closely resembles conjunctivitis. It should be borne in mind that conjunctival injection at the limbus (corneoscleral junction) is also a feature of iritis and glaucoma.

Triangular yellow deposits (*pingueculae*) with their base at the limbus may

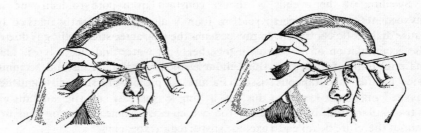

FIG. 6   Eversion of the Upper Lid.

develop with advancing years beneath the conjunctiva between the inner canthus and the edge of the cornea. In the same area a progressive fibrosis may develop and encroach upon the cornea (*pterygium*), particularly in tropical countries.

Oedema of the conjunctiva (*chemosis*) results from a variety of causes, but particularly brings to mind the possibilities of malignant exophthalmos, superior vena caval obstruction or chronic respiratory failure, according to the individual context.

*Subconjunctival haemorrhage* may obscure the greater part of the sclera and alarm the patient. It is usually due to rupture of a local blood vessel in the course of a bout of coughing or for no obvious cause. Occasionally it may be due to bleeding from a fractured skull. A bright red colour persists for several days until the blood is absorbed.

**The Sclera.** Normal sclera is uniformly white in colour and is the most suitable site for the early detection of jaundice. It appears blue in the rare hereditary disorder of connective tissue called fragilitas ossium, since the sclerae are thin and the blue colour is caused by the choroidal pigment beneath. In elderly patients scleromalacia often allows the choroidal pigment to be seen as small brown patches on either side of the iris.

**The Cornea.** Normal cornea is perfectly transparent, and even considerable damage to its surface or small embedded foreign bodies may be difficult to recognise without the assistance of a stain such as fluorescein; with this any breach of the surface will be readily visualised. Opacities of the cornea consisting of fibrous tissue may occur for many reasons, including trauma and infection and if large and centrally placed they interfere seriously with vision. A white ring at the outer margin of the cornea (arcus senilis) is commonly *arcus* present in elderly patients. If it is observed in young subjects it may indicate *cornealis* premature degenerative changes usually associated with ageing. A yellow or brown Kayser-Fleischer ring at the periphery of the cornea is pathognomonic of hepatolenticular degeneration (Wilson's disease).

**The Iris.** This is inspected while the pupillary reactions are tested, but requires closer scrutiny if iritis is suspected. Symptoms of iritis include pain in the orbit or over the nose or forehead, photophobia and excessive watering of the eye. The vessels of the bulbar conjunctiva at the limbus are dilated, the detailed pattern of the iris is blurred and the pupil may be irregular, especially when dilated by treatment with atropine, or if a mydriatic such as Mydrilate or homatropine has been instilled for purely diagnostic purposes. This is due to adhesions of the iris to the lens (posterior synechiae) which are likely to be permanent.

Examination of the *lens, vitreous body* and *retina* is described on page 419.

**Intraocular Tension.** This can be tested digitally but at the best only a very approximate assessment can be made without using a tonometer. The importance of detecting the rise in pressure in acute glaucoma is emphasised by the fact that vision is likely to be lost permanently unless treatment is instituted rapidly. The discovery of a low intraocular pressure, though of no importance as regards the eye itself, is useful confirmatory evidence of dehydration (p. 66). The middle, ring and little fingers of both hands of the examiner should be placed on the patient's brow in order to steady the hand in relation to the patient's eye, and the two index fingers are used to test the tension of the globe by eliciting fluctuation (Fig. 7). Unless this is done gently, there is some danger of causing retinal detachment, especially if the pressure is high.

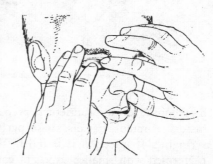

Fig. 7  Testing Intra-ocular Tension.

## The External Ears

The size, the shape and some details of the form of the auricle normally vary widely between individuals. Congenital deformities involving the ears occur, some of which are of genetic origin. In Down's syndrome the auricles are usually small and the lobule may be rudimentary or absent. The helix of the ear is a recognised site of gouty tophi, consisting of sodium biurate crystals deposited in the cartilage; these may eventually form white chalky nodules which ulcerate and discharge on the surface of the skin.

**Auriscopic Examination.** The external auditory meatus and the tympanum may be inspected through an electrically lit auriscope (p. 413). An improved view of the drum and the meatus will usually be obtained if during inspection the auricle is drawn upwards, backwards and slightly laterally in order to straighten the external meatus as much as possible (Fig. 8). Wax is commonly encountered, and must be removed if the drum is to be examined adequately. Provided there is no history or sign of infection or of perforation of the ear drum, the wax may be removed by syringing with warm water. To soften the wax preliminary treatment with warm water containing sodium

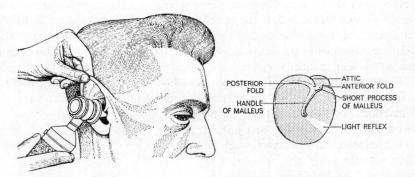

Fig. 8    (*a*) Auriscopic Examination.    (*b*) The Tympanic Membrane.

bicarbonate or a proprietary preparation (Cerumol) may be required. A history of middle ear disease or perforation of the drum, however, precludes syringing. If infection is found in the external meatus, mopping should be performed with small pledgets of cotton-wool applied through the speculum with appropriate fine dissecting forceps. Thus the way should be cleared for inspection of the drum. The normal drum appears pearly-grey in colour, with the handle of the malleus visible and lying almost vertically near the centre of the tympanic membrane. A cone of light is reflected from its lower end downwards and forwards to the periphery of the drum (Fig. 8b).

Acute otitis media can usually be suspected in the presence of earache. In infants the diagnosis will have to be made without the help of this useful localising symptom in what may present simply as an acute febrile illness. The common abnormalities on inspection of the drum are acute inflammation and perforation (p. 388). Foreign bodies lodged in the external meatus are not uncommon in children, and may require instrumental removal.

## The Nose and Sinuses

In spite of its conspicuous position and excepting the overlying skin, the information to be gathered from inspection of the nose as part of a general examination is limited. It may be deformed as a result of an old fracture, or enlarged, red and bulbous (rhinophyma) in the late stages of rosacea. The nose may be narrowed when there is chronic obstruction of the airway in childhood and this associated with mouth breathing produces the 'adenoid facies'.

Each nostril should be closed in turn by finger pressure, and the patient asked to breathe through the other with the mouth closed. The airways should then be examined by direct inspection, preferably with the aid of a nasal speculum. The state of the mucosa and the anterior ends of the inferior turbinates can be visualised; the pearly-grey smooth surface of a polyp or a bleeding point on the nasal septum are two common abnormalities which may be seen.

Infection of the frontal air sinuses may cause a headache which characteristically reaches a peak within two or three hours of rising and then spontaneously subsides as the day proceeds. Involvement of the maxillary sinuses may simulate toothache. A purulent nasal or post-nasal discharge is often present and there may be tenderness on pressure over the affected sinus. The diagnosis may be confirmed by radiological examination.

## The Mouth

Routine examination of the mouth must include inspection of the lips, teeth, gums, tongue, palate, tonsils, mucosa of the cheeks, floor of the mouth and the oropharynx. Any of these structures may be involved by local disease or may show lesions which are part of a systemic disorder. If a mirror is required to examine the nasopharynx and the larynx, then this procedure should be postponed until near the end of the physical examination. The technique of indirect laryngoscopy is described on page 170.

**The Lips.** Exposure to cold commonly causes dryness followed by desquamation and cracking of the lips. Somewhat resembling this is the much rarer cheilosis of riboflavine deficiency causing red, denuded epithelium at the line of closure of the lips, peeling towards the mucocutaneous junction. A similar appearance may follow the use of lipstick to which the patient is allergic.

Angular stomatitis, consisting of painful inflamed cracks at the corners of the mouth, is often caused by ill-fitting dentures allowing saliva to dribble out of the corners of the mouth, followed by infection with *Candida albicans*; this condition may also be due to deficiency of iron or riboflavine.

A fissure of the lower lip particularly, and especially in an older type of patient, which fails to heal within two weeks in response to treatment, should always be regarded as a possible epithelioma. Intractable lesions of this type may require excision for microscopic examination.

**The Teeth.** The deciduous teeth are discussed on page 389. Only too often the 32 so called 'permanent teeth' also have a relatively short life. Inspection of the teeth will give some indication of the patient's attitude to hygiene in general, as well as to that of his teeth. The three principal findings are discoloration, caries and missing teeth. Discoloration is usually due to staining from tobacco or from poor hygiene, but devitalised teeth also gradually become grey. Caries or decay may be kept in check for many years by regular conservation treatment with fillings. Missing teeth are most commonly the molars, and as these are used for grinding rather than biting, their absence is important in connection with dyspepsia. If dentures are worn, enquiry should be made as to whether they are used for eating or only on social occasions. Elderly patients often discard their dentures because they have become ill fitting as a result of atrophic changes in the gums. They often think it is not worth while obtaining a new set and the repercussions on digestion or nutrition may be considerable.

The teeth may be notched and peg-shaped in congenital syphilis (Hutchinson's teeth), pitted and mottled yellow in colour in fluorosis, and poorly developed (hypoplastic) in juvenile hypoparathyroidism. Eruption of the teeth may be retarded as part of any disorder responsible for delayed development, especially rickets.

**The Gums.** In highly civilised communities, gingivitis is very common. It may be due to Vincent's infection (p. 82). At first bleeding is apt to occur, and a narrow line of inflammation can be seen at the free border of the gum, and the interdental papillae are swollen. If the condition progresses, food debris, bacteria and pus tend to accumulate between the teeth and the gum margin (pyorrhoea alveolaris). Halitosis may be apparent and the teeth may become loose. Infection in these sites is a particular danger to patients with valvular heart disease as from it *Streptococcus viridans* may enter the blood stream to cause bacterial endocarditis. A further hazard is that pus may be aspirated into the bronchial tree and initiate pneumonia.

Phenytoin (Epanutin) used for the treatment of epilepsy gives rise in some cases to a firm hypertrophy of the gums which may make it desirable to change to some other anticonvulsant. Other abnormalities due to systemic disease are rare, but examples include the soft, spongy, haemorrhagic gums of scurvy, the hypertrophied bleeding gums of acute leukaemia, the blue line of chronic lead poisoning and the tumour (epulis) which may draw attention to hyperparathyroidism.

**The Tongue.** Inspection of the tongue has probably always been a rite with doctors and their patients. The layman frequently attaches great weight to the appearance of his tongue and may readily develop obsessions about its cleanliness and the significance of any real or imagined changes. These convictions in turn can lead to forms of self-medication which may be harmful, for example, frequent and persistent purging which can even produce potassium deficiency. It is well, therefore, to listen carefully to any comment that a patient may make in this regard, not so much for any value it might have regarding the interpretations usually offered, but because of the implications described, recognition of overt or surreptitious self-medication, and also for the insight that it may provide about obsessional traits and other disorders of this type.

MOVEMENT AND SIZE OF THE TONGUE. The response to the command 'put out your tongue' may provide information about much else besides the movement of the tongue and mandible; for example, in a stuporous patient a normal response would also indicate integrity of hearing and comprehension. Even the extent to which a tongue can be protruded may be important; neurological disease, tight frenulum, modesty or indeed any painful condition of the mouth may restrict the movement of the tongue. At this point the symmetry, the size and the shape of the tongue should be noted. Fasciculation (p. 275) may be seen in lower motor neurone disease such as progressive bulbar palsy and should be observed as the tongue lies at rest within the mouth. Wasting of the tongue occurs with lesions of the hypoglossal nerve (p. 276) and if, as is likely, only one nerve is affected, the appearance of unilateral wasting of the tongue may be very striking. The tongue is enlarged in some cases of primary amyloidosis, in acromegaly and in myxoedema, and in the latter especially it may interfere with articulation. Undue emphasis should not be placed on abnormalities of shape, since many normal tongues are rounded anteriorly, while others are obviously pointed. If on the other hand the organ is asymmetrical, then the possibility of a unilateral intrinsic swelling would have to be considered.

THE SURFACE OF THE TONGUE. This usually receives the most attention, particularly from devotees of self-examination. The tongue normally varies greatly both in regard to colour and to the appearance of the surface. Shades of pink and red, with a range of grey or even yellow or brown towards the centre, may be acceptable as normal. Variations in colour may be due to foods, particularly coloured sweets, or they may be due to quantitative or qualitative changes in the haemoglobin. *Cyanosis* can best be assessed clinically by inspection of the tongue (p. 110). Small, red, flat elevations can be seen on the surface, especially at the tip and edges; these are the fungiform papillae. The filiform papillae are situated in parallel rows across the tongue and give rise to the fur. Transient disappearance of patches of papillae leaving islands of fur between is termed the *geographical tongue,* usually a symptomless change and of no known significance. Diffuse atrophy of the filiform papillae results in the smooth clean-looking tongue of *iron or vitamin B deficiency.* Complaints of pain are not uncommon in these circumstances, or the tongue may be noted to be unduly sensitive to discomfort from hot fluids or food, or from highly flavoured articles. It is important to distinguish this appearance from *leukoplakia,* in which smooth grey opaque areas may be interspersed with a few red inflamed patches; this may be due to syphilis or to chronic irritation and is a pre-cancerous condition.

*Excessive furring,* by contrast, is of little diagnostic significance. It occurs when a soft or milky diet is eaten, and in fever or dehydration.

Separating the anterior two-thirds from the posterior third of the tongue are the *circumvallate papillae* (p. 264) set in a wide V with its apex pointing backwards and originating at the foramen caecum. Patients who discover these relatively prominent papillae for themselves are often alarmed by the thought that they might be cancerous. *Congenital fissuring* of the tongue occurs in varying degrees but has no pathological significance.

**The Palate.** This component of the mouth is usually described in two parts, the hard palate consisting of the anterior two-thirds, and the soft palate with the uvula lying posteriorly. Deformity such as cleft palate may be noted, and a narrow high arched palate may be found. The latter is of little importance by itself, but may be associated with other varieties of congenital abnormality. Apart from examination of the surface the movement of the soft palate should always be checked. The uvula varies much in size and shape; it seldom presents clinical problems except as a source of offence to the patient with obsessional disorders focused in the mouth. The examination of movement of the soft palate is described on page 273.

**The Tonsils.** The tonsils can be recognised as masses of lymphoid tissue which lie beneath the mucous membrane between the pillars of the fauces. In common with lymphoid tissue elsewhere, the tonsils enlarge to reach a maximum between the ages of 8 and 12 years, after which involution takes place. There can be little doubt that failure to recognise this normal phase of lymphoid hyperplasia has led to many erroneous recommendations for tonsillectomy. The distinction between streptococcal tonsillitis and less common causes of sore throats such as infectious mononucleosis, Vincent's infection (p. 82) or diphtheria (p. 82) is very important. In making the examination the points to be noted are the exact extent of the inflammation, the presence of exudate and whether it can be readily removed. Soft, white, solid material is sometimes found exuding from one or more of the tonsillar crypts and should not be mistaken for evidence of infection.

Tumours of the tonsils may also occur either in isolation or as part of lymphatic leukaemia, lymphosarcoma or another reticulosis.

**The Pharynx.** The oropharynx can be seen behind the soft palate and the tonsillar fossae. To do so adequately it may be necessary to depress the tongue with a spatula and ask the patient to say 'ah' in order to elevate the soft palate. The gag reflex (p. 272) may be induced incidentally or deliberately at this point in the examination. Small lymphatic nodules can normally be observed on the posterior wall. Mucus or pus consequent on infection in the nose may sometimes be visible trickling down the back of the throat. The nasopharynx can be inspected only with the aid of a suitable mirror and good illumination. After these areas of the mouth and pharynx have been examined, the remainder of the buccal cavity should be checked. Any dentures should, of course, be first removed. A good light or a torch is essential and a spatula is required to separate cheeks and tongue from the teeth and gums.

**The Salivary Glands.** In the course of the examination of the mouth the opening of the parotid duct may be seen on the buccal mucosa as a small papilla opposite the second upper molar tooth. The openings of the ducts of the submandibular salivary glands seldom require identification, but may be found near the midline in the sublingual papilla, adjoining the root of the frenulum of the tongue. Each of these openings is more readily seen if a free flow of saliva is provoked by something tasty. Purulent infections of glands served by these ducts may be marked by pus exuding from the orifices.

Salivary calculi may obstruct the outlet from the ducts or cause transient swellings and pain in the line of the ducts or in the salivary glands themselves. Examination of the glands is conducted as for any other swelling (p. 48) when there is an abnormality in the appropriate area as, for example, in mumps, sarcoidosis and tumour.

### SOME GENERAL AFFECTIONS OF THE MOUTH

*Carcinoma* occurs in the region of the mouth, and may be found for example on the lips, the tongue, the fauces, or the floor of the mouth, usually in the form of an ulcer, infected to a greater or lesser extent. The only compelling evidence in favour of the diagnosis of neoplasm may be the chronicity of the lesion. In the later stages of disease, enlargement of the regional lymph nodes, fixation of the mass, and other signs of malignant disease may appear, but in the earlier stages any indolent ulcer for which an adequate explanation is not forthcoming provides a clear indication for biopsy examination.

The term *stomatitis* is used to describe a number of conditions affecting the mouth, having in common some features of inflammation. The signs may be restricted to the mouth, but in other conditions the lesions in the mouth may represent only one aspect of a general disease with much more widespread manifestations.

Stomatitis commonly complicates acute leukaemia or agranulocytosis, since these deprive the patient of the normal cellular defence mechanism against infection. In leukaemia the gums often bleed and may be so swollen that the teeth may be largely obscured. Agranulocytosis may present as a sore throat which may progress to an ulcerative form of stomatitis. Unless vigorously treated with antibiotics, a fatal pneumonia is likely to supervene.

In *aphthous stomatitis* ulcers occur on the inner sides of the lips, the edges of the tongue, the insides of the cheeks or on the palate. In the earliest stages a small vesicle forms which is quickly destroyed, leaving a shallow ulcer usually surrounded by a red margin. Such ulcers are characterised by the intensity of the discomfort they create, and while they may heal quickly in the course of a day or two, they may progress to form multiple deep indurated ulcers which heal slowly, and may then leave a small scar. The lesions tend to occur in crops; a patient may be free of ulcers for months at a time, only to suffer a relapse. The cause is obscure. They are often seen in patients with ulcerative colitis.

*Ulcerative stomatitis* (Vincent's infection) is due to two organisms, a spirochaete and a fusiform bacillus which can be seen in a smear taken from one of the ulcers. The condition is painful and foul smelling.

*Thrush* may occur in the infants of mothers who carry infection with *Candida albicans* in the vagina; it also occurs, particularly in the elderly, in association with febrile or debilitating diseases. The fungus may be seen as individual or coalescent white deposits adhering lightly to the mucous membrane of any part of the mouth. There is very little evidence of inflammation unless bacterial infection has been superimposed.

*Syphilis,* in the secondary stage, causes highly infective mucous patches consisting of shallow ulcers with a narrow red edge and a surface covered by a thin white membrane described as resembling snail tracks. The primary ulcer or chancre of syphilis may also occur on the lips or on the tongue rather than on the genitalia.

*Specific fevers* with associated skin rashes often also show lesions of the oral mucosa. In measles particularly these signs are of diagnostic value as they appear before the skin rash. Small erythematous macules with white centres called Koplik's spots are distributed over the mucosa of the cheeks opposite the molar teeth and sometimes spread widely throughout the mouth.

The lesions of smallpox and chickenpox in the mouth rapidly ulcerate, so that their appearance, unlike the skin eruption, is not specific. The breaches in the mucosa may, however, enable superimposed bacterial infection to gain a footing.

The membrane of diphtheria is liable to form on any part of the mucous membrane of the mouth, nose, pharynx, larynx or trachea and particularly in the region of the tonsils. The affected area bleeds if attempts are made to remove the patch of membrane by swabbing. The causative organism can be readily identified by bacteriological examination.

*Pigmentation in the Mouth.* Melanin deposition in the buccal mucosa is normal in negroes and is proportionally less common as the skin becomes lighter, so that usually it is not seen at all in fair-skinned, fair-haired subjects. Pathological pigmentation in the mouth occurs in Addison's disease. If there are no other suggestive features of this rare condition, the most likely cause in patients with black hair and brown eyes is still congenital. Other causes which would have to be considered, particularly in fair persons, are chronic cachexia, the malabsorption syndrome, haemochromatosis or the rare Peutz-Jegher's syndrome of polyposis of the small intestine with pigmentation around and in the mouth and particularly on the lips and fingers.

# THE NECK

Physical abnormalities in the neck are so common that it is essential that careful inspection and palpation should be undertaken in any systematic physical examination.

While it is necessary to examine the neck by inspection from the front, palpation is often more readily and more effectively performed by examining the patient from behind, preferably in the sitting position.

In the first instance, inspection of the neck will show deformities, abnormal movements, or restriction of movement. Any changes there may be in the skin, such as scars, unusual pigmentation, rashes, telangiectases, spider naevi, abnormal growth of hair, arterial or venous pulsations, or tumours will be noted. Systematic palpation should then be carried out, bearing in mind the salivary glands, the lymph nodes and the thyroid gland. From the front the examiner can palpate the back and sides of the neck. The patient should then sit up and the examination continues from behind. Palpation is carried out successively beneath the mandible, over the tonsillar lymph nodes, over the anterior triangles, above the clavicles and especially deep to the sternoclavicular attachments of the sternomastoid muscle where lymph node enlargement may be associated with disease particularly in the chest, and occasionally in the abdomen or pelvis. Finally, the thyroid gland should be examined. The necessity for auscultation in the neck, especially over the great vessels, should not be overlooked.

## The Thyroid Gland

An enlarged thyroid gland is one of the most common abnormal swellings in the body. Any enlargement of the gland is described as a *goitre,* and while this should be examined like any other mass as described on page 48, there are certain features of an enlarged thyroid gland which merit a fuller description.

Unless the patient is very thin and has a longer neck than usual, and unless the sternomastoid muscles are atrophied, a normal thyroid gland will usually escape detection on inspection or palpation. The isthmus consists of a relatively slender band of tissue joining the two lobes across the front of the trachea, and these in turn are closely applied to either side of the trachea and the thyroid cartilage. The importance of the position of the patient and the observer during the examination of the thyroid gland should be emphasised. The ease with which a small swelling in the gland can be seen and felt depends very much on the degree of flexion or extension of the neck. Kocher, a pioneer of thyroid surgery, ensured adequate extension of the neck by insisting that the gland should be examined with the patient supine and the neck extended over a pillow (Fig. 9a). This however prevents examination of the neck from behind, and is not essential if the examiner remembers that moderate extension of the neck will make a swelling lying in front of the cervical spine more prominent on inspection and palpation. While the thyroid gland is being examined, the patient should be asked to swallow at appropriate intervals, and if necessary should be given a drink to facilitate this. The examination is best performed with the patient seated in a good light, with the neck partly extended as described, and with convenient access for the observer so that he can continue his examination from behind when the preliminary inspection and palpation of the gland have been completed from in front (Fig. 9b).

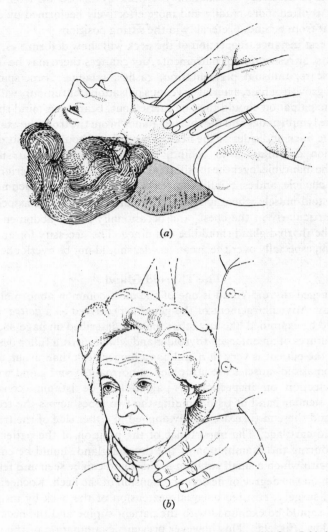

(a)

(b)

Fig. 9    Palpation of the Thyroid Gland    (a) from the Front and (b) from Behind.

The *position* of a goitre is usually characteristic, but it should be recalled that it may extend into the superior mediastinum, or indeed may be entirely retrosternal, and so be overlooked on clinical examination. Rarely, too, the gland may be located, in separate parts or as a whole, along the line occupied by the thyroglossal duct. When it is situated near the origin on the dorsum of the tongue, the structure is referred to as a lingual goitre. In this situation its nature may be puzzling until this is confirmed by biopsy or histological examination after the swelling has been removed, or by the ability of the swelling to concentrate radioiodine.

*Colour changes* over a thyroid swelling are most unusual, unless it is very big, when distended veins may be responsible for a dusky blue discolouration of the skin. After exceptionally large doses of radioiodine, thyroiditis occurs and may be associated with slight reddening of the skin, tenderness and perhaps transient dysphagia.

Other forms of thyroiditis, particularly the subacute or giant cell variety, may be associated with transient episodes of fever, and *pain* and *tenderness* in a goitre. The pain characteristically tends to radiate from the site of the gland upwards and backwards on either side towards the mastoid processes. Dysphagia may also be present.

The *size* of a goitre is impossible to define with any precision, a difficulty which is particularly unfortunate in view of its importance in the choice of a suitable therapeutic dose of radioiodine for a patient with hyperthyroidism. The dimensions as determined by palpation can only be roughly estimated, but changes in the circumference of the neck measured over the point of maximum swelling may be used as an indication of alterations in the size of the gland.

The *shape* of the gland is usually asymmetrical, though less so in a primary toxic goitre than in a secondary or nodular toxic goitre. Simple goitres may be relatively symmetrical in their earlier stages, but usually become irregular with time. As a rule, except with thyroid adenomas, it is possible to define the two lobes of any goitre.

The *mobility of the gland* is a characteristic feature. The fact that the thyroid gland is ensheathed by the pretracheal fascia determines its movement on swallowing and distinguishes a goitre from most other tumours of the neck. Invasive thyroid carcinoma may lead to fixation of the gland to surrounding structures and very large goitres may be immobilised because they expand to occupy all the space available in the root of the neck.

The *consistency* of a goitre may vary from soft to 'stony hard', the latter usually attributable to carcinoma, calcification in a cyst, or intense fibrosis of the type found in Riedel's goitre. Furthermore the texture of the gland may vary from one part to another, just as does the smoothness of its surface. Nodules in the substance of the gland may be large or small, single or multiple, and these variations should always be noted in assessing any goitre.

The presence of *enlarged lymph nodes* near a goitre will suggest the possibility of carcinoma of the gland but they may of course be due to some unrelated cause.

*Auscultation* as a rule should also be performed, since it provides useful information about the degree of vascularity of the gland, a bruit indicating an abnormally large blood flow. In the untreated state this usually implies hyperthyroidism, but the use of antithyroid drugs may promote an increase in the blood supply sufficient to produce a murmur. Precautions should be taken to ensure that a murmur arising in the carotid artery or transmitted from the aorta, or a venous hum originating in the internal jugular vein is not mistaken for a bruit in the thyroid gland.

*Radiological examination* of a goitre may reveal calcification in the substance of the gland, narrowing or displacement of the trachea or a retrosternal goitre; rarely, obstruction of the oesophagus will be demonstrated when the lumen is outlined with barium.

*Isotope Studies.* Identification of a mediastinal swelling as of thyroid origin may be obtained by administering a suitable dose of radioiodine and observing the uptake of the isotope if any, in the region of the swelling. Scanning of the thyroid gland in this way is useful not only in identifying and locating thyroid tissue, but also in estimating the amount of tissue present, and in detecting 'hot' or 'cold' nodules in the gland which concentrate radioactive iodine more or less than the surrounding tissue.

## THE LYMPHATIC SYSTEM

The lymph nodes should be palpated as a routine in the course of each regional examination. The usual sites which should always be examined include the following: pre- and post-auricular, submental, tonsillar, occipital, and posterior and anterior triangles of the neck as described on page 168. The epitrochlear lymph nodes are conveniently felt under the thumb if the patient's right elbow is grasped from the front by the examiner's right hand and vice versa for the left (Fig. 10). The procedure is facilitated if, with his other hand, the examiner suspends the patient's arm by the wrist and flexes it to a right angle at the elbow. The examining hand should then be slid up the

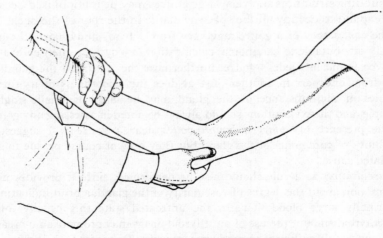

FIG. 10    Palpation of the Epitrochlear Lymph Node.

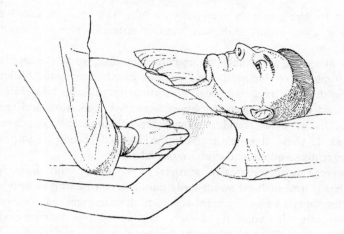

Fig. 11  Palpation of the Axilla.

inner side of the arm to the axilla, for some lymph nodes lie along the brachial vessels. The right hand should then be used to palpate the vault and medial wall of the left axilla and vice versa for the right axilla (Fig. 11). Lymph nodes in the groin and those extending a short distance with the femoral vessels must also be palpated, though interpretation of the findings in this region is dubious unless enlargement is considerable or change in consistency is gross. While palpating the abdomen it may sometimes be possible to feel enlargement of para-aortic or iliac lymph nodes.

Apart from enlargement, there is much diagnostic information to be gained by noting the consistency of the nodes and the presence or absence of tenderness or fixation in accordance with the scheme for the examination of any mass (p. 48).

When there is no obvious local cause for enlarged lymph nodes, it may be helpful to review the lymphatic system as a whole, including palpation of the liver and spleen. If the outcome points to diffuse involvement of lymphoid tissue, radiological examination of the chest will be essential and microscopical examination of the blood and bone marrow and section of an excised lymph node may also be required. Needle biopsy of an enlarged gland is used in the diagnosis of bubonic plague, trypanosomiasis and sometimes in kala azar.

## THE BREASTS

**General Considerations.** The female breast is liable to be affected by a variety of disorders including, for example, acute pyogenic abscess, fibrocystic disease and simple and malignant tumours. Since the breast is the most frequent single site of carcinoma in women of all age-groups, a general examination is incomplete unless both breasts have been examined, whether called for by the patient's symptoms or not. Any mass detected must be regarded as a potentially malignant tumour until this presumption has been excluded.

Breast abscesses are usually accompanied by damage to the nipple during the early phase of lactation and seldom cause diagnostic difficulty. In fibrocystic disease, irregular areas of nodularity, usually bilateral, may be detected and these are often combined with cyst formation and tenderness either locally or over a wider area. Fibro-adenoma will also have to be considered. If these changes are sharply localised it may be impossible to exclude carcinoma on clinical examination alone.

Carcinoma characteristically consists of a solitary and often irregular nodule that is firm or hard and usually painless, contrasting sharply with the surrounding breast tissue. In more advanced disease there may be evidence of infiltration into the adjacent tissues, fixation to the overlying skin and underlying muscles and enlargement of the regional lymph nodes. A blood-stained discharge from the nipple may be the only detectable feature of an intraduct tumour which may be so small as to be impalpable. Inversion of the nipple is a common abnormality but is usually bilateral. Retraction or deformity, especially when associated with an eczematous change, developing in a previously normal nipple, is a diagnostic feature of carcinoma.

In males it should be recognised that carcinoma of the breast occurs at a rate equivalent to about 1 per cent of that in women. Gynaecomastia is frequently seen in Klinefelter's syndrome. It may also be caused by drugs such as spironolactone or when oestrogens are used in the treatment of prostatic carcinoma.

**Anatomical and Physiological Considerations.** For the purposes of examination and description, the breast may be divided into the following components: the nipple, the areola and four quadrants, upper and lower, inner and outer, with the axillary tail projecting from the upper and outer quadrant. The adult nipple consists of erectile tissue covered with pigmented skin which is shared with the areola. The openings of the lactiferous ducts may be seen near the apex of the nipple. The breasts are normally symmetrical. The size and shape of the breast in healthy women vary widely in accordance with hereditary factors, sexual maturity, the phase of the menstrual cycle, parity, pregnancy and lactation, and the general state of nutrition. The amount of fat surrounding the glandular tissue largely determines the size of the breast except during lactation, when the temporary enlargement is almost entirely glandular.

Swelling and some tenderness of the breasts commonly occur in the week before and at the time of menstruation. This engorgement is sometimes attributed to water retention associated with the fluctuations in the secretion of ovarian oestrogens and progesterone occurring at these times. Palpation may show that the glandular elements of the breasts are more readily detected in these circumstances than at other times, and they give an impression of radiating strands of firm tissue with a variable degree of granularity. The ease with which the glandular elements of the breast can be felt varies with the age of the patient, the prominence of the glandular tissue and the quantity of the surrounding fat. There is also a tendency for the strands to be less obvious towards the periphery.

A complete examination of the breast must include systematic palpation of the regional lymph nodes draining the area of the breast. The groups of nodes in both axillae and in both supra-clavicular fossae must be examined. The other breast of course must also be scrutinised.

**Procedure for Examination.** Whenever the presence of a carcinoma is suspected, the full procedure detailed below should be used. If the breast is being examined as part of a general systematic examination, it may be acceptable to use a less complete procedure, bearing in mind that many an early carcinoma has first been recognised in the course of a thorough routine examination and before the patient has been aware of any abnormality.

An adequate examination of the breasts requires that the patient should be completely undressed to the waist and initially should be seated on a chair. The doctor should sit opposite the patient with his back to the light. Occasionally special care may be required to avoid offending the unduly modest patient, but this should never prevent a complete examination.

Before proceeding to palpation, a systematic inspection of both breasts should be undertaken. Any degree of asymmetry between the two sides should be sought, together with changes in the skin, the nipple and the presence of any local swelling. In order to emphasise any local change of this type, and in particular the presence of a mass or an area of fixation, the patient should be asked to take up each of several positions in turn.

1. The patient's hands are resting on her lap so that the pectoral muscles are relaxed as shown in Figure 12a, page 90.

2. The hands are firmly pressed on to the hips ensuring contraction of the pectoral muscles (Fig. 12b).

3. The arms are raised above the head, stretching the pectoral muscles as well as the skin overlying and surrounding the breast (Fig. 12c).

4. The patient leans well forward so that the breasts are pendulous (Fig. 12d).

5. Finally, the breasts are examined while the patient is lying flat on a couch or bed, with the side under review raised by a pillow (Fig. 12e). This can be the opportunity also for an abdominal examination with particular reference to enlargement of the liver.

In each of these positions the breast is inspected, followed by palpation of the four quadrants and the axillary tail in turn. The breast should be examined with the palm of the hand and the tissue rolled gently against the chest wall. This will have the effect of accentuating a local lesion such as a tumour, while the diffuse nodularity of fibrocystic disease becomes barely palpable. If a mass is noted or suspected it should also be felt with the

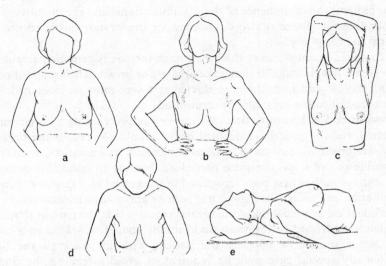

FIG. 12    POSITIONS FOR THE EXAMINATION OF THE BREASTS

Note in (*b*) that the patient is not symmetrically positioned and that this is reflected in an apparent difference in the breasts.

finger-tips so as to elicit the other characteristics of any lump, as described on page 48. Apart from the size, texture and consistency of any swelling, particular attention should be paid to mobility of the mass, any infiltration there may be into the surrounding tissue and whether there is fixation of the tumour to the pectoral fascia or to the skin. One of the most characteristic features of carcinoma of the breast is 'tethering' of the skin. This may not be obvious at first, but if the breast is elevated gently by the hand, the area of dimpling overlying the tumour becomes visible immediately.

Finally the examination of the axillae should be performed as described on page 87. This should be undertaken first with the arms relaxed in order to explore the apex of the axilla and then with the hands on the hips in order to tense the axillary fascia and to contract the pectoral muscles.

The nature of a lump in the breast can often be determined with reasonable certainty by the application of these methods, but in spite of this, it is unusual for a final decision to be reached on clinical grounds alone. On most occasions operation and histological examination will be required.

# THE SKIN

## Structure and Functions

The skin consists of a thin superficial, avascular cellular layer (the epidermis) and a deeper tough, fibro-elastic layer (the dermis). In addition to its main constituents, the latter also contains nerves, blood vessels, sweat glands, sebaceous glands and hair follicles. Beneath the skin there is a layer of areolar tissue containing fat. The amount of fat varies widely in different parts of the body and from one individual to another.

The skin protects the deeper parts from trauma, from infection and from extremes of heat and cold. Vitamin $D_3$ is formed in the skin from 7-dehydrocholesterol in response to ultra-violet light, and possible harmful effects of this form of radiation are reduced by the melanin pigment also formed in the skin. Animals are insulated against cold and wet by hair and by the secretions of the sebaceous glands, and heat loss can be minimised by erection of the hairs consequent on contraction of involuntary muscle fibres—the arrectores pilorum. A vestige of this reaction is seen in man in the form of 'goose-flesh'. The skin is also of vital importance in dissipating heat by vasodilation and sweating, and it conserves heat by vasoconstriction aided by the insulating effect of the subcutaneous fat. It serves also as a channel for the excretion not only of water and electrolytes, but also of normal and abnormal metabolites and drugs.

Disease ensues if any of the main structures of the skin are missing or cease to function. Thus breaches of the surface are liable to infection; ultra-violet light causes sunburn in unpigmented skins; failure of sweating results in death from hyperpyrexia in hot climates; vasodilation in a cold atmosphere may result in death from hypothermia, a combination which is apt to occur in coma from excess of alcohol; loss of nerve function may result in trophic ulcers; cuts and burns of the skin of the hands accompany the absence of pain and temperature sense in syringomyelia. In addition there is a wide variety of primary disorders of the skin and there are many dermal manifestations of systemic disease.

## Examination

When examining the skin, attention must be paid to abnormalities of its structure and function and to any pathological lesions present. The discovery and differentiation of disorders affecting the skin depend largely upon inspection, though palpation sometimes has a useful part to play. Normal practice should include examination of the whole body surface. This is usually carried out piecemeal as the various systems are being examined, but the skin should be scrutinised as a whole when the main complaint appears to be a dermatological disorder.

**Colour.** Localised or generalised variations in colour are similar to those already discussed for the complexion (p. 59). *Pigmentation* may be particularly significant. Pregnancy and Addison's disease have already been discussed in this context (p. 60). The body may also be somewhat pigmented in the unclean, especially in those instances, now fortunately uncommon, in which there is infestation with body lice (*Pediculus corporis*). Chronic inflammation, as is often seen in varicose eczema, may give rise to pigmentation. Some localised colour changes are produced by fungal infections and numerous other skin diseases. In a patient who has been resident abroad the possibility of leprosy should be entertained if depigmented anaesthetic patches are found.

The necessity for local heating in the climatic and domestic conditions prevailing in Britain leads to another striking form of pigmentation, *erythema ab igne,* or, more colloquially, 'Granny's tartan'. This is commonly seen on the legs of women who sit close to a fire for long periods, and is therefore more commonly found in the elderly and in the inactive. The pigmentation is at first red and later brown in colour, and follows the distribution of cutaneous venous plexuses, thus providing the appearance of a coarse net. Even patients with hypopituitarism whose facial pallor is so characteristic, are liable to this form of pigmentation, and indeed these and hypothyroid patients may be specially susceptible beca_se of their sensitivity to cold. The discovery of a similar pattern on the skin of the abdomen or elsewhere, due to the local application of heat, should lead to enquiry about the possibility of pain.

**Texture and Sebaceous Secretion.** Normal skin has a fine texture and a slightly moist surface. At one extreme is the dry scaly skin of congenital ichthyosis, and at the other is the greasy skin often noted after puberty with its liability to acne vulgaris. Over-active and hypertrophied sebaceous glands become blocked by comedones (blackheads) which consist of plugs of semi-solid secretion capped by horny debris darkening on oxidation. This may be succeeded by an inflamed papule and then by a pustule which ultimately bursts. Larger lesions result in permanent scarring. Acne is characteristically distributed over the face, back of the neck, and the front and back of the chest. The hypertrophy of the skin and subcutaneous tissues, particularly of the face, the hands and feet, is often a striking feature of acromegaly.

**Sweating.** Diffuse sweating counters the rise of body temperature liable to occur in hot atmospheres, during exercise, in fevers or in hyperthyroidism and failure to sweat in a hot climate may cause death from hyperpyrexia (heat stroke). Episodes of sweating occur in fainting, with severe pain, during menopausal flushes, in acute hypoglycaemia or during acute hypertensive episodes caused by a phaeochromocytoma. Sweating on the face, palms of the hands, soles of the feet and in the axillae is often due to nervousness. Interruption of the sympathetic nerve supply, as in Horner's syndrome (p. 257) or following sympathectomy causes a local loss of sweating. Rarely there may be a congenital absence of sweat glands.

Sweat contains most of the solutes of blood, but their concentration is much less than in a filtrate of serum. In cystic fibrosis (mucoviscidosis) a characteristic increase can be demonstrated in the concentration of sodium chloride in the sweat (p. 411). In diabetes mellitus the glucose content of sweat is high, and this predisposes to skin infections, particularly with fungi and pyogenic organisms.

A febrile patient, though not sweating visibly, may lose a considerable amount of water. Even more serious account must be taken of visible sweating, which may be responsible for the daily loss of several litres of water containing electrolytes in a concentration of about one-third of that in the plasma.

Hyperhidrosis, or excessive and inappropriate sweating, is usually confined to the axillae, the palms of the hands, and the soles of the feet. In individuals severely affected, hyperhidrosis may not only cause considerable embarrassment and discomfort, but may predispose to fungal infection between the toes characterised by painful cracks in thick, white, sodden skin.

**Skin Temperature.** Differences in temperature between symmetrical regions can be detected with remarkable accuracy by the backs of the examiner's fingers, providing that the hand is not cold. Excluding the recent application of heat to the part, a local rise in temperature is due to an increased blood flow. This may be due to inflammation, to Paget's disease of underlying bone, or to tumours with a large blood supply. It may also be due to a recent deep venous thrombosis with a shift of circulation into the skin vessels, or to chronic arterial block which has resulted in the opening up of collateral circulation through the skin.

In contrast to local increases of temperature, local cooling, particularly of a limb or part of a limb, may be of supreme importance since it implies recent interference with the circulation in the part involved. Arterial embolism or thrombosis will need to be considered in these circumstances, when colour changes and pain are likely to be prominent features (p. 140). In some circumstances, for example with a 'saddle embolus' lodged on the bifurcation of the aorta, both lower limbs might be equally cool.

**Hair.** The circumstances in which the growth and distribution of the hair are disturbed are described on page 70.

**Nails.** Abnormalities of the nails are discussed on page 68.

**Lesions of the Skin.** The skin is no exception to the rule that method is necessary for the study and description of its pathological lesions. The history is obtained in the usual way, but specific points may require special attention, for example, the possibility of contact with infectious diseases like childhood fevers, scabies, syphilis or leprosy. Contact with animals or occupations involving the handling of animal products introduces the possibility of unusual infections of the skin such as animal ringworm, orf, erysipeloid and anthrax. The distribution of the lesions may suggest contact dermatitis, when special enquiry must be made about work, the purchase of new clothing, jewellery, or the application of new cosmetics or hair dyes. Another important factor may be the potential effects for good or ill of a variety of medicaments which may have been applied with or without medical advice. To add to the problem, many variants of the typical appearance and distribution of the lesions may be seen and further difficulties may arise from the effects of scratching or secondary infection.

When examining the skin and assessing the significance of the abnormalities noted, not only must account be taken of their type and distribution but also whether associated lesions are to be found, for example on the mucous membrane of the mouth or nose, the conjunctiva, or even the vagina. The presence of enlarged lymph nodes in the appropriate drainage area should be sought in all inflammatory or potentially neoplastic conditions of the skin.

For descriptive purposes certain definitions are necessary. Most abnormalities can be defined by one or more of the following terms.

*Erythema* means reddening of the skin, and the term is usually qualified by an adjective such as diffuse, punctate, macular or papular. A *macule* indicates a small circumscribed discoloration of the skin, i.e. a 'spot' such as a freckle. *Papular* lesions are by definition raised above the surrounding surface of the skin and this can easily be confirmed by running the finger-tips over the affected area. *Vesicular* lesions (blisters) may be superimposed on the changes already mentioned, and consist of collections of fluid in the epidermis or the dermis. Vesicles vary in size, the larger varieties being described as *bullae*. If the fluid within vesicles becomes purulent the lesions are known as *pustules*. *Urticaria* is a raised pale area of skin, varying in width from the size of a pin head to many centimetres, caused by an increase in interstitial fluid with a high protein content due in turn to increased capillary permeability. The lesions are surrounded by a flare resulting from arterial dilation through an axon reflex. A similar mechanism affecting the subcutaneous tissues gives rise to the less well-defined swelling of *angio-oedema*.

Visible *scaling* or *desquamation* due to abnormal growth of the skin is a feature of most chronic eczematous lesions. The superficial keratin layer remains nucleated and no longer rubs off imperceptibly. Removal of the epidermis when the lesion is scaly may help to distinguish between psoriasis which leaves a dry surface with bleeding points, and eczema in which a moist, weeping area is exposed.

Linear markings known as *cutaneous striae* may sometimes be seen around the abdomen, shoulders, buttocks and thighs. Those of recent origin are pink, while older striae are white or opalescent. They are found in healthy adolescents after sudden increments in weight, in pregnancy and in obesity. In Cushing's syndrome the striae tend to be darker red in colour and more conspicuous than in other conditions.

The observation of *scars* may remind patients of operations which have been forgotten. Puncture marks of hypodermic injections may be noted in diabetics, but, if not adequately accounted for, should raise suspicions of addiction to drugs such as heroin or cocaine.

## Some Common Abnormalities and their Significance

Examination of the skin seldom fails to reveal some abnormality. Many are of limited significance, for example callosities, moles, freckles, erythema ab igne, warts and acne. The importance of some of these is in the eye of the beholder. A few acne pustules on the face of a teenage girl is of no relevance from the point of view of physical health, and the doctor is aware that the condition will clear up spontaneously in a few years. From the girl's view-point, however, this disfigurement is a social embarrassment which may well influence her behaviour and colour her whole outlook on life. Medically trivial skin lesions should be treated with a respect and sympathy which may seem disproportionate to their gravity. The student can and should soon become familiar with changes of this type by paying attention to the skin in every patient. By so doing, the less usual and sometimes far more important conditions will also be noticed. Some of the more common lesions encountered are discussed separately but briefly under the headings of vascular abnormalities, infections, allergic reactions, cutaneous manifestations of generalised disease, and primary skin disorders, including tumours. Such an outline provides a general perspective of the range to be covered and gives some indication of what can be learned from a careful study of the skin. The importance of this examination in childhood is discussed on page 383. For a detailed description of individual lesions, the student should consult a textbook of dermatology.

## VASCULAR ABNORMALITIES

**Purpura.** Spontaneous bleeding into the skin may be manifest as purpura of various sizes and shapes, or in the subcutaneous tissues it may be visible as bruises (ecchymoses). Such a liability to bleed may be due to one of many defects in the process of blood clotting, to a vasculitis as in Henoch's purpura, to inadequacy of the capillary intercellular cement substance as in scurvy or to toxic damage to the small blood vessels. The last may occur in uraemia, from drugs such as phenylbutazone, or in infections such as infective endocarditis, meningococcal meningitis and septicaemic plague. The size and the distribution of the lesions may be very useful guides to the cause of the bleeding. Thus generalised bruises and petechiae, combined perhaps with evidence of bleeding elsewhere in an otherwise fit patient, are suggestive of thrombocytopenic purpura. Petechiae in a patient who is obviously unwell might suggest leukaemia, infective endocarditis or uraemia. A raised purpuric eruption usually distributed symmetrically and mainly over the extremities suggests the Henoch-Schönlein syndrome if associated with abdominal pain or arthralgia. Massive painful bruising of the legs with induration of the muscles, and perifollicular haemorrhages, in an old man living by himself, are almost pathognomonic of scurvy.

Purpura most commonly takes the form of *petechiae,* i.e. small irregular blue lesions of about 1 to 3 mm in diameter visible in the skin deep to the epidermis. Since they consist of extravasated blood they fail to disappear on pressure or on stretching the skin in the affected areas. By contrast, lesions with an intact vasculature can be made to fade and on release of the pressure the colour gradually returns. Contrary to expectations however it is often difficult or impossible to blanch a haemangioma completely, such as a

Campbell de Morgan spot (p. 97), owing to the complexity of the vascular channels involved. Petechiae tend to occur in crops, and unless replaced by fresh lesions, disappear in three or four days or less. They should be regarded as evidence of abnormal capillary fragility, and special tests are sometimes used to demonstrate that this is so. In Hess's test a sphygmomanometer cuff is applied to the upper arm and maintained at a pressure of 80 mmHg for five minutes. Many purpuric spots appear on the forearm when capillary fragility is increased.

*Senile purpura* is common in elderly patients and is usually confined to the dorsal surfaces of the forearms and hands. The lesions are purple in colour and remain so until they disappear; they may be as much as 2 cm or more in diameter, and persist for many days or even weeks before they are absorbed. Thereafter a small white scar usually persists permanently, and sometimes many of these are to be seen on the forearms. The lesions are produced by shearing strains on the skin, associated with loss of elastic tissue from the affected skin. Similar changes occur in patients on long-term treatment with corticosteroids.

*Ecchymoses* or bruises usually result from trauma, but their significance increases in proportion to the triviality of the injury which has produced them. Spontaneous bruising for no demonstrable reason occurs more often in women than in men. An acquired liability to bruising from minor injury, as in the case of petechiae, indicates the necessity for a full investigation of the blood clotting mechanism. Ecchymoses persist longer than petechiae and usually undergo a series of colour changes in the skin from blue to green, yellow and brown as the extravasated blood is broken down.

**Dilation of Blood Vessels.** Obstruction of the blood flow through main vessels may be compensated for by the development of a *collateral circulation*. Venous collaterals are observed much more frequently than arterial because they are relatively common and are usually visible (p. 143). Arterial collaterals are seldom detected in conditions other than coarctation of the aorta (p. 141). Dilation of the small veins (*telangiectasia*) of the face is not necessarily pathological; such an appearance is, however, liable to develop in chronic alcoholics and in those exposed constantly to the rigours of the weather. Small irregular telangiectases also accompany the pigmentation and scarring which follow radiation damage to the skin, and they may be a feature of a number of skin disorders.

*Arterial spider telangiectases* (spider naevi) are characterised by a central arterial dot from which radiate numerous dilated vessels, all of which are readily obliterated by pressure. Refilling commences from the central dot, and the whole system can be emptied by pressure with the point of a pin on the central arteriole feeding the vessels. These lesions occur on the face, arms and upper part of the body and are particularly common in patients with hepatic cirrhosis, though they may also be seen frequently in pregnancy and hyperthyroidism and occasionally in normal people.

*Hereditary haemorrhagic telangiectasia* is a rare hereditary disease. The dilated blood vessels present as punctate red or purple spots or larger swellings up to 1 or 2 mm in diameter. They occur especially about the face and on the mucuous membranes of the mouth and nose, and also at the finger-tips. Epistaxis is common and anaemia of sufficient severity to require blood transfusion may develop.

*Haemangiomas* on the skin of the chest and abdomen commonly develop with advancing years. They consist of firm, bright red to purple swellings, about 1 to 2 mm in diameter, usually standing up slightly above the surface of the skin, and are know as Campbell de Morgan spots. Only with difficulty can they be obliterated or made to fade on pressure, and they have no recognised significance as indication of other disease, nor are they in any way harmful themselves.

## INFECTIONS

The *exanthemata* such as scarlet fever, measles, rubella and chickenpox have characteristic skin eruptions. This is also true of *syphilis* in its secondary stage.

·*Herpes simplex* consists of one or more vesicles which usually form on the mucocutaneous junction round the mouth but which may occur occasionally anywhere on the skin or mucosae, for example on a finger or on the penis. The condition is due to a virus infection and in susceptible subjects may recur during trivial fevers or common colds or even as a result of excessive exposure to sunlight. The lesions of herpes simplex are a frequent accompaniment of pneumococcal and meningococcal infections and malaria. A dark coloured crust may follow on the site of the vesicles as the latter dry.

*Herpes zoster,* 'shingles', is caused by infection of the posterior root ganglion with the virus of chickenpox. The thoracic nerves or the ophthalmic division of the trigeminal nerve are commonly affected and the latter may lead to corneal ulceration. There may be a prodromal period of several days characterised by pain in the distribution of the appropriate nerve mimicking conditions such as pleurisy, cholecystitis or sinusitis. Thereafter the skin in the same area develops an irregular erythema upon which groups of vesicles appear. These in turn may ulcerate, but in the course of two weeks or more they dry up and are replaced by crusted lesions which finally separate. Permanent scarring of the skin is common and may be the only sign in patients with post-herpetic pain, which is sometimes severe and persistent, particularly in the elderly. The incidence of herpes zoster is unusually high in malignant conditions, particularly leukaemia and Hodgkin's disease. Occasionally it may cause a lower motor neurone paralysis, and in herpes of the geniculate ganglion, facial palsy sometimes develops, together with a collection of the typical vesicles in the external auditory meatus.

*Bacterial infections* of the skin are common and those due to the *Staphylococcus pyogenes,* like impetigo and furuncles (boils), are potent sources of cross infection. Such infections may readily become disseminated among debilitated persons.

*Infestation of the skin* and hair by lice and other insects is not uncommon, and is easily overlooked. The hosts are often careless of their hygiene, or unable to care for themselves because of their youth, senility, mental deficiency or poverty. Mites and fleas may be acquired from contact with crops or with domestic animals, and their presence should be suspected if bites or itching follow such exposure. One species of flea, *Pulex irritans,* is fully adapted to man. Infected fleas from rodents are responsible for transmitting plague and endemic typhus fever. In *scabies,* a mite (*Sarcoptes scabiei*) burrows beneath the epidermis, particularly into the fine skin of the web of the fingers, the wrists, feet and penis, and often leaves a shallow linear track. Itching, especially at night, is a cardinal feature of this form of infestation, and scratch marks are common, sometimes in turn becoming infected. The parasite can be identified under the low power of a microscope if it is picked out of the burrow in the skin with a needle and placed in a drop of 5 per cent. potassium hydroxide on a microscope slide.

Infestation with *Pediculus capitis* (the head louse) is most readily recognised by the presence of the eggs (nits) on the hair of the host. These superficially resemble flakes of dandruff, but are found to be fixed to the hair, and rub off only with difficulty. Once suspected, the lice can usually be found with ease.

*Pediculus corporis* (the body louse) is found upon the trunk and in the axillae, whereas *Phthirius pubis* (the crab louse) may be found on the pubis, in the axillae, on the chest wall or in the eyebrows. This organism burrows into the epidermis and may easily be overlooked because of this and also because it remains virtually immobile. Undisturbed, it presents after feeding on blood as a blue spot, and when fasting as a light brown spot about 1 mm in diameter, and may need to be dislodged with a needle or dissecting forceps for microscopic examination. Infestation with crab lice is transferred only by close contact, and its acquisition can be classed almost as a venereal infection.

## ALLERGIC REACTIONS

The agent responsible for sensitisation may reach the skin by the blood stream or may react with the skin through external contact. Both immediate and delayed types of hypersensitivity occur, as exemplified by urticaria and dermatitis. A specific food such as shellfish may occasionally be incriminated, but nowadays drugs are more usually responsible. A wide variety of rashes may result including most commonly a punctate, macular or papular erythema, but also urticaria or purpura. Careful enquiries should therefore be made about pills, mixtures, injections, lotions or ointments which the patient may have been using. It is insufficient simply to ask the patient about medicines. At the same time, other possible manifestations of adverse reactions to a drug should be sought such as fever, lymphadenopathy, proteinuria, hepatitis, anaemia, leucopenia or thrombocytopenia. An external irritant should be suspected from the distribution of a rash at its onset; it may be detected by considering the patient's occupation or by obtaining a history of contact with a new garment, cosmetic, soap, watch strap, etc., in accordance with the possibilities raised by the areas involved. An example of contact dermatitis due to sensitivity to a hair dye is shown in Plate III. Curious linear urticarial lesions (creeping eruptions) are also provoked by the larvae of *Strongyloides stercoralis,* an intestinal helminth acquired in the tropics.

### CUTANEOUS MANIFESTATIONS OF GENERALISED DISEASE

It will be clear from the foregoing that some vascular, infective and allergic lesions will be part of a general rather than a local disturbance. A few examples will be given of other disease processes in which the importance of the dermatological changes lies in the information they give about disease elsewhere. Skin manifestations often supply part of the evidence of *vitamin deficiency,* as for example follicular hyperkeratosis (vitamin A), cheilosis, angular stomatitis and glossitis (riboflavin), pellagra (nicotinic acid) and scurvy (vitamin C).

In *poisoning,* particularly from barbiturates, tense bullae may appear on sites such as the fingers or over the malleoli within 24 hours of ingestion of the drug, probably due to a direct effect on the metabolism of the skin. The skin is frequently involved in the *connective tissue disorders,* for example scleroderma (p. 69), dermatomyositis and lupus erythematosus. In the last named condition an erythematous eruption may be present over the bridge of the nose and adjacent parts of the cheeks (butterfly rash, Plate III). *Sarcoidosis* may involve the skin producing papules, nodules or plaques, and is also one of the causes of *erythema nodosum*—a series of red, painful, tender, indurated swellings, varying in size from a few millimetres to several centimetres in diameter. They are to be found most constantly over the front of the legs, though they may also extend over the knees and on to the thighs, and may even be found on the extensor surface of the arms or forearms. The tenderness may sometimes be sufficiently marked to make even the weight of bedclothes intolerable. In the adult, sarcoidosis is a common cause, but in children and young adults primary tuberculosis or streptococcal infection is more often responsible. This condition, like *erythema multiforme* (Plate IV), may also be produced by drugs such as sulphonamides.

*Xanthomatosis* is characterised by pink or yellow lesions of varying size, distributed widely on the trunk and limbs often over tendon sheaths. Hypercholesterolaemia and hypertriglyceridaemia are usual and the condition may be associated with diabetes mellitus.

*Dermatitis artefacta* (Plate III) is characterised by lesions with an artificial appearance; they are usually linear and sharply defined at accessible sites in patients with personality disorders.

These few examples may serve to demonstrate that cutaneous lesions are often present in systemic disorders representing almost every aspect of medicine. In some cases the skin manifestation actually provides the main diagnostic clue. This may be equally true of common conditions such as the rashes of the usual infectious diseases of childhood and of rare disorders like xanthomatosis. The important lesson is to learn to look at the skin and to question the significance of every abnormality that can be observed.

## PRIMARY SKIN DISORDERS

*Psoriasis* is an important example of one of the most common forms of primary skin disorder. The characteristic lesions are usually clearly defined, scaly, erythematous patches with a predilection for the extensor surfaces of the elbows or knees. When the patches are scratched numerous distinctive silvery scales are produced. Involvement of the finger-nails (p. 69) occurs in some cases, while in others psoriasis may be associated with a form of rheumatoid arthritis.

Both benign and malignant *tumours* may occur. In the *papilloma* (wart) all elements of the skin are involved, while other benign tumours may be derived from the individual tissues comprising skin, for example sebaceous cysts, lipomas, neurofibromas and naevi. *Sebaceous cysts* can be distinguished by the fact that they arise in the dermis and therefore the skin cannot be moved over them. In addition, a central comedo (blackhead) may be present, and the swelling, if not too tense, may be indented by pressure. *Neurofibromas* are relatively rare, and may occur as isolated nodules distributed with the branches of cutaneous nerves (Plate IV). They are usually associated with scattered patches of brown pigmentation. They may be important not only because of the disfigurement they cause, but also because they are occasionally associated with tumours of nervous origin elsewhere, for example, in the posterior mediastinum, 'dumb bell tumours' on spinal nerve roots, acoustic neuromas, meningiomas or even the tumours of chromaffin tissue responsible for phaeochromocytomas. *Naevi* include congenital lesions such as *angiomas* (port wine stain) and *melanomas* (moles). The latter may undergo malignant change especially those which are deeply pigmented, coal black and shiny (Plate IV . Very malignant melanomas may lose their colour

The *basal cell carcinoma* or *rodent ulcer* is a locally malignant tumour which is very frequently seen about the face in elderly persons. These growths start as pearly-white nodules which slowly enlarge until the centre becomes crusted or ulcerated. The *squamous cell carcinoma* or *epithelioma*, in contrast, is a rapidly growing tumour which may spread to adjacent tissues and to the lymph nodes at an early stage. *Metastases* from distant sites such as the lung, the breast, or the kidney may be of passing interest only when the primary diagnosis has already been made. Sometimes, however, a carcinoma will first present as a cutaneous metastasis, and if this

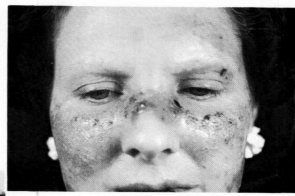

Systemic lupus erythematosus

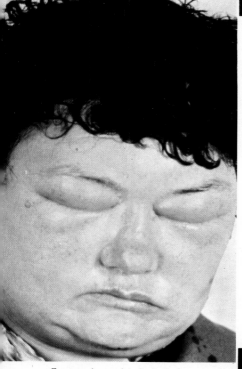

Contact dermatitis (hair dye)

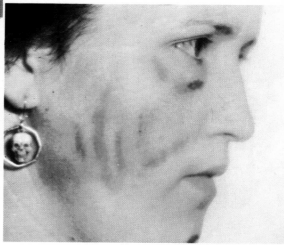

Dermatitis artefacta (Note also the ear-ring)

PLATE III.    THE SKIN AS A DIAGNOSTIC AID

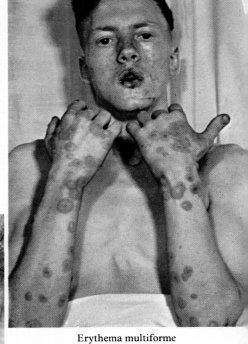

Erythema multiforme

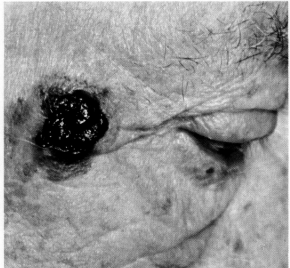

Malignant melanoma

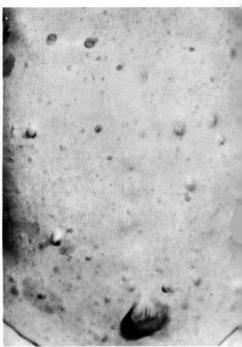

Neurofibromatosis

PLATE IV.   THE SKIN AS A DIAGNOSTIC AID

is suspected with a swelling of recent origin, biopsy should always be undertaken.

## THE METHODS IN PRACTICE

### The Recognition of Drug Addiction

This example is chosen because of the growing prevalence of drug addiction. The increasing variety of preparations on which patients become dependent, coupled with the implications that this carries for the doctor who may encounter such patients unexpectedly, make it important that the few signs which may be present are recognised without delay. Drug addicts commonly are sociopathic (p. 26) and particularly when supplies are short or when for medical or economic reasons, withdrawal is in progress, disorders of behaviour may be apparent. This is most familiar in the patient dependent upon alcohol, but similar features may be seen in withdrawal of many other drugs, particularly narcotics, cannabis, barbiturates and amphetamines. These may be used in isolation or in various combinations; unusual features not seen with single preparations may originate in this way.

An overdose of a powerful narcotic such as heroin may lead to coma with constricted pupils, depressed or periodic respiration, hypotension, and with recovery, vomiting. If withdrawal continues, irritability, restlessness, tremor, sweating, lacrimation, nausea and abdominal pain may be apparent. Depending on the route of administration normally adopted, there may be for example evidence of needle puncture, thrombosed veins, ulcers at injection sites, skin sepsis and lymphadenopathy or hepatitis transmitted by infected needles.

With recovery, the state the addict seeks to achieve may last for some hours, followed by a period of increasing restlessness and purposeful activity aimed at obtaining the next dose. For example feigned illness may mark the patient's arrival at a doctor's surgery or at the hospital casualty department. Individuals in this category are often very knowledgeable about medical and hospital procedures and, like the patient with Munchausen's disease (p. 3), pass from one doctor or hospital and one town or city to another taking advantage of whatever opportunities they can contrive to obtain even single doses of their requirements. Nowadays all clinicians should be on the alert for such patients and if suspicion is aroused, careful scrutiny should be conducted for the external manifestations of this disease.

## CONCLUSION

The general examination provides a wealth of opportunity for diagnosis by the simple techniques of inspection and palpation alone. These basic procedures are also fundamental components of the examination of the individual systems. Where supplemented by auscultation and, to a lesser extent, by percussion, they meet the needs of many clinical problems. With easy access to ancillary methods of diagnosis, the doctor may tend to limit the use of his special senses and fail to base his diagnostic decisions on information gained by taking a patient's history with care and thereafter performing a thorough physical examination. It is only on such a background that logical and economical use can be made of the methods now widely available to confirm clinical diagnoses or to investigate an enlarging category of patients with symptoms only and without physical signs of disease.

# CHAPTER 5
# The Cardiovascular System

'All of him sees, all of him listens and all of him thinks'.
XENOPHANES
*Greek Philosopher* 500 B.C.

Xenophanes could have been speaking of any good physician. Only the rather tenuous excuse that the cardiologist listens twice over—once to the history and again with particular attention through the stethoscope—gives this chapter a special claim to his aphorism. However, the looking, listening and thinking can be done with much greater insight nowadays as a result of new information obtained in the clinical laboratory from investigations such as cardiac catheterisation, angiocardiography and phonocardiography.

Although basic techniques in history taking and examination are little different from those employed 100 years ago and more, both processes, and particularly the examination, have been more quickly refined in the last 25 years than at any previous time. Thus few physicians trained before this period were correctly taught how to measure jugular venous pressure, which is now accepted as one of the most important observations in any patient with heart disease. The less obvious auscultatory signs were not appreciated until phonocardiography had defined them accurately and enabled them to be interpreted. The advances made by cardiac surgeons have taught physicians to realise that new and higher standards of diagnostic accuracy are required. Overall, a clearer understanding has emerged of the physiology of the heart and circulation and of the deviations which occur in disease. As a consequence of these and other contributions in recent years the student's work at the bedside has been made more rational and hence more enjoyable. The author will have failed in his object if at the end of this chapter the reader is left with the impression that the examination of the cardiovascular system is a wearisome task. Nothing could be further from the truth.

## THE HISTORY

The main value of the history in disorders of the cardiovascular system is in providing a measure of functional capacity. Dyspnoea, pain and oedema are the cardinal manifestations of heart disease, and are discussed in detail as their analysis depends on an understanding of their origin and significance. However, it is important to appreciate that severe heart disease may be asymptomatic, and only come to light when a complication arises, as, for example, when an arterial embolism occurs.

The general principles which are involved in the assessment of the severity of a symptom have been described in Chapter 1. It is a common practice in the field of cardiology to use the term 'functional grade' to denote the degree of incapacity caused by pain or dyspnoea (p. 47). Though such a classification may be a useful abbreviation it is no substitute for a succinct record of the patient's description of his symptoms. Questions which often prove helpful include the following: 'What do you now find difficult that you used to be able to do easily?'; the housewife generally gives up scrubbing and polishing first—but in an age of mechanisation there may be other reasons for this! 'When you are walking, can you talk at the same time?'; or 'Do you now keep others back?'; or, when there is difficulty in establishing when a symptom occurs (e.g. cardiac pain), it is often useful to say—'Suppose I wanted to see you with the pain, what could you do that would be most likely to bring it on?'.

### Dyspnoea

The analysis of breathlessness is discussed on page 41, but some recapitulation is necessary here.

*Dyspnoea on effort* is usually the first symptom of left heart failure, but does not differ significantly from breathlessness on exertion due to other diseases. Dyspnoea of cardiac origin is almost invariably relieved by rest, but may occasionally proceed to pulmonary oedema after severe unaccustomed exercise.

Various types of dyspnoea may occur at rest. *Paroxysmal nocturnal dyspnoea* (p. 44) is the most characteristic symptom of left ventricular failure, as a result of hypertension, or of aortic stenosis for example. The breathlessness, which usually subsides in about 10 minutes after sitting up, is due to the flooding of alveoli with oedema fluid, for the horizontal position favours such transudation in the lung. This symptom can appear quite suddenly in a patient who was apparently normal on the previous day. It requires a special search for a cause of increased left ventricular work; or in the absence of such a cause it is usually an indication of disease of the left ventricle. It is a rare symptom in mitral stenosis, except during pregnancy and with the onset of atrial fibrillation, for over the years thickening of the alveolar walls and dilatation of the pulmonary lymphatics preserve the patient from sudden flooding of the alveoli. Abrupt blockage of the mitral valve by a left atrial thrombus or myxoma can cause this symptom, but this is very uncommon. The distinction between attacks of pulmonary oedema and of bronchial asthma is sometimes difficult and is discussed on page 44.

Breathlessness demanding the upright position, *orthopnoea*, when due to heart disease, is a symptom of persistent pulmonary oedema and indicates that the heart disease is far advanced. With improvements in therapy it is now much less commonly seen than it used to be. In attacks of *acute pulmonary oedema* there is persistent severe breathlessness of sudden onset. The accessory muscles of respiration are used, and there is generally considerable accompanying alarm and anxiety. Unless treatment is prompt and effective, the cough, initially repetitive and unproductive, may produce copious watery, frothy and often blood-tinged sputum.

In *Cheyne-Stokes or periodic breathing* (p. 174), there are alternating phases of apnoea and hyperpnoea. It is normal in the elderly during sleep, and may persist for years. In contrast, the development of this type of breathing during the waking hours in patients with cardiac failure is often a pre-terminal event. Accurate recording methods show that periodic variation in the depth of breathing is common in cardiac failure from all causes, although frequently overlooked on clinical examination.

## Pain

The most common pain is that due to myocardial ischaemia. Less frequently pain may arise from the pericardium or as a result of aortic disease.

### Angina Pectoris

Cardiac pain arising on exertion, angina pectoris, may occur without other symptoms and without abnormal physical signs. Under these circumstances precise evaluation is vitally important. The method of analysis of a pain has already been indicated (p. 29), and this pain may be appropriately used as an example of the use of the method.

**Site.** In describing the symptom the patient often places both hands on the chest with fingers meeting on the lower sternum, or uses other characteristic gestures (p. 31).

**Radiation.** A feeling of heaviness or uselessness in one arm, usually the left, or both arms often accompanies the sensation in the chest. Aching in the wrists, or in the jaw or neck, and less often in the back of the chest may be volunteered or elicited in cross-examination. Any of these places of reference may be involved without discomfort in the chest, and the relationship to exertion is then the indication that the pain is probably of cardiac origin. It is under these circumstances that precise diagnosis is most likely to be delayed, as in the patient with an aching jaw when walking up hill who seeks dental rather than medical advice.

**Character.** The pain is characteristically described as like a tight band round the chest, or as a feeling of constriction or of heaviness. The phrasing of the description depends so much on the personality of the patient that this is less reliable than other features, such as the circumstances under which the symptom occurs and its radiation, if any. The pain is often attributed wrongly to indigestion. The patient may deny that the sensation is painful, and may regard it as a form of breathlessness; indeed sometimes the distinction cannot be made even by his doctor.

**Severity and Duration.** Cardiac pain produced by exertion usually begins at about the same place in the course of a regular walk. It generally demands a rest, or the adoption of a slower pace, so that the patient does not allow it to become severe. With rest the pain usually disappears in two or three minutes.

**Aggravating Factors.** Walking uphill, particularly in a cold wind, or exercise after meals is often noted as likely to result in angina pectoris, or to bring it on more easily. Confusion may arise in the phenomenon of so-called 'second wind angina', for example the patient who develops the symptom during the first hole in a game of golf but does not have it later despite steeper hills. This is a fairly common variant, but is sometimes erroneously considered to exclude a cardiac origin for the pain. Angina pectoris is often produced by excitement, stress or fear. Boxing matches on television, sexual intercourse, marital rages or after-dinner speaking by those who do not enjoy it, are examples of situations which may provoke angina pectoris.

**Relieving Factors.** Pain persisting significantly longer than about five minutes after the end of exercise is very unlikely to be angina pectoris. Nitrites hasten the relief of the pain, but occasionally rare forms of oesophageal pain may also be helped, thus underlining the potential fallacies of uncontrolled therapeutic trials.

**Associated Phenomena.** Dyspnoea is a usual accompaniment, as can be readily appreciated by walking with a patient who has angina pectoris, but is scarcely ever mentioned by the patient. The dyspnoea may result in the patient, and his doctor, wrongly attributing the symptom to disease of the lungs. Belching is common, and often appears to relieve the pain; it may similarly misdirect medical interest towards the stomach.

Angina pectoris can be provoked by anaemia, obesity or hyperthyroidism; it can also occur even in early middle age with severe anaemia in the absence of coronary artery disease. In some cases it may be a symptom of aortic stenosis or syphilitic aortitis.

### OTHER CHEST PAINS OF CARDIOVASCULAR ORIGIN

The pain of *cardiac infarction* generally differs from that of angina pectoris in that it is more severe and oppressive and occurs or persists at rest; its type and radiation are similar. The pain or discomfort is often accompanied by a sense of apprehension or of impending death, sometimes called angor animi. The patient tends to lie still and is generally quiet and pale, and often sweats. The pain usually reaches a maximum in minutes, or over an hour or so, and is then persistent for hours until relieved by effective analgesics. Occasionally the pain is intermittent or remittent even without treatment. A severe infarction may be accompanied in addition by vomiting and even haematemesis. Cardiac infarction is not invariably painful, and evidence that it has occurred may be found in many sufferers from angina pectoris either from electrocardiographic or postmortem examination.

Prolonged cardiac pain at rest mimicking that of myocardial infarction may result from tachycardia in patients with diseased coronary arteries; in such cases the patient may be aware of palpitations, or the tachycardia may be detected if he is seen during the attack. In some patients cardiac pain occurs mainly in the recumbent position and it is then called *decubitus angina*. Persistent disabling cardiac pain, sometimes termed *coronary failure*, may precede myocardial infarction.

The pain of *pericarditis* is often mistaken for that of cardiac ischaemia. The features in common are that it is retrosternal and may radiate to shoulders, neck or upper arms. However, it is usually accentuated, or may be present only during inspiration; this is not a feature of pain arising from the myocardium, but pericarditis follows a few days after a myocardial infarction and at this stage there may be pain associated with breathing. The pain of pericarditis may also be provoked by swallowing or by change of position.

Rapid accumulation of fluid in the pericardial space gives rise to a sense of retrosternal oppression, usually indistinguishable from that of myocardial ischaemia. The development of a haemopericardium in a patient with myocardial infarction, and under treatment with anticoagulants, may be mistaken for a further episode of infarction. Other signs of acute cardiac tamponade (p. 149) may allow a distinction to be made on clinical grounds. If there is doubt a radiograph of the chest may be helpful and should be obtained.

*Syphilitic aneurysm of the aorta*, which is now uncommon in Britain, may produce pain when there is erosion of bone, usually a persistent interscapular or upper retrosternal ache, often worse at night. Pain from *dissecting aneurysm of the aorta* is usually of dramatically sudden onset and in the upper chest posteriorly more often than anteriorly. Spread of the dissection to the abdominal aorta may account for abdominal pain. *Massive left atrial enlargement* is a rare cause of pain in the back, variable in quality but often an ache made worse by, and persisting long after, exertion. A momentary jab of pain at about the site of the cardiac apex is a common experience in normal subjects and is sometimes called *precordial catch*; it never indicates organic heart disease.

Various bizarre discomforts are described by those subject to *anxiety* and can usually be readily distinguished. However, patients who have organic pain and are prone to use colourful descriptions may demand considerable patience and sympathy if the symptom is to be interpreted correctly.

## Oedema

Oedema is the most characteristic feature of fluid retention in cardiac failure; together with ascites and pleural transudates, it is dealt with more fully on pages 52 and 148.

## Miscellaneous Symptoms

A repetitive, dry, unproductive *cough*, accompanied by tachypnoea, is the herald of pulmonary oedema in some cases. Cough may also be a symptom of aneurysm of the aorta. Compression of the trachea or a main bronchus sometimes gives this a trumpeting quality, and may be described as a brassy cough. *Haemoptysis* is a particularly common symptom of mitral stenosis. It may also be a feature of pulmonary infarction (p. 159) which is a very common complication of mitral stenosis or of cardiac failure, particularly in the bedridden; evidence of deep venous thrombosis in the legs (p. 143), and of pleurisy or pleural effusion should then also be sought. *Syncope* may be prolonged in circulatory catastrophes such as severe myocardial infarction or pulmonary embolism, or intermittent and benign in simple fainting attacks (p. 38).

*Palpitations*, or awareness of the heart beat, is a common feature of anxiety and can be produced by sympathomimetic drugs such as adrenaline, ephedrine or isoprenaline; panic attacks are commonly confused with paroxysmal tachycardia. Patients can often say whether the heart beat seems to be regular or irregular, and by tapping with the finger can sometimes indicate the approximate heart rate. Such evidence is occasionally of help in diagnosing paroxysmal tachycardias when normal rhythm has returned before the patient is seen.

*Tiredness* is a common symptom in severe heart disease, particularly in the presence of cardiac failure. Its unexpected appearance in a patient with congenital or rheumatic heart disease should arouse suspicions of infective endocarditis. However it is a common symptom of other disorders; for example the patient with mitral valve disease who complains of tiredness is more likely to be depressed than to have infective endocarditis.

The *eyes* may be affected in various forms of circulatory disease. Sudden impairment of vision may be a feature of retinal haemorrhage in severe hypertension, or of embolism in rheumatic heart disease, and is more likely to occur when there is atrial fibrillation, or in infective endocarditis. It may also occur with retinal arterial thrombosis or cranial arteritis. Generally, however, such incidents do not impair vision, but are revealed on routine examination with the ophthalmoscope. Impairment of vision may also result from the development of a visual field defect due to occlusion of a cerebral artery (p. 246). *Renal function* is disturbed in severe cardiac failure. The patient frequently rises at night to pass urine and diurnal oliguria may also occur. There may be polyuria during an attack of paroxysmal tachycardia. In terminal cardiac failure, particularly with a persistently very high venous pressure, *hepatic failure* with or without jaundice, *gastro-intestinal failure* with malabsorption and *renal failure* can all add to the severity of the illness and contribute to apathy, malaise and anorexia. The sudden appearance of drowsiness, weakness and ptosis may be expressions of *electrolytic disturbance* due to inappropriate use of powerful diuretics.

## Previous Medical History

About half of those with chronic rheumatic heart disease know that they have had either acute rheumatic fever or chorea, and it is important to ask about this if the information is not volunteered. Diphtheria may cause severe cardiac failure, but if the patient survives, the heart returns to normal.

The progress of heart disease should also be analysed as accurately as possible, i.e. 'When was heart disease first suspected?'; 'When was the rhythm first noted to ϴe irregular?' (first treatment with digitalis often indicates this point); and 'When did symptoms first develop, and what were they?' With experience it will be learned that symptoms are relatively early in some diseases, e.g. mitral stenosis, and almost terminal in others, e.g. aortic stenosis.

Certain medical contexts have also to be recognised, such as the liability of patients with Marfan's syndrome (p. 64) or coarctation of the aorta to acute dissection of the aorta, or of patients with Friedreich's ataxia or dystrophia myotonica to cardiomyopathy. Arterial occlusion, whether peripheral or coronary, is abnormally frequent in diabetics, and in patients with hypercholesterolaemia (e.g. with xanthomatosis). Recurrent urinary infections may lead to chronic pyelonephritis and explain the development of hypertension. The rare carcinoid tumour with hepatic metastases can produce unusual flushing of the skin and signs of tricuspid and pulmonary valvular disease.

**Obstetric History.** In the assessment of the female patient with heart disease, of which mitral stenosis is the most common, any development or exacerbation of symptoms during past pregnancies should be carefully noted. This information is of course of particular relevance when deciding on the medical management of a subsequent pregnancy.

**Family History.** In rheumatic heart disease, premature arterial disease, and hypertension, a family history of the same complaint is very common.

**Social History.** Precise information about the amount of physical effort demanded of the patient by the home (or, in the case of a flat, by the stairs) and by his work or the journey to it, is essential in deciding on the patient's rehabilitation and after-care. When the patient is a housewife, details of the help available at home, and of her commitments, need to be known.

Ischaemic heart disease and chronic cor pulmonale are much commoner in cigarette smokers, so that the smoking habits must be recorded. Cardiomyopathy can result from an excessive consumption of alcohol, so that enquiries must also be made in this area.

# THE PHYSICAL EXAMINATION

The routine examination should start with a general inspection of the patient, particular attention being paid to any cyanosis or breathlessness. The arterial and venous pulses are next assessed. Oedema should be sought, particularly at the ankles, in those who are ambulant, and over the backs of the thighs and over the sacrum in those who are confined to bed. Then the heart is examined by inspection, palpation, percussion (when indicated) and auscultation. The recording of the blood pressure is usually postponed to the end of the examination in the hope that the patient will become more relaxed. The optic fundi must also be examined. In this way it should be possible to decide whether or not any significant abnormality is present. Any more detailed investigation can then be planned in the light of these findings.

### General Inspection

The opportunity of making a prolonged, careful and critical scrutiny of the patient must be exploited to the full while the history is being taken, for it is at this stage that conditions such as hyperthyroidism, hypothyroidism, or severe anaemia, if one of these is present, should be detected. This scrutiny will provide valuable evidence to the trained observer, while one less skilled is delving prematurely for his stethoscope. Thus, for example, it is often necessary deliberately to ask oneself whether there is evidence of hyperthyroidism, particularly in the elderly female patient with cardiac failure and atrial fibrillation. In this type of patient, one should not expect the exophthalmos and full neck of the younger thyrotoxic subject but should seek especially the staring look, the agitation and, later, the warm hands.

Changes in the complexion should be studied, as described on page 59, particular attention being paid to the colour of the skin.

**Skin Colour.** The colour of unpigmented skin depends on the quality and quantity of the blood in the subpapillary venous plexuses. In anaemia or if there is vasoconstriction as may occur under emotional stress or with nausea, the skin will be pale. High colour over the cheek bones (malar flush) may be seen in adults with mitral stenosis, particularly in those with severe pulmonary hypertension. The skin will have a purplish tinge if there is an excessive amount of reduced haemoglobin. This colour is known as cyanosis. Its origin may be peripheral, in which a low blood flow leads to an unusually high proportion of reduced haemoglobin, or central, in which arterial blood is incompletely saturated with oxygen.

**Peripheral Cyanosis.** This will be a familiar sight in the hands, cheeks, lips and ears in cold weather; it is due to the vaso-constrictor effect of cold upon blood vessels. Whether the part looks cyanosed or white depends upon the amount of blood in the veins. In most forms of heart failure the cardiac output is reduced and the blood flow to vital organs, such as the brain and heart, can be maintained only by differential vasoconstriction at the expense of the skin and other less important organs. Widespread peripheral cyanosis then occurs and even the tongue may be involved in severe cases; cyanosis of the tongue is more usually due to arterial undersaturation, i.e., central cyanosis.

**Central Cyanosis.** There are two groups of causes:

1. Acute or chronic disorders of lung function sufficiently severe to impair the oxygenation of the blood. The commonest chronic disorder in Britain causing central cyanosis is bronchitis with emphysema. The

respiratory causes of central cyanosis are discussed further on page 166.

2. When venous blood bypasses the pulmonary circulation and is shunted into the systemic circulation (right to left shunt). This is seen in arteriovenous shunts associated with hepatic cirrhosis, in pulmonary arteriovenous fistulae and in Fallot's tetralogy and other rarer forms of congenital heart disease where systemic venous blood bypasses the lungs. Exercise may increase the proportion of blood shunted and so remove doubt about the presence of cyanosis. When the shunt is severe, clubbing of the fingers and toes (p. 167), injection of the conjunctivae, and polycythaemia are common accompaniments. Breakdown of the abnormally numerous erythrocytes may lead to gout in severe cases.

Methaemoglobin or sulphaemoglobin may occasionally cause cyanosis. The presence of these abnormal pigments in the blood can be detected by spectroscopic examination.

## Respiration

The rate, depth and rhythm of breathing and any evidence of respiratory distress should be observed. If the patient is breathless, he will usually dislike having to lie flat on a bed or couch, and adding a pillow or raising the head of the couch may be welcomed both for its relief from discomfort and as a sign of understanding on the part of the examiner.

## Pulsations in the Neck

An arterial or a venous pulse may be visible in the neck and if this is the case an abnormal rhythm may be detected during the initial inspection. In the young, an obvious arterial pulse in the suprasternal notch or a very prominent carotid pulse should immediately suggest coarctation of the aorta, or aortic incompetence. In elderly women, the pulsation of a 'kinked' atheromatous carotid artery is often seen, almost invariably on the right side and often accompanied by hypertension. This is often mistaken for an aneurysm, and has gained the (rather unkind) name of 'student's aneurysm'. If the patient lies supine, a venous pulse is usually visible even in normal subjects. The further study of the jugular venous pulse is described on page 120.

## Examination of the Arterial Pulse

The pulse wave which is felt by the examining finger is imparted to the column of arterial blood by the contraction of the left ventricle and takes between 0·2 and 0·3 sec to reach the feet; the blood takes 10 times as long to make the same journey. The form of the pulse wave is largely determined by the quantity of blood ejected into the aorta, the speed of ejection and the rigidity of the arterial system.

The arterial pulse is examined for *rate, volume, tension, form of the wave* and *rhythm*. The peripheral pulse most commonly used for clinical examination is the radial at the wrist; examination of other arterial pulses is described on page 141. Its absence from the normal site may be due to an anatomical variant, as a result of which the artery crosses laterally over the lower end of the radius to pass through the 'anatomical snuff-box'. If the radial pulse cannot be felt there or at its usual site, the ulnar and brachial pulses (p. 142) should then be sought. Rarely the radial artery may be palpable, but the pulse may be absent as a result of its occlusion; there are usually no symptoms because the ulnar artery is able to supply the hand through the arteries of the palmar arch.

The student is generally told to report also on the state of the arterial wall. All that he needs to know is that in general the artery is liable to be thicker, to become tortuous and to undergo medial calcification with the passage of years. These changes are not related to atheromatous change, and are benign. Feeling the artery does not provide information about atheroma, and it is the incidence of this which mainly determines the inadequacy of an artery.

**Pulse Rate.** The pulse rate can, with practice, be estimated with fair accuracy without the use of a watch. With a watch it should be possible to count the pulse to a heart rate of about 200; at faster rates some find reasonable accuracy can be achieved, as judged by an electrocardiogram, by counting alternate beats. Some find it easier to count the heart rate by auscultation, and in infants this is essential. *Sinus tachycardia,* or a rapid heart rate, is normal in infants and small children; it is an accompaniment of anxiety at any age, and it is a feature of shock, haemorrhage, fever and many other conditions. *Sinus bradycardia,* or a slow heart rate, is often found in athletes in training; it may also result from elevation of the intracranial pressure. Extrasystoles, when they alternate with normal beats and produce no palpable pulse, may cause an illusion of bradycardia, but auscultation will reveal them.

In *complete heart block* the pulse rate is usually less than 40, and may fall as low as 20. Independent pulses of atrial origin may be detectable in the jugular veins (p. 120). In 2:1 heart block the venous is twice the arterial pulse rate.

With *paroxysmal atrial tachycardia* the heart rate usually lies between 140 and 180 (it may be as much as 300 in infants), is regular in time, and constant in rate to within one or two beats per minute as long as the attack lasts. It results from the spontaneous development of an ectopic pacemaker in the atrium and the abnormally rapid atrial contractions are often visible in the jugular pulse. In *paroxysmal ventricular tachycardia* the ectopic focus is in the ventricle, but the heart rate is similar to that in atrial tachycardia. The atria usually contract at a normal rate, and this may be identified in the jugular venous pulse; varying relationship between atrial and ventricular contraction results in a beat to beat difference in stroke volume which may be reflected in a beat to beat variation in the pulse volume and in the intensity of the first heart sound (p. 130). However, only an electrocardiogram can make the distinction with certainty.

*Atrial fibrillation* is considered under pulse rhythm (p. 116). With *atrial flutter* the pulse rate depends on the degree of atrio-ventricular block; when the block is constant the rhythm is regular and the pulse rate bears a mathematical relationship to the atrial rate. Small waves, transmitted from atrial contractions, at a rate of about 5 per sec may be visible in the jugular venous pulse. Carotid sinus pressure, by increasing atrioventricular block, may in some cases reduce the pulse rate, e.g. a change from 2: 1 to 3: 1 block will suddenly reduce a pulse rate of 150 to 100 beats per minute.

**Pulse Volume.** The term 'pulse volume' is used to indicate the movement imparted to the finger by the pulse; it varies with the pressure applied by the finger. In general, there is a relationship between left ventricular stroke volume and pulse volume if no abnormal obstruction intervenes; in the elderly, thickening, and particularly calcification of the arterial wall, will reduce the pulse volume. Emotion, exercise, heat and pregnancy are among the physiological factors which increase the pulse volume. A rapid run-off from the arterial system will produce a high pulse volume, whether due to dilatation of systemic arterioles, as in chronic severe anaemia and thyrotoxicosis, or due to an incompetent aortic valve or a patent ductus arteriosus. Pulse volume in large arteries has nothing to do with local blood flow, as can be easily confirmed by feeling the large pulse in the stump of a femoral artery above an amputation site. Small arteries may undergo vasoconstriction; for example, in swimmers the radial pulse may be impalpable after prolonged immersion in cold water, even though the blood pressure and stroke output are normal.

A small volume in a single peripheral pulse indicates local obstruction to blood flow; under these circumstances the arrival of the wave is also delayed when compared with the contralateral pulse. Unless delay is present an anatomical variant should be suspected and sought. The radial and femoral arteries, where they are usually palpated, are about equidistant from the aortic valve and the pulses are synchronous. In coarctation of the aorta the pulse wave travels from the arch of the aorta via collateral vessels and its arrival at the femoral artery is therefore delayed. Feeling the radial and femoral pulses simultaneously will show that the femoral pulse is weak and its arrival is delayed after the radial pulse. When there is severe reduction in cardiac output all the peripheral pulses are small; this is the case in nearly all forms of cardiac failure due primarily to heart disease, the main exception being aortic incompetence.

Various factors cause a variation in the pulse volume from beat to beat. The most common one is a variation in rhythm, for after a longer diastole there is an increase in left ventricular stroke volume and pulse volume. Variation in pulse volume is therefore characteristic of the arrhythmias to be dealt with later (p. 116).

*Pulsus paradoxus* (Fig. 13) is a clinically detectable exaggeration of the normal condition, and hence is a misnomer. It refers to the increase in arterial

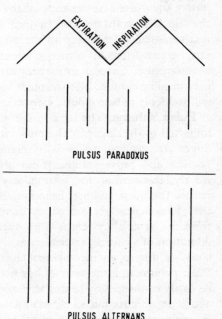

FIG. 13  PULSUS PARADOXUS AND
PULSUS ALTERNANS
In these diagrams, redrawn from continuous intra-
arterial pressure recordings, each pulse beat is
indicated by a vertical line representing the pulse
pressure. In pulsus paradoxus, note that the
mean pressure and the pulse pressure fall during
inspiration.

PULSUS PARADOXUS

PULSUS ALTERNANS

pressure during expiration, and reduction during inspiration. This is partly because physical changes in intra-thoracic pressure are transmitted through the arteries and partly because during expiration the squeeze on the lungs increases left ventricular filling and therefore left ventricular ejection. In health the variation in arterial blood pressure with breathing is not detectable in the pulse tension (p. 115) felt with the finger, but it is this change in pressure which triggers sinus arrythmia (p. 116) through the baroreceptors. The pressure change may however be detectable during the measurement of blood pressure by the cuff method, for if the cuff pressure is arranged to fall slowly enough the Korotkov sounds may be heard only on expiration over a few mmHg at the top of the range.

The most common cause of pulsus paradoxus is an increased amplitude of intrathoracic pressure change with breathing; consequently it is noted in airway obstruction, particularly with asthma. It is also a characteristic sign of pericardial effusion and constrictive pericarditis. In these circumstances the pulse may be felt to be very weak or to disappear in inspiration; then too the presence of pulsus paradoxus should be confirmed during the blood pressure measurement, and expressed as, for example, 'paradox over the upper 35 mmHg'.

*Pulsus alternans* (Fig. 13) is a sign of left ventricular failure in which alternate pulses are less strong; it may be persistent, or intermittent and appear only after an extrasystole or after the Valsalva manoeuvre (p. 118); as with pulsus paradoxus, minor degrees are best detected with the sphygmomanometer.

The *tension,* reflected by the pressure needed to abolish the pulse, relates to the systolic pressure within the artery. Low arterial tension is a feature of many emergency situations. The blood pressure record is a much more reliable way of demonstrating this.

**The Form of the Pulse Wave.** The form of the pulse wave may be of diagnostic value. The throttle effect of *aortic stenosis* makes the arterial upstroke slow, and there is often a so-called anacrotic peak on the upstroke; this first peak is due to the percussion wave of ventricular systole transmitted through the valve to the aortic blood, and the second is imparted by the delayed jet of blood passing through the stenotic valve.

In combined *aortic stenosis and incompetence* the stenosis is not so severe and the stroke volume is larger; under these circumstances the two peaks are

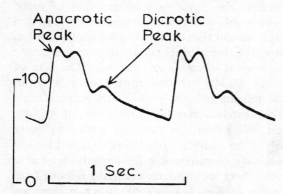

Fig. 14  Bisferiens Pulse
Intra-arterial tracing from a patient with aortic stenosis and regurgitation. The two palpable elements in this pulse are the anacrotic peak and the second peak. In contrast, in the dicrotic pulse the anacrotic peak is absent and the dicrotic peak is exaggerated.

more clearly defined and a double impulse may be felt in the arterial pulse, preferably by feeling the carotid artery with the thumb. This is the so-called bisferiens pulse (Fig. 14) and is almost pathognomonic of aortic stenosis and incompetence. Although it is usually a 'makeweight' sign, i.e. sought after the diagnosis has been made in other ways, it often obtrudes on the consciousness and indicates the diagnosis before the stethoscope is used.

In *aortic regurgitation without stenosis* the pulse is of high volume and the upstroke is sharp, due to a large stroke volume being ejected into a low pressure system. This pulse is most readily appreciated by placing the palm of the hand on the patient's forearm while his arm is elevated. The blood in the arteries of the elevated arm drains in a retrograde direction during diastole so that the increase in pulse pressure is enhanced. This type of pulse is often called 'collapsing'. (The term 'water hammer' is better reserved for the Victorian toy of that name, for few physicians have ever seen one.)

The *dicrotic pulse* refers to a double impulse in which the dicrotic elevation of pressure, at the time of aortic valve closure, is increased. It is found in conditions in which there is reduced peripheral vascular resistance, e.g. fever, particularly in the young whose arteries are more elastic.

**Pulse Rhythm.** The normal pulse is usually regular, but *sinus arrhythmia,* which is a slowing of the pulse in expiration, is physiological and is a particularly common finding in children. The explanation is that there is an increase in left ventricular filling and ejection during expiration (p. 114). The blood pressure rises, the baroreceptors and the vagus nerves are stimulated, and reflex slowing of the heart results. When a large atrial septal defect allows the filling of the two ventricles to remain more constant throughout the respiratory cycle, sinus arrhythmia is absent or slight and this is therefore a minor sign of atrial septal defect, particularly in children.

*Ectopic beats* (extrasystoles) should be recognised by their prematurity, the compensatory pause which follows them, and their reduction or abolition by exercise. The premature beat is often unusually loud on auscultation because the atrioventricular valves are wide open at the onset of systole. When very numerous the pulse may mimic that of atrial fibrillation, but exercise should enable a distinction to be made. Though generally unimportant they are a useful sign of early digitalis intoxication, and are then of ventricular origin. Ectopic beats occurring every alternate beat cause *pulsus bigeminus, coupled rhythm,* or *coupling.* The site of origin of an ectopic beat can usually be determined only with an electrocardiogram (ECG). When an ectopic beat occurs soon after a normal beat, the filling of the ventricle may be insufficient for a pulse to be produced; auscultation will reveal this cause of a missing pulse at the wrist as the extra beat will be audible. Heart block, in addition to producing regular bradycardia, may be responsible for irregularity, e.g. in 3 : 2 *atrio-ventricular block* when there are regularly occurring missing beats on auscultation and at the pulse; in *Wenckebach's phenomenon* there are cycles of steadily increasing intervals between atrial and ventricular contraction from beat to beat culminating in a dropped ventricular beat and pulse. These rhythms can be identified with certainty only by ECG, or by clear demonstration of the atrial pulse in the jugular veins.

With *atrial fibrillation* the pulse is totally irregular, although when the ventricular rate is slowed with digitalis the pulse may in some cases seem to be regular if felt only for a short time. With most other disturbances of rhythm the pulse is basically regular. The pulse beat may be missing at the wrist at faster ventricular rates and it is then necessary to count the heart rate by auscultation. The difference between heart rate and pulse rate is called the *pulse deficit;* simultaneous examination by two observers is required if accuracy is to be obtained.

## Blood Pressure

The technique of recording blood pressure by the cuff method is generally learned in the physiology department, but some of the more important practical aspects merit repetition here. The manometer most widely used in Britain is the mercury-filled instrument; the aneroid is more convenient and compact, but a suspicion of inaccuracy has led to a widely held prejudice against its use. Engineers however have long realised the robustness and reliability of a well-made aneroid pressure gauge. It is an easy matter to establish its accuracy by checking against a mercury instrument from time to time if this is doubted. The normal width of the cuff for adult use is about 12 cm; a wider cuff is employed for the leg and a narrower one for infants and children. A cuff of given size compresses a fat arm less efficiently than it does a thin arm, and this accounts for artificially high records of blood pressure obtained with standard cuffs in obese subjects, when compared with intra-arterial pressure records. The arm blood pressure should be recorded with the subject lying flat; the leg pressure must be so recorded in order to avoid the increment of pressure due to the height of the column of arterial blood between the heart and the cuff. Care must be taken that the brachial artery is not compressed by vigorous hyperextension at the elbow or by pressure with the stethoscope bell, for either may cause sounds and introduce errors in the measurement of diastolic pressure. The cuff should be carefully and smoothly applied. It should then be inflated until the radial pulse is obliterated and the pressure allowed to fall until the pulse returns (*systolic pressure*) and in this way it is possible to avoid mistakes due to the 'auscultatory gap', i.e. the phenomenon in which Korotkov sounds are heard over the brachial artery at, say, 220 mm Hg, disappear when the cuff pressure falls to 200 mm Hg and reappear at 180 mm. The silent interval between, in this case, 200 mm and 180 mm is the '*auscultatory gap*'. The unwary may record the systolic pressure well below the true figure, in this case 40 mm lower.

The pressure is allowed to fall slowly while the stethoscope is applied over the brachial artery at the elbow. The point at which the sounds fade sharply is generally considered in Britain to be the nearest approach to the *diastolic pressure*. This correlates better with direct intra-arterial recordings of the diastolic pressure than does the point at which the sounds disappear completely. In some normal persons, indeed, sounds may still be audible at zero pressure. Occasionally, the physician is requested, for example by some insurance companies, to record three levels, namely, the systolic pressure, the point at which the sounds become muffled and the point at which they disappear.

When a difference in the pulse in the two arms is suspected the blood pressure should be recorded on each side; when a weak delayed femoral pulse is associated with hypertension in the arms the blood pressure in the legs should also be recorded (see coarctation of the aorta, p. 113 ). The cuff is applied to the thigh, with the patient lying prone, and the stethoscope is placed over the popliteal artery.

Casual records of blood pressure are less valuable than repeated records with the patient at rest. Emotional factors may elevate the blood pressure mm Hg, and the diastolic more than 20 mm Hg higher than in subsequent records when the patient has become accustomed to the procedure. Such falls in pressure on repeated examination are often erroneously attributed to treatment provided for hypertension. Devices which record blood pressure continuously demonstrate the temporary hypertensive effect of doctors approaching a patient's bed.

### Vasomotor Reflexes

Vasomotor reflexes are among the many factors which control the blood pressure. Baroreceptors in the aorta and at the carotid bifurcation (carotid sinus), when stimulated by a rising arterial pressure, initiate afferent impulses; the efferent pathway is through the vagus nerve, and the heart rate is slowed. Conversely, falling arterial pressure results in sympathetic stimulation which improves the efficiency of the myocardium and increases the peripheral arterial resistance. Precise observations on these reflexes required an electromanometer and continuous records of arterial pressure. However, there are some simple bedside tests which allow some of the faults to be detected without the use of special equipment. When a normal subject adopts the vertical from the horizontal position, reflex vasoconstriction maintains the arterial blood pressure, and venoconstriction contributes to maintenance of the venous return. These adjustments do not take place when there is vasomotor paralysis from neuropathy or when ganglion or α-sympathetic blocking drugs are being used; then the assumption of the vertical position causes a fall in blood pressure which in turn may result in syncope. This variety of hypotension can be detected if the blood pressure is recorded when the patient is erect.

Slowing of the heart usually follows when the *carotid sinus* is compressed with the thumb. Pressure should be exerted on one side only, and should be released as soon as the reduction in heart rate has been detected. Rarely the carotid sinus is unusually sensitive; extreme bradycardia then follows carotid sinus pressure, and occasionally syncope may ensue. The increased vagal tone produced by carotid sinus pressure is made use of when attempting to arrest an attack of paroxysmal atrial tachycardia. When the reflex is impaired there may be no alteration in heart rate when the carotid sinus is compressed.

**The Valsalva manoeuvre.** This is a forced attempt at expiration when the mouth is shut and the nose held closed, and is also employed to test vasomotor reflexes (Fig. 15). During the straining period the high intrathoracic pressure impairs the venous return and the cardiac output falls. Syncope would result were it not for the fact that there is a reflex arteriolar vasoconstriction which maintains the blood pressure despite the reduction in cardiac output. When the Valsalva manoeuvre ends, there is a rapid increase in the cardiac output, which, combined with an intense arterial vasoconstriction, results in a significant rise in arterial blood pressure; the vasomotor reflexes are triggered again, and bradycardia and peripheral vasodilatation follow. The tachycardia

VALSALVA   MANOEUVRE

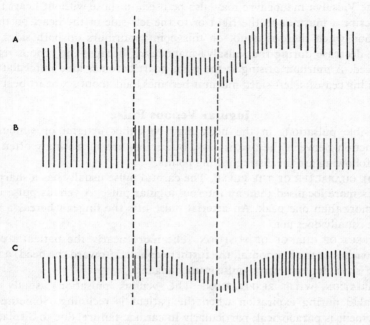

FIG. 15   VALSALVA MANOEUVRE

The interval between the dotted lines indicates the period of forced expiration against resistance. The pressure of each pulse beat is represented by a single line as in Fig. 13.

(A) Normal subject. Note that the fall of arterial pressure during the Valsalva manoeuvre is arrested as a result of a reflex increase in vasomotor tone; afterwards there is an 'overshoot' in arterial pressure. Tachycardia develops during the straining period, and bradycardia follows the 'overshoot'. These are readily appreciated with a finger on the pulse. (B) Cardiac failure, the 'square wave' response. The cardiac output is maintained during the straining period so that the baroreceptors are not stimulated. (C) Vasomotor paralysis. The 'overshoot' is absent and there is no bradycardia.

during the Valsalva manoeuvre, and the bradycardia after it, are easily detected with the finger on the radial artery; both depend on the integrity of the vasomotor reflexes, and are absent when there is vasomotor paralysis.

The Valsalva manoeuvre may also be useful in the detection of heart failure, for under these circumstances, unlike the normal, the cardiac output is not reduced; there is therefore no fall in arterial pressure during the manœuvre, and no bradycardia after it. This results in a so-called 'square wave' response in the arterial pulse; the increment in arterial pressure transmitted through the arteries from the elevation of intrathoracic pressure is not detectable at the radial pulse; in the *absence* of both the normal tachycardia and subsequent bradycardia the presence of cardiac failure can usually be inferred. This test is positive in all forms of cardiac failure, and may be useful in distinguishing the subject of bronchial asthma from the subject of pulmonary oedema if the patient is seen at a time when he is not breathless.

The Valsalva manoeuvre may also be used, in those without heart failure, to ascribe a murmur to the right or to the left side of the heart on the rare occasion when there is doubt on this point; murmurs on both sides of the heart decrease during the Valsalva manoeuvre, because the venous return is reduced. A murmur arising in the right heart becomes loud immediately the straining ceases; a left-sided murmur becomes loud about six heart beats later.

### Jugular Venous Pulse

Visible pulsations in the neck may be either arterial or venous. The distinction between the two is easy, but errors are surprisingly often made. The following are the distinguishing points.

THE CHARACTER OF THE PULSE. The carotid pulse usually has a sharp onset and is more localised than an internal jugular pulse. A venous pulse usually has more than one peak. An arterial pulse lifts the finger whereas a venous pulse usually does not.

EFFECT OF CHANGE OF POSITION. The more nearly the patient's position approaches to the horizontal, the further cephalad (toward the head) a venous pulse is visible. An arterial pulse is unchanged.

VARIATION WITH RESPIRATION. The venous pulsation usually moves cephalad during expiration when the patient is reclining. Sometimes this movement is paradoxical, particularly in cardiac failure, due to displacement of blood from the abdomen by descent of the diaphragm, so that the venous pressure rises during inspiration.

EFFECT OF PRESSURE AT THE ROOT OF THE NECK. Moderate pressure above the clavicle by the finger can obliterate a venous pulse; an arterial pulse is unchanged.

EFFECT OF ABDOMINAL PRESSURE. Pressure on the abdomen will displace the venous pulse cephalad both in normal subjects and in cardiac failure. This so-called *hepato-jugular reflux* is useful in enabling the distinction to be made between an arterial and venous pulse. It is not, however, a reliable test for cardiac failure, for the difference from the normal is quantitative rather than qualitative, and simultaneous changes in intrathoracic pressure, on which jugular venous pressure partly depends, are unpredictable. Abdomino-jugular reflux would be a better name, for it is not necessary to press in the area of the liver, and in patients with heart failure pressure on the liver may cause pain.

**Inspection.** When a patient lies relaxed supported by a pillow, or by the elevated end of a couch, the jugular venous pulse can readily be examined. In the normal subject it can usually be seen only when the patient is almost horizontal. The internal jugular veins lie deep to the sternomastoid muscles,

·remarkably in some patients, and the systolic pressure may be more than 50 whereas the external jugular veins can be seen lying just beneath the skin. It is essential, therefore, that the patient's head lies relaxed, supported by a pillow, so that movements of the skin overlying the internal jugular veins can be seen; if the sternomastoid muscles are active this is not possible. The most convenient method is to examine the profile of the side of the neck overlying the internal jugular vein, and to time the venous events against the arterial pulse in the patient's carotid artery which is simultaneously palpated by the examiner's thumb (Fig. 16).

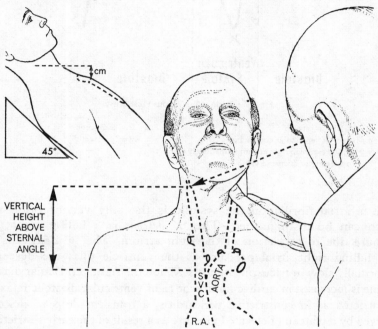

FIG. 16   ESTIMATION OF THE JUGULAR VENOUS PRESSURE

The observer is looking for pulsation of the skin transmitted from the uppermost point of distension of the right internal jugular vein. Alternatively the examiner may stand on the patient's right side with his left thumb on the patient's right carotid and inspect the pulsation of the skin on the left side of the neck.

However the left internal jugular vein may be a less reliable manometer than the right (p. 123).

Normally an '*a*' *wave* resulting from right atrial systole can be detected in the venous pulse just before the carotid pulse, and also a '*v*' *wave* of right atrial filling when the triscuspid valve is shut during ventricular systole (Fig. 17). The 'a' wave is of unusually large amplitude when there is right atrial hypertrophy, for example when there is an abnormally high resistance to right atrial discharge from tricuspid stenosis or from a hypertrophied right ventricle. The 'v' wave is enhanced and earlier in onset when there is tricuspid valvular regurgitation from dilatation of the right ventricle in cardiac failure, or from disease, generally rheumatic, of the tricuspid valve. When

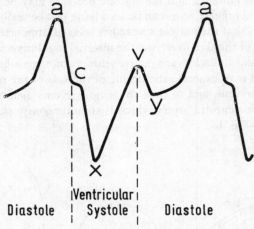

FIG. 17    Form of the Venous Pulse Wave.

a = atrial contraction                                    a − x = 'x descent'
c = onset of ventricular contraction                      v − y = 'y descent'
v = peak pressure in right atrium immediately prior
      to opening of tricuspid valve

there is atrial fibrillation the systolic is the only venous pulse wave which can be distinguished. The *'x' descent* is a falling right atrial pressure due to relaxation of the right atrium. The *'y' descent* is due to a falling right atrial pressure as the ventricle fills; the descent is abnormally slow in tricuspid stenosis. When the right ventricular diastolic volume is increased in cardiac failure, or right ventricular diastolic relaxation is restricted as in constrictive pericarditis, a transient deep 'y' descent is followed by a plateau of elevated pressure as a result of the early restriction of diastolic discharge of the right atrium. The observation of what must seem at first sight formidable minutiae, and their proper interpretation, may provide valuable clinical evidence.

In atrial fibrillation the 'a' wave is of course absent. Striking venous pulsations are seen when the right atrium contracts against a closed tricuspid valve as in nodal rhythm, when a premature ventricular systole produces premature arrest of right atrial discharge, or, phasically, in complete heart block. These are known as *venous cannon waves*.

## Jugular Venous Pressure

Central venous pressure can be measured by inspection alone in most patients (Fig. 16) The principle involved is that the internal jugular veins act as manometer tubes in continuity with the right atrium. The veins are distended with blood only when the pressure within the vein is higher than atmospheric pressure. The vertical height of the 'point of collapse', as Sir Thomas Lewis called it, or uppermost point of distension of the vein above the sternal angle, is the venous pressure and is measured in centimetres of blood. Although there is, of course, blood passing through the vein above this point, the vein is not distended with blood. The external jugular veins are less reliable as manometers, partly because they are liable to kinking, which may be recognised by absence of pulsation. However, they may also give a falsely low pressure record. This occurs particularly in severe cardiac failure when the skin blood flow is small, and the probable mechanism is that the vein is emptied by a Venturi effect where it joins a larger vessel through which there is a greater flow; whenever possible the internal jugular veins are to be preferred as manometers. Occasionally there is a discrepancy in the height of the point of collapse in the two internal jugular veins. In this case the left will be the higher, and is falsely elevated due to intermittent compression of the internal jugular vein by the left subclavian artery. It follows that under these circumstances the right side gives the true jugular venous pressure (J.V.P.).

This clinical technique of estimating jugular venous pressure is the simplest method available, is repeatable, and is more accurate than measuring venous pressure at the elbow because the pressure difference between antecubital vein and right atrium may be considerable. However, the technique requires practice; the most usual error is a failure to determine the point of collapse correctly. With such a large column of blood the system is considerably 'damped', so that peaks of pressure are not faithfully recorded. By taking the midpoint between the maximum and minimum pressures a close approximation to mean pressure is however achieved. In some emergency situations it may be impossible to measure J.V.P., e.g. when the patient has to be horizontal. Then measurements of central venous pressure (C.V.P.) by intravenous catheter and manometer may be necessary.

The importance of the jugular venous pressure is that persistent elevation of the venous pressure is one of the earliest and one of the most reliable signs of cardiac failure. Normally the jugular veins are distended to a height of not more than 2 or 3 cm above the sternal angle with the patient at 45°. Anxiety can produce an elevation of venous as well as of arterial pressure; it is therefore important to check more than once before concluding that a J.V.P. of 3 cm or more is evidence of cardiac failure. The jugular veins can be used as manometers only when the upper level of filling is pulsatile. When the venous pressure is very high, i.e. more than 15 cm, as occurs in tricuspid valvular incompetence and constrictive pericarditis, the upper level of venous pulsation will be seen behind the angle of the jaw or even in front of the ears when the patient is sitting upright, and often the venous pulse moves the ear lobes. In such cases cardiac failure should be easily and immediately recognised from the foot of the bed. Extreme distension of the venous system restricts pulsation and may, paradoxically, lead to the venous hypertension being overlooked.

It may be impossible to measure J.V.P. in an infant, or in an adult who is very breathless, if the accessory muscles of respiration are in use. It may also prove difficult or impossible if there is a very much increased difference between inspiratory and expiratory J.V.P., such as may occur when the fluctuation of intrathoracic pressure is much increased. A vigorous arterial pulse may obscure a venous pulse.

Superior mediastinal obstruction can cause overfilling of the jugular veins, but the upper level of filling is not pulsatile, and abdominal pressure does not cause further overfilling. It is usually accompanied by some swelling of the face and neck, particularly below the eyes, and suffusion of the conjunctivae (p. 166).

## Examination of the Heart

### Inspection

A careful scrutiny of the chest should aim principally at detecting deformity and both normal and abnormal pulsation.

Skeletal abnormalities such as pectus excavatum or kyphoscoliosis may be part of Marfan's syndrome in which congenital abnormalities of the heart and aorta are common. In those forms of congenital heart disease in which gross pulmonary arterial hypertension is a feature during the growing period, e.g. in some large ventricular septal defects, there may be prominence of the left chest over the hypertrophied right ventricle, and a bilateral Harrison's sulcus (p. 172) may be seen. The tense pulmonary arteries reduce lung compliance, the pull of the diaphragm is increased and the chest wall may be distorted at its attachment to the ribs just as it is in the severe asthmatic who suffers from this disease during the growing period. Emphysema may be suspected, and severe kyphosis or scoliosis diagnosed, by inspection alone and both these conditions can lead to heart failure.

The forceful apex beat of left ventricular hypertrophy, the left parasternal impulse of right ventricular hypertrophy, and the pulsation of a hypertensive pulmonary artery in the second left intercostal space may all be detected on inspection. An aneurysm of the aorta may produce a pulsation in the second right intercostal space or of the upper sternum. When the heart is much enlarged the whole anterior chest wall may be seen to move with each heart beat.

Epigastric pulsation transmitted from the abdominal aorta is a normal finding, particularly in thin people. Pulsation in this region may however also be abnormal due to enlargement of the right ventricle, abdominal aneurysm or to pulsation of the liver as a result of tricuspid regurgitation.

### Palpation

Discriminating palpation of the chest is one of the most valuable methods in the examination of the heart, and can often narrow down the diagnosis in such a way as to enable prediction of some at least of the findings on auscultation. The right hand is first placed on the left chest wall with the middle finger lying in about the fifth intercostal space in the anterior axillary line. The position of the apex beat is then defined, if possible, and its quality noted. Abnormal vibrations (see thrills below) are also sought and noted. The hand is then placed to the left of the sternum and then on the manubrium and pulsations and thrills again noted.

**Apex Beat.** The position of the apex beat is best defined as the furthest point downwards and outwards on the chest wall where the finger is lifted by the cardiac impulse. Many students are puzzled by the fact that the finger is lifted during systole, when the ventricle is contracting. This is due to the complex rotatory movement of the heart with systole, one effect of which is a forward movement of the apex. Sometimes the apex beat cannot be felt. The common causes of this are obesity or emphysema, and in the latter case the heart sounds may be faint or inaudible. More rarely the heart beat may be impalpable, due to displacement by disease of the lung or pleura, which should be detected by the finding of deviation of the trachea or by examination of the chest. A pericardial effusion may also make the heart beat impalpable. Very rarely as a congenital abnormality the heart lies on the right side (dextrocardia), but this rarity should be revealed if due attention is paid to the site of maximum intensity of the heart sounds.

The normal apex beat is within the mid-clavicular line in the fifth interspace. The second costal cartilage is at the level of the manubriosternal angle whence the interspaces can readily be identified. When displaced, the site of the apex beat should be described in terms of intercostal space and with reference to mid-clavicular, anterior axillary and mid-axillary lines. Such descriptions should be made with the patient semi-recumbent, for the heart moves to a variable extent on standing or turning to one side.

The apex may be displaced because the heart is displaced, in which case examination of the chest should reveal the cause of this, or it may be displaced because of cardiac enlargement. In the latter case alterations in the praecordial pulsations may enable the examiner to determine which ventricle is mainly responsible. The apex beat is abnormally forceful in left ventricular hypertrophy, and the terms *heaving, thrusting* or *sustained* are commonly used to describe it. In mitral stenosis, on the other hand, the abnormally increased shock of closure of the mitral valve may be palpable in which case the sensation is like that of an unusually hard knock on the other side of a closed door.

The best evidence of right ventricular hypertrophy is a diffuse impulse to the left of the sternum. As already described, these physical signs may be partially or completely obscured by obesity or emphysema. In emphysema there may be considerable right ventricular hypertrophy at post mortem, and yet this may not have been appreciable by palpation in life, because the over-inflated lung intervenes between the heart and the chest wall.

**Thrills.** Murmurs (p. 34) may be so loud as to be palpable as thrills, the most common examples being the apical diastolic thrill of mitral stenosis and the basal systolic thrill of aortic stenosis (often accompanied by a suprasternal thrill and carotid 'shudder'). Thrills are best appreciated when the patient leans forward with the breath held in expiration, with the exception of the thrill of mitral stenosis which is most easily felt when the patient turns on to the left side. The back of a purring cat traditionally and accurately provides the nearest palpable equivalent to the diastolic thrill of mitral stenosis; systolic thrills are more nearly imitated by a bluebottle trapped in the hand. The upper left parasternal systolic thrill of pulmonary stenosis, and the lower left parasternal systolic thrill of a ventricular septal defect, are the most common examples among the congenital abnormalities. A diastolic thrill at the base of the sternum is very uncommon, occurring only with rupture or eversion of an aortic valve cusp with gross aortic regurgitation. A suspected thrill is denied by the subsequent finding that there is either no murmur or only a very quiet one.

**Other Palpable Abnormalities.** When the semilunar valves close under an abnormally high pressure there may be a palpable shock at the upper end of the sternum. When this is due to closure of the pulmonary valves, it is often most readily appreciated to the left of the sternum. An aneurysm of the arch of the aorta may produce a pulsation which is generally maximal in the second right intercostal space, but which may also lift the sternum. Likewise, a dilated pulmonary artery may give a palpable pulse to the left of the sternum at about the second left intercostal space. Occasionally pericardial friction (p. 140) is palpable.

## Percussion

There is usually an area of dullness to percussion to the left of the sternum where the heart lies against the chest. This area is reduced or absent in many cases of emphysema. There may be abnormal dullness to percussion to the right of the sternum when a pericardial effusion is present; massive enlargement of the left atrium occurs rarely in rheumatic disease of the mitral valve, usually with gross mitral incompetence, and this may also produce dullness to the right of the sternum. A large aneurysm of the aorta may produce an area of abnormal dullness to the right of the upper sternum. Percussion is usually employed only when these conditions are suspected. When a radiograph is available the value of percussion is very limited.

## Auscultation

The promotion of the stethoscope from the status symbol of the early clinical years to the refined diagnostic tool of the practised auscultator is hard won. Most students pass through a phase, the length of which is usually inversely proportional to the skill of their teachers, in which they doubt whether they will ever acquire a mastery of the stethoscope; yet the principles which guide its use are fairly straightforward.

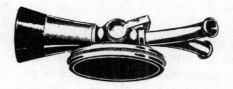

FIG. 18    The Sprague-Bowles Stethoscope.

**Type of Stethoscope.** There is no need to put oneself at a disadvantage by purchasing an inefficient stethoscope. The bell, with the chest piece *lightly pressed* against the skin, is best for conducting low pitched sounds and murmurs and the diaphragm, *firmly applied,* is used for detecting high pitched sounds or a very quiet early diastolic murmur; both are therefore required and experience has proved that the Sprague-Bowles stethoscope (Fig. 18) is the best available at the present time. In the genuine instrument when the diaphragm is removed, the metal grooves are seen to be separated by sharp ridges. The St George's stethoscope is a more elaborate but a very efficient instrument. The Littman stethoscope is certainly very convenient but repeated testing has convinced the author that it is not as good as the Sprague-Bowles in conveying a quiet early diastolic murmur. However it is used by many cardiologists and must be regarded as an acceptable alternative.

In all stethoscopes the ear pieces must fit comfortably and the spring must be strong enough to hold them in place. The tubing should be about 25 cm in length, thick enough to reduce external noise and of similar bore to the metal parts, i.e. about 3 mm.

**Method in the Use of the Stethoscope.** Leatham in his monograph *Auscultation of the Heart and Phonocardiography* advises the clinician to start auscultation with the diaphragm chest piece in the pulmonary area (p. 128) where the two components of the normal second sound provide a reliable point of orientation in the cardiac cycle. Others prefer to listen first at the apex with the bell chest piece. A form of catechism such as the following should then be used:

1. What is the quality and intensity of the first and of the second heart sound?

Normally the first heart sound is louder than the second at the apex, whereas the reverse is true at the base.

2. Are there any added sounds?

This will demand listening for (*a*) high-pitched or clicking sounds such as the opening snap (p. 133) and ejection sounds (p. 133), associated with opening of atrioventricular and semi-lunar valves respectively, and (*b*) low pitched sounds such as the third and fourth sounds (p. 131), which result from blood entering the ventricles, and which are often accompanied by a palpable impulse.

3. Are there any murmurs?

This will require a deliberate analysis of systole and diastole, and a realisation that murmurs may be low pitched (e.g. the mitral diastolic murmur, p. 138) or high pitched (e.g. the aortic diastolic murmur, p. 137).

If there is a murmur:

(a) Is it systolic or diastolic?
(b) What part of systole or diastole does it occupy?
(c) What is its quality and pitch?
(d) What is its intensity?
(e) Where is it loudest and what is its radiation?

4. Are there any other unusual adventitious sounds, e.g. of friction (p. 140), or the clicking sound sometimes associated with a pneumothorax (p. 188)?

There may be difficulty, particularly in the early stages, in deciding whether a murmur is systolic or diastolic. The following points will enable this decision to be made:

1. An identification of each heart sound; the higher pitched and more abrupt quality of the second heart sound at the base of the sternum should settle this point. Once the rhythm is established the bell can be moved inch by inch on the chest to where the murmur is heard and the relationship of the murmur to the sound now specified as the second heart sound can be established.

2. Lifting of the stethoscope by the apical impulse during systole will often be helpful.

3. The identification of systole by the simultaneous palpation of the patient's carotid artery is found useful by some.

4. The best method in practice is from recognition of the murmur. For example, the low-pitched rumbling murmur of mitral stenosis is not only pathognomonic of that condition, but indicates diastole. Similarly, the harsh saw-like murmurs of aortic and pulmonary stenosis indicate systole as well as their cause. Sir Thomas Lewis's advice still applies today, to know the murmurs 'as one learns to know a dog's bark'.

When these questions have all been answered while listening at the apex, the same questions should then be asked while listening to the *right* and to the *left of the sternum* in the second intercostal space. Aortic valve closure and aortic ejection murmurs are usually loudest in the first of these positions, and comparable events for the pulmonary valve at the second. These two areas are commonly referred to as the *aortic* and *pulmonary areas* respectively, but it must be appreciated that they are 5–8 cm from the surface projection of these valves, and indicate rather the surface area to which these murmurs and sounds are preferentially conveyed. At these sites most trained auscultators prefer to use the diaphragm chest-piece of the stethoscope. The pulmonary element of the second heart sound is heard after the aortic element during inspiration; at this time venous return to the right ventricle increases due to the fall in intrathoracic pressure, and left ventricular filling is reduced due to an increase in capacity of the readily distensible pulmonary veins. Conversely, during expiration right ventricular filling is impaired and left ventricular filling is increased; the closures of the pulmonary and aortic valves then coincide to produce a single second heart sound. *Splitting of the second heart sound* can therefore be regarded as a normal finding during inspiration; abnormal splitting is described on page 130.

The diaphragm chest-piece should then be placed at the lower left sternal edge, in about the fourth intercostal space, for it is at this site that aortic and pulmonary diastolic, and also tricuspid systolic and diastolic murmurs, are usually loudest. This area is referred to as the *tricuspid area*. An aortic diastolic murmur is sometimes audible only when the patient sits up and leans forward, with the breath held in full expiration. This manœuvre brings the heart nearer to the chest wall, and eliminates breath sounds which may be closely similar in pitch to an aortic or pulmonary diastolic murmur. It is wrong to state that there is no aortic diastolic murmur unless this manœuvre has been employed; a quiet room and a good diaphragm stethoscope favour its detection. Similarly, it is not possible to decide that there is no mitral diastolic murmur unless it has been listened for around the apex with the patient half on the left side, and with the bell stethoscope lightly applied to the skin. The area in which a mitral diastolic murmur can be heard is sometimes little larger than the stethoscope chest-piece. One of the causes of failure to find it, is not searching precisely at the apex, e.g. far round into the axilla when there is great cardiac enlargement. If the cardiac output is increased by exercise, e.g. by asking the patient to touch the toes a few times, the murmur of mitral stenosis may be more easily heard.

When these areas have been examined any murmur found should then be followed to the point at which it is maximal, and the site of maximal intensity should be recorded. Too rigid a habit of listening only in the classical areas—mitral, aortic, pulmonary and tricuspid—is a potent cause of failing to detect significant auscultatory abnormalities.

In practice, the employment of a system such as this takes a much shorter time than would seem possible from the length of this description. The junior student, having read the foregoing, will no doubt feel that the learning of auscultation constitutes a task beyond his capacity. The best plan is to learn the technique in stages. First he should familiarise himself with the normal heart sounds by listening to the normal hearts of colleagues and patients. He can then proceed to the analysis of murmurs. Finally, he will be able to grapple with the added sounds. The beginner may find difficulty when he compares notes with his teacher because the latter has trained himself to listen to the various parts of the cardiac cycle independently, and has reached a point where he may concentrate on something which is quiet, e.g. an elusive aortic diastolic murmur, in preference to louder but, for him, less important auscultatory features. An appreciation of this difference in interpretative emphasis may assist understanding.

## HEART SOUNDS

**First Heart Sound.** This is mainly due to mitral valve closure, the contribution of tricuspid valve closure in health being small. It follows that it is loudest at the apex, for the sound is conveyed best to the only surface projection of the left ventricle. It is louder than usual if the normal partial valve closure has not occurred as left ventricular filling approaches completion, e.g. when diastole is short as a result of tachycardia, a premature beat, or atrial fibrillation, or when there is a short interval between atrial and ventricular contraction; in the last the electro-cardiogram shows a short P-R interval. It is characteristically sharp and loud with mitral stenosis when the high left atrial pressure delays mitral valve closure and the diseased antero-medial cusp closes with a snap which may be palpable—the so-called closing snap of the mitral valve or sharp first heart sound.

The first heart sound is unusually quiet when the mitral valve does not close normally, as in cases of mitral incompetence in which the antero-medial cusp is diseased, when the valve is heavily calcified and immobile, or in conditions accompanied by a low blood pressure, e.g. myocardial infarction and shock.

**Second Heart Sound.** This is best heard at the upper sternum at the level of the second intercostal space and is due to aortic and pulmonary valve closure. *Normal splitting* of the second heart sound during inspiration has already been described (p. 129), i.e. in inspiration the pulmonary element of the second heart sound is heard after the aortic element. The aortic component is reduced in intensity when the aortic valve is calcified, as in some cases of aortic stenosis, and increased by diastolic hypertension. In syphilitic aortitis, with widening of the aortic ring, the sound is often low pitched and ringing.

*Fixed splitting.* Abnormally wide splitting is heard throughout the cardiac cycle when there is delay of the pulmonary component of the second heart sound (Fig. 19). This occurs (1) when the right ventricle ejects more than the left, for example in atrial septal defect (2) when delay in conduction makes right ventricular systole late, for example with right bundle branch block; or (3) with mechanical delay in emptying of the right ventricle in some cases of pulmonary stenosis or pulmonary hypertension.

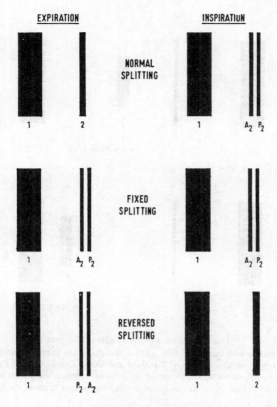

FIG. 19   Splitting of the Second Heart Sound.

*Reversed splitting.* If left ventricular ejection is delayed by left bundle branch block or prolonged by aortic stenosis or hypertension reversed splitting is common, i.e. the split is heard during expiration instead of inspiration.

**Third Heart Sound.** Phonocardiograms in normal persons reveal two sounds which cannot usually be detected by the ear. These are the third and fourth sounds and they are thought to be due to sudden stretching of the ventricular walls in the same way as a noise is produced by the wind when it fills an empty sail. In certain circumstances, these vibrations become audible and a 'triple' or 'gallop' rhythm is heard.

The third heart sound is caused by ventricular filling at the time of opening of the A.-V. valves (Fig. 20). The sound is loudest at the apex, is low pitched, and is best detected with the bell stethoscope lightly applied. It is a normal finding in childhood. A third sound is also heard when left ventricular filling is increased as a result of mitral incompetence, a patent ductus arteriosus or a ventricular septal defect for example. It also occurs in left ventricular failure when the left atrial pressure is increased. In right ventricular failure,

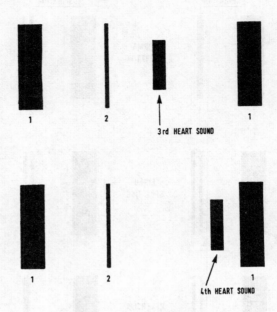

Fig. 20   Third and Fourth Heart Sounds

The third sound coincides with the onset of ventricular filling, and the fourth sound with the ventricular filling which results from atrial contraction. The third and fourth sounds are heard at the cardiac apex when they arise in the left ventricle, and to the left of the lower sternum when their origin is in the right ventricle. (*N.B.* Figs. 20–25 are diagrammatic representations of phono-cardiograms.)

particularly when there is tricuspid incompetence, a third sound may be heard over the right ventricle. A third heart sound is also heard in constrictive pericarditis when this limits ventricular filling.

**Fourth Heart Sound.** This is due to ventricular filling as a result of atrial contraction (Fig. 20) and is an accompaniment of atrial hypertrophy without stenosis of the relevant A.-V. valve. When a ventricle is hypertrophied, its resistance to filling is increased, and hypertrophy of the corresponding atrium follows. A fourth heart sound is therefore heard at the apex in many cases of aortic stenosis and systemic hypertension, and over the right ventricle in pulmonary stenosis and pulmonary hypertension; the right atrial fourth sound is generally accompanied by an abnormally large 'a' wave in the jugular venous pulse. Often a presystolic impulse at the apex is visible, and it may be readily palpable even though the fourth heart sound is audible only on careful listening with the bell stethoscope lightly applied on the apex.

**Triple and Gallop Rhythms.** Triple rhythm with tachycardia is sometimes referred to as gallop rhythm; when due to a third sound it is described as protodiastolic gallop, while a fourth sound produces presystolic gallop.

When diastole is very short the distinction between these types may be impossible and the rhythm is then called summation gallop on the supposition that the third and fourth sounds both contribute to the added sound.

**Opening Snap.** This added sound, which occurs soon after the second sound, is almost pathognomonic of mitral stenosis, is clicking in quality, and is best heard along a line between the cardiac apex and the lower left sternal edge. It is of similar significance to the closing snap, or sharp first heart sound, already described (p. 130), and it heralds the onset of the mitral diastolic murmur. It is best heard with the diaphragm of the stethoscope, and its presence implies that the anteromedial cusp of the mitral valve is pliant. The higher the left atrial pressure, the sooner this sound follows the second heart sound. When it is heard it should lead to a careful search for the characteristic murmur of mitral stenosis.

**Ejection Sound.** This high-pitched clicking sound arises from the semilunar valves, and its mechanism of production is comparable to that of the opening snap; it is caused by an abnormal semilunar valve becoming tense

TABLE I

*Normal and Added Sounds Related to Events and Timing of the Cardiac Cycle*

| Sound | Event | Timing |
|---|---|---|
| First Sound Ejection Sound | Closure of A-V Valves Opening of Aortic and Pulmonary Valves | SYSTOLE |
| Second Sound | Closure of Semilunar Valves | |
| Opening Snap | Opening of Abnormal A-V Valves (e.g. in mitral stenosis) | |
| Third Sound | Ventricular Filling Begins | DIASTOLE |
| Fourth Sound | Ventricular Filling Increases With Atrial Contraction | |

under systolic pressure, e.g. in some cases of aortic stenosis and pulmonary stenosis. It occurs at the onset of the systolic murmur, and is heard in the same place as the murmur (p. 135). It may also be found with systemic and with pulmonary hypertension, to the right or to the left of the upper sternum respectively.

A small and usually left-sided pneumothorax may cause a systolic clicking sound, so-called *clicking or noisy pneumothorax* (p. 188).

The relationship of the normal and added sounds to the events and timing of the cardiac cycle is illustrated in Table 1.

## THE MURMURS

Murmurs arise from turbulent blood flow and they tend to be propagated in the same direction as the flow. Obviously, the louder a murmur is, the further it will be propagated, irrespective of its site of origin. In the analysis of a murmur its timing and quality are its most important distinguishing features, and the latter has to be learned from experience, although recordings may be of help. The features required for proper analysis have already been described (p. 128).

The significance of a systolic murmur depends mainly on its intensity, for when quiet it may be due only to an increased blood flow. In pregnancy or anaemia, for example, a murmur of this type is often heard in the pulmonary area. A diastolic murmur is invariably significant however soft it may be.

The intensity of a murmur is often described in terms of grades, as follows:

GRADE 1. Just audible in a quiet room, with the patient's breath held and using a good stethoscope.

GRADE 2. Quiet.

GRADE 3. Moderately loud.

GRADE 4. Loud, and accompanied by a thrill.

GRADE 5. Very loud.

GRADE 6. Audible without a stethoscope and with the head away from the chest. Such a murmur may sometimes be heard with the stethoscope chest-piece on top of the patient's head, on the sacrum or even at the wrists! It is often heard by the patient's spouse.

Murmurs of Grade 4 and louder are accompanied by a palpable thrill. It is unusual for competent observers to record more than one grade difference after listening to the same murmur. The record should state, for example, Grade 5/6 murmur, i.e. fifth out of six grades, so that the number of grades used is made clear.

**Systolic Murmurs.** These are divided into *ejection murmurs* and *pansystolic murmurs*. The first appear 'diamond shaped' in phonocardiographic records, i.e. maximal in mid-systole (Fig. 21); ejection murmurs result from increased blood flow through normal semilunar valves, or normal (or increased) blood flow through distorted semilunar valves. Their 'shape' is

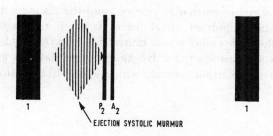

P₂ A₂

EJECTION SYSTOLIC MURMUR

FIG. 21   AORTIC STENOSIS
The aortic element of the second heart sound is delayed and a split second heart sound results.

determined by the moment-to-moment pressure gradient across the valve. *Pansystolic* murmurs are so called because they extend throughout systole, and they are the result of escape of blood from a ventricle into an area of low pressure, as with a leaking atrio-ventricular valve, or a small ventricular septal defect. The murmur has little mid-systolic accentuation, and, unlike the ejection murmur, starts immediately after the first heart sound and may spill over into early diastole, for the pressure gradient responsible for the abnormal flow persists after closure of the semilunar valves. The distinction between an ejection type systolic murmur and a pansystolic murmur can usually be made with the stethoscope, but occasionally may be impossible even with a phonocardiogram.

EXAMPLES OF EJECTION-TYPE SYSTOLIC MURMURS. The murmur of *aortic stenosis* was called a 'bruit de scie' by Laënnec, the founder of the stethoscopic art. This is an admirable name, for the acceleration and deceleration of the saw provide a precise analogy. It is usually loudest in the second right intercostal space or suprasternal notch, and radiates to the neck. With calcific aortic stenosis it sometimes has a mewing quality like the cry of a seagull. If the aortic stenosis is severe, and left ventricular function well preserved, there is usually an accompanying thrill, and in the carotid arteries the turbulence is felt as a carotid shudder. With the onset of cardiac failure the murmur may become surprisingly soft. The murmur is generally better heard at the apex than it is over the right ventricle, and occasionally may be louder at the apex than it is at the base. An ejection sound strongly favours valvular stenosis; in every other respect the murmur of the much rarer subvalvular stenosis is clinically similar.

The murmur of *pulmonary stenosis* is of similar quality, and at the same level, but loudest in the second left intercostal space. The murmur radiates towards the left shoulder. The increased pulmonary blood flow of an *atrial septal defect* also may produce a pulmonary ejection systolic murmur but this is not usually of more than grade 3/6 intensity. The flow of blood through the defect itself does not produce a murmur. The second sound may be split throughout the respiratory cycle in both conditions, due to delay in onset, or a prolongation, of right ventricular ejection, and the distinction between mild pulmonary stenosis and an atrial defect is often impossible on clinical examination alone. A mid-diastolic murmur in the tricuspid area indicates turbulent flow at the tricuspid valve and strongly favours an atrial septal defect; it is the only diastolic murmur which sounds like a systolic murmur. It never rumbles.

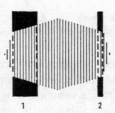 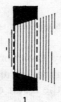

FIG. 22   Pansystolic Murmur.

EXAMPLES OF PANSYSTOLIC MURMURS (Fig. 22). *Mitral regurgitation* of significance usually produces an apical pansystolic murmur, radiating to the axilla and often heard over the lower left chest at the back. It may be as loud as grade 5/6. The increased forward flow through the valve in diastole often produces a low-pitched short mid-diastolic murmur of abrupt onset, or a third heart sound, but when some mitral stenosis coexists atrio-ventricular flow is less rapid, and the murmur is longer and less abrupt in onset.

*Tricuspid regurgitation* usually produces a pansystolic murmur audible over the right ventricle to the left of the sternum in the fourth intercostal space. A much enlarged right ventricle may extend to the left anterior axillary line, and under these circumstances the murmur is often mistaken for that of mitral regurgitation. The explanation already given for the diastolic murmur or third sound of mitral regurgitation applies to a similar murmur or sound at the left sternal edge in the fourth interspace accompanying tricuspid regurgitation. A tricuspid regurgitant murmur is usually accompanied by a systolic jugular venous pulse wave and often by systolic expansion of the liver. These are common findings in heart failure from rheumatic or ischaemic heart disease, or with chronic cor pulmonale.

A pansystolic murmur to the left of the sternum is the characteristic murmur of a jet of blood through a *ventricular septal defect*. It has a characteristic rough quality, like the tearing of fabric, and is usually accompanied by a thrill. When the defect is small this is the only physical sign. When it is larger the greater shunt of blood is responsible also for an apical mid-diastolic murmur of increased mitral valve flow.

**Diastolic Murmurs.** The three main types of diastolic murmur are (1) those of leaking semi-lunar valves, which are loudest in early diastole when the pressure gradient is highest, and which are decrescendo; these are termed *early diastolic murmurs*; (2) the murmurs of turbulent blood flow at the atrio-ventricular valves, which start slightly later in diastole and are therefore sometimes called *mid-diastolic* or *delayed diastolic murmurs*; and (3) murmurs due to turbulence at one of the A.V. valves and resulting from atrial contraction, so-called *presystolic*, or *atrial systolic* murmurs.

EXAMPLES OF DIASTOLIC MURMURS. *Aortic regurgitation* produces a bellows-like murmur of all grades of intensity (Fig. 23). When very soft it resembles a breath sound, and can then be detected only when breathing is arrested in expiration, and with the patient leaning forward. In aortic regurgitation of rheumatic origin the murmur is usually loudest to the left of the sternum in the fourth intercostal space; in syphilitic aortic regurgitation the murmur is

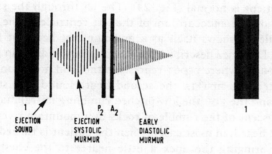

1
EJECTION
SOUND

EJECTION
SYSTOLIC
MURMUR

P₂ A₂

EARLY
DIASTOLIC
MURMUR

1

FIG. 23 AORTIC STENOSIS AND INCOMPETENCE
The diamond-shaped systolic murmur is preceded by a clicking ejection sound. A high-pitched decrescendo murmur immediately follows the aortic second sound; this murmur is usually blowing in quality and best heard at the left sternal edge in the fourth intercostal space.

often louder to the right of the sternum. Even the quietest aortic diastolic murmur cannot be ignored, and finding it may be of great clinical importance when infective endocarditis is suspected. In practice the murmur is often overlooked, and if the proper steps have been followed this is usually because the listener has not attuned his hearing to the necessary high pitch.

The murmur of *pulmonary regurgitation* is similar in quality and site to that of aortic regurgitation. A loud second heart sound to the left of the sternum or other evidence of pulmonary arterial hypertension (p. 151) favour pulmonary regurgitation as the cause of the murmur. Pulmonary regurgitation is much less common than aortic regurgitation. The murmur of pulmonary regurgitation is often called the *Graham Steell* murmur after the cardiologist who first described it; he called it the *murmur of high pressure in the pulmonary artery* long before it was possible to measure this pressure in man. It occurs with pulmonary arterial hypertension, e.g. in some cases of mitral stenosis or pulmonary arterial thrombo-embolism.

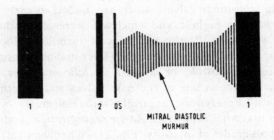

1         2   OS                  1

MITRAL DIASTOLIC
MURMUR

FIG. 24   MITRAL STENOSIS

The opening snap (O.S.) is high-pitched and usually best heard to the left of the lower sternum. The long low-pitched mitral diastolic murmur has a mid-diastolic and ɔre-systolic accentuation.

*Mitral stenosis* betrays itself to the stethoscope even when in all other respects the patient is normal (Fig. 24). The jet through the stenosed mitral valve impinges on the endocardium of the left ventricle at the apex, and the resulting turbulence shows itself as a murmur best heard at the site of the apical impulse. Duroziez described the auscultatory findings in mitral stenosis as FFOUT-TA-TA-ROU, where FFOUT represents the loud first sound (though LUP might be better), the first TA the second heart sound, the second one the opening snap, and the ROU the low-pitched rumbling mitral diastolic murmur which is reminiscent of the rumble of rocks in a mountain river in flood. The murmur is best heard, in most cases, when the patient is turned half on to the left side, thus bringing the apex a little nearer to the chest wall, and by increasing the turbulence of mitral valve blood flow by slight exertion. When the reduction of the mitral valve orifice is only slight, the characteristic rumbling murmur is heard only during the increased blood velocity of atrial systole—the so-called presystolic murmur. The murmur of mitral stenosis causes a low-pitched vibration of the chest wall which can often be damped out by pressure with the bell of the stethoscope. It is not generally appreciated that two people can listen to the same area, in the same patient, with the same bell stethoscope, and yet disagree because one person presses the bell harder against the skin than the other. A short rumbling apical presystolic murmur is often heard in patients with gross aortic regurgitation but without mitral stenosis, and is called after *Austin Flint*, who first described it. It is said to be due to the aortic regurgitant jet interfering with the normal opening of the antero-medial cusp of the mitral valve. The label is usually reserved for patients who have aortic regurgitation which is not due to rheumatic heart disease, for in the latter case mitral stenosis would be the more likely cause of the murmur. The murmur of *tricuspid stenosis* is similar in timing to that of mitral stenosis, loudest to the left of the lower sternum, and in quality is higher pitched and harsher, and hence more like a systolic murmur. Its intensity usually increases during inspiration.

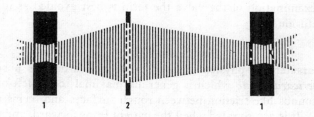

FIG. 25    Continuous Murmur.

**Venous Hum.** A continuing roaring noise, colourfully called the *bruit de diable*—(top, not devil!)—is often audible above either clavicle, and only if the head and shoulders are higher than the heart (i.e. when the patient is sitting, standing or reclining against pillows). It is audible in most children when sitting. It is due to blood flow through the jugular veins, and is abolished by pressure with the hand against the side of the patient's neck above the stethoscope, or by the patient assuming a horizontal or head-down position. It alters in intensity with changes in position of the head, and when loud may be heard surprisingly far away, e.g. to each side of the lower sternum. Its importance rests on the fact that it is extremely common, and often gives rise to a mistaken belief that there is a patent ductus arteriosus. However, a venous hum lacks the late systolic accentuation characteristic of the murmur of a patent ductus (Fig. 25).

**Arteriovenous Murmurs.** The characteristic murmur of an arteriovenous fistula is continuous throughout systole and diastole, but with a diamond-shaped accentuation reaching a peak at the time of the second heart sound (Fig. 25). A patent ductus arteriosus, though not strictly an arteriovenous fistula as it joins the aorta to the pulmonary artery, provides a good example of this murmur, and in this case it is maximal in the second left intercostal space and generally accompanied by a thrill.

**Exocardiac Murmurs.** This term is applied to murmurs which appear to result not from turbulent blood flow but from some cause outside the heart. They are best regarded as being of unknown aetiology, as no explanation has generally been found in those few cases in which a post mortem examination has been made. Exocardiac murmurs are characteristically musical or scratchy and almost always systolic. Their intensity, which may be of any grade, varies with change of position and with respiration more than is usually the case with murmurs due to turbulent blood flow. They are sometimes intermittent. Exocardiac murmurs are not a feature of heart disease and accordingly are of no importance to the patient unless mis-diagnosed.

**Functional Murmurs.** The term 'functional' has been used to describe murmurs arising from turbulent blood flow, but without disease of the relevant heart valve. As this situation can be established with certainty only

by direct examination of the valve the term is best avoided as it is liable to
lead to confusion.

### PERICARDIAL FRICTION

The characteristic physical sign of acute pericarditis is a systolic and
diastolic *pericardial rub* which is generally maximal to the left of the lower
sternum, sounds like friction between rough surfaces and seems near to the
stethoscope. It is accentuated when the patient leans forward, and by pressure
with the stethoscope. Pleura overlies some of the heart and a pleural rub at
this site may be indistinguishable from pericardial friction. If there is an
independent left-sided pleural friction, apparent pericardial friction is more
likely to be *pleuro-pericardial* (p. 193).

## The Peripheral Vascular System

### The Arteries

The symptoms of arterial disease arise from partial or complete occlusion,
most commonly in the larger arteries as a result of atheroma or embolism.
The clinical manifestations depend on the site and extent of the obstruction
and the adequacy of the collateral vessels. For example, in children and
healthy young adults ligation of the femoral artery in the thigh or the
brachial in the arm will generally give rise to no serious symptoms, whereas in
the elderly the collateral flow is less good and severe ischaemia and even
gangrene are likely to result.

### THE HISTORY

Intermittent claudication (from the Latin, *claudicare*—to limp) is usually
the first symptom of chronic arterial inadequacy in the legs. The complaint is
of discomfort, cramp or pain in the calf provoked by exercise, and relieved by
rest. The patient may be observed to limp if asked to exercise to the point of
pain. The 'claudication distance' should be noted, i.e. how far the patient can
walk on level ground at a steady set pace before pain develops. This can be
used as a basis for measuring progress. Claudication may also occur in the
buttocks, from occlusion of the internal iliac artery, and in the thigh from
occlusion of the common femoral artery; pain in the calf is much more
common than these. Ischaemic pain in the forearm as a result of exercising
the limb is rare but may follow occlusion of the axillary or brachial artery.

Rest pain may occur in a severely ischaemic limb and the patient may be
forced to sleep in a chair or with the leg hanging over the side of the bed in an
attempt to obtain relief.

### THE PHYSICAL EXAMINATION

**Inspection.** (*a*) *Signs of Arterial Insufficiency*. The signs of impairment of
arterial flow are pallor, coldness and nutritional changes and are most marked
at the periphery. If the blood supply is suddenly and critically reduced, the

limb becomes cold, pale and later bluish, and gangrene may ensue. Chronic ischaemia results in nutritional changes, such as failure of growth of nails and of hairs on the dorsum of the phalanges, and atrophy of the skin and subcutaneous tissues of the finger-tips.

Arterial insufficiency in the lower limbs can be demonstrated by elevating the legs to 90° with the trunk. The veins and capillaries empty rapidly and, if the distal arterial pressure is then too low to keep the vessels filled against gravity, pallor of varying degree develops within a few seconds. If there is considerable impairment of arterial flow, the foot may take on a cadaveric appearance. If the limbs are then lowered by changing the patient to the sitting position, as with the legs dangling over the side of the bed, colour returns slowly and irregularly with a patchy distribution of increasing intensity until the forefoot assumes a deep reddish colour (reactive hyperaemia). The rate at which these colour changes take place and their degree give an indication of the severity of the arterial insufficiency. They are most obvious when one limb is normal and can be used as a control. Similar changes can less commonly be demonstrated in the upper limbs. Normally the veins of the feet fill about five seconds after changing from an elevated to a dependent position. Poor arterial flow causes delay in venous filling.

Raynaud's disease occurs most commonly in young women in whom the main arteries to the limb are apparently normal. The small arteries of the fingers may close from undue sensitivity to moderate cold. The fingers become white, cold and insensitive. This is followed by cyanosis from circulatory stasis and by painful rubor from increased blood flow with recovery. Similarly, 'Raynaud's phenomenon', may occur at any age in connective tissue disorders or after trauma to a digital artery.

(b) *Visible Pulsation*. Arterial pulsation in the neck is discussed elsewhere (p. 111). In coarctation of the aorta, arterial pulsation may be seen in the scapular areas and is best detected when the patient is leaning forward with his arms in front. Pulsation of the brachial arteries may be visible as a result of sclerotic changes in the media and loss of elasticity (brachial dance or locomotor brachialis). Aneurysms of the limb arteries are uncommon and are readily identified by their expansile pulsation.

**Palpation.** When there are manifestations of arterial insufficiency in a limb, it is essential to determine whether there is any alteration in the pulses or of the temperature.

(a) *Normal Pulses*. The pulse can be felt in most of the main arteries of the limbs and neck in the normal subject. The *common carotid* artery is easily palpable with the thumb placed medially to the sternomastoid muscle at the upper end of the thyroid cartilage, the left thumb being used for the patient's right side. This manœuvre is also used for carotid sinus pressure. The *temporal artery*, commonly used by the anaesthetist, is palpable anteriorly to the upper margin of the pinna. The *subclavian artery* is felt by standing behind the patient and pressing downward with the forefinger above the middle of the clavicle (first part) or, standing in front of the patient, feeling below the junction of the middle and lateral thirds of the clavicle (third part). The *brachial artery* can be felt along the medial border of the humerus and at the elbow medial to the biceps tendon. The *radial and ulnar arteries* are both palpable at the wrist. There is a simple and efficient test for the patentcy of these arteries. Ask the patient to clench the fist. Compress each artery simultaneously with a thumb against the bone behind it. The patient then unclenches the hand; the skin will be pale. On releasing the pressure over one artery, the skin of the hand blushes if the artery is patent. The process is repeated for the other vessel. This test is valuable when one of the arteries is to be used for some investigative purpose; occlusion of the other precludes its use if the test carries any risk of producing thrombosis. The *digital pulses* are often palpable in a warm hand.

The *abdominal aorta* can be felt in the epigastrium, and particularly easily in a thin elderly subject. The *femoral arteries* are palpable at about the midpoint of the inguinal ligament. The *popliteal artery* is felt by placing the tips of the fingers of the right hand in the middle of each popliteal fossa in turn, while the patient lies supine with the knees straight or slightly flexed. Learning to feel this pulse requires practice, particularly in regard to the correct amount of pressure to use; lack of experience accounts for a widespread and erroneous impression that this pulse is only rarely palpable. The *posterior tibial artery* is felt behind the medial malleolus, and the *dorsalis pedis* is palpable lateral to the extensor hallucis tendon. Often in the elderly one or both of these vessels cannot be detected.

If the dorsalis pedis pulse is not palpable in a young subject the blood flow may be mainly through the perforating peroneal artery the pulse of which may be palpable.

(*b*) *Temperature.* When the blood flow to a limb is impaired, the normal gradual decline in temperature towards the periphery becomes abrupt at the level where significant ischaemia begins. This change can readily be detected by touch when comparison is made with the other limb.

**Auscultation.** A systolic bruit may be audible over and distal to the site of stenosis of an artery, but producing the murmur by pressing too hard with the bell of the stethoscope must be avoided. The internal carotid, renal and iliac arteries are most commonly affected. Sudden distension of a large artery, as in aortic incompetence, may produce a snapping sound like a pistol shot in the peripheral arteries. The characteristic murmur of an arteriovenous fistula has been described on page 139.

**Supplementary Examination.** Atheroma of the limb arteries is usually accompanied by similar changes elsewhere, and in such patients the examination is not complete until symptoms and signs of coronary artery disease, in particular, have been sought.

## The Veins

The most important causes of impairment of the efficiency of the venous circulation are (1) obstruction to the flow by thrombosis, phlebitis or external pressure, and (2) incompetence of the valves in varicose veins. Evidence of these processes is sought by means of *inspection* and *palpation*. Thus the classical signs of inflammation may be detected, a thrombosed vein may be palpable or there may be evidence of venous obstruction.

### THE MANIFESTATIONS OF VENOUS OBSTRUCTION

As in the case of the arteries the clinical manifestations of venous obstruction depend on its site and extent together with the adequacy of the collateral vessels. Distal to the obstruction there may be distension of the veins, cyanosis and oedema.

When obstruction of a main vein is established, for example, by thrombosis or tumour, an alternative route must be found for the venous return along collateral channels. These may become visible in the subcutaneous tissues at characteristic sites in relation to the primary lesion. Thus a marked circulation may be established over the anterior chest wall when the superior vena cava is occluded (p. 166), and over the lower abdomen when the inferior vena cava is involved (p. 210). At the umbilicus, a caput Medusae (p. 211) may occasionally be seen in the presence of portal obstruction, and in the lower limbs the recognition of a well developed collateral circulation may direct attention to the presence of thrombosis of a deep vein of the leg (see below).

The direction of the blood flow can be demonstrated by emptying one of the anastomotic veins by running two fingers along it until they are a few centimetres apart and then releasing the pressure on each point in turn. When one finger is raised, inflow of blood into the occluded segment of vein is relatively slow and will be halted at the first valve situated in that segment, whereas lifting of the other finger will allow rapid and complete inflow of blood.

**Thrombosis of the Deep Veins of the Leg.** This is of great medical importance, and is a common clinical finding, particularly in those who are confined to bed, and after operations or childbirth. Its significance lies in the risk of pulmonary embolism (p. 150) which is an all too frequent cause of sudden and unexpected death, or of morbidity from pulmonary infarction and obstructive pulmonary arterial disease. Prompt recognition and anticoagulant treatment may be life saving.

Although the medical profession is well aware of the importance of venous thrombosis, the frequency of clinical diagnosis of the condition is far short of the finding, in unselected post-mortem material, that one-half of all patients dying in hospital have evidence of venous thrombosis in the legs, and one-quarter have evidence of pulmonary infarction. The symptoms cannot be relied upon to draw attention to the process, for there are usually no symptoms or only slight discomfort in the calf, or oedema of one ankle. Unexplained fever, a small rise in pulse rate or a slight deterioration in well-being may alert the observant to the possibility of venous thrombosis.

The crucial examination is a careful scrutiny of the exposed lower limbs while the patient lies supine on the bed. The reliable signs are swelling and slight duskiness of the skin of the calf, and pitting oedema at the ankle on the affected side. Dilatation of small veins passing over the shin of one leg is almost pathognomonic. The affected calf is nearly always warmer to the touch than the unaffected one. When the affected limb is raised the dilated superficial veins do not empty normally. Gentle palpation of the calf will often show that it is tenser than its normal fellow, and tenderness may be elicited. It is generally taught that measurement of the two calves is useful in establishing that one side is swollen. When the eyes cannot detect the difference in size, measurement is of little practical value. Forceful dorsiflexion of the foot may produce pain in the calf (Homan's sign); this test is non-specific and has the serious disadvantage that a thrombus may be dislodged in the process. Tests with a recorded mortality are best avoided in clinical practice.

It is important to realise that obstruction of a large vein, e.g. the common iliac vein, may occur without any abnormal physical signs. Instruments may be helpful, for example the ultrasound method of detecting blood flow, or the clearance of radioactive material from the leg.

### THE ASSESSMENT OF VARICOSE VEINS

Varicose veins are evidence of a progressive and often genetically determined condition in which there is dilatation and elongation of venous channels. The course of the vessels becomes tortuous and there is thickening of the walls together with some degree of fixation to the surrounding tissues. The nutrition of the part becomes impaired by venous stasis and hypoxia. Partly because of their length and partly because of an inherent weakness in their walls, the veins most commonly affected are the long saphenous, and, to a lesser extent, the short saphenous in the leg. At an early stage there is incompetence of the valves, both in the superficial veins and later in their communications with the deep system. Contrary to the normal, blood then flows from the deep to the superficial systems, and a further increase in the degree of dilation and stasis results. The early symptoms of varicose veins are generally discomfort and fatigue in the leg, brought on by standing and relieved by elevation.

**Examination.** Gross varicosities, or the presence of secondary complications such as varicose ulceration, usually present no difficulty in diagnosis. Minor, or early dilation, however, is often overlooked as a cause of symptoms and the examination must be capable of demonstrating this degree of abnormality.

The patient should be standing and the site and extent of the varicosities identified by inspection and palpation, the latter being of particular value in the fat leg. It is usual to see the maximal dilatation in the region of the inner side of the calf or above the ankle. This may well be the only evidence of varicosities affecting the entire vein. Dilated segments may also be seen at several sites on one or both of the major veins separated by apparently normal segments.

The competence of the valves, an assessment of which is essential to the correct management of the case, may be demonstrated by the *Trendelenburg test*. This requires the 'emptying' of the veins of the leg by elevation of the limb. The long saphenous vein is then compressed by a finger or by a light tourniquet at the saphenous opening, and the patient stands. If the vein fills from below while the finger is in position the valves in the communicating veins are incompetent. If there is little or no filling within half a minute the finger should be removed and an immediate filling from above indicates incompetence at the sapheno-femoral junction. In the event of filling of the system from below, a more accurate estimate of the site of the incompetent communicating veins can be obtained by repeating the test using multiple points of compression, either with the fingers or several simultaneous tourniquets at various levels on the leg. Filling of any individual segment of vein indicates that this area is related to an incompetent deep communicating vein.

In those patients in whom there is difficulty in demonstrating the exact extent of the incompetence, or in whom there is some doubt as to the state of the deep venous system, it may be necessary to complete the investigation with a venogram.

## FURTHER INVESTIGATIONS

The standard aids to the diagnosis of disorders of the cardiovascular system are radiography, fluoroscopy and electrocardiography.

**Radiography.** A standard film of the chest, namely a posterior-anterior exposure with at least six feet in distance between the X-ray tube and the film, provides valuable information, in particular about the size of the cardiac shadow, and of the main pulmonary artery and aorta. Enlargement of the left auricle (also called the left atrial appendix) appears as a bulge on the left border of the heart and is a usual feature of mitral stenosis; the left atrium may often be seen as a dense almost circular opacity within the cardiac outline, and the shadow of the right atrium characteristically encroaches upon the right lung field, abnormally so as this chamber becomes enlarged. The relative contribution of each of the two ventricles is often impossible to determine in a posterior-anterior film, although the apex tends to be more rounded in left than in right ventricular hypertrophy. Lateral and oblique radiographs, with the oesophagus outlined by barium, may provide further evidence as to which chambers contribute chiefly to cardiac enlargement.

Usually, however, both electrocardiography and clinical examination are better tools for this purpose.

A standard radiograph is also particularly valuable in indicating that a pericardial effusion has developed. Pulmonary oedema, pulmonary infarction and hydrothoraces may be more certainly established by radiography than by clinical examination. Pulmonary arterial hypertension, and both increased and reduced pulmonary blood flow may also produce characteristic radiographic changes.

**Fluoroscopy.** In general, fluoroscopy has no advantage over the radiograph, and the short distance between the source of X-rays and the screen distorts the cardiac outline. The method is, however, useful for detecting intracardiac calcification, particularly in diseased mitral and aortic valves. The movement of calcified cusps helps to identify the valve. An image intensifier is more efficient than the standard fluoroscopic screen for this purpose.

**Electrocardiography.** The electrocardiograph is invaluable for certain specific purposes, namely the elucidation of an arrhythmia, the detection of hypertrophy of each of the cardiac chambers, and, above all, for evidence of acute injury to heart muscle from ischaemia or metabolic disturbances. The electrocardiograph is the only reliable method which can indicate the site of a myocardial infarction in life.

**Miscellaneous.** The phonocardiograph has sharpened auscultatory practice and is occasionally helpful in diagnosis.

The echocardiograph, which is a record of the reflection of ultrasound directed at the heart, is making a growing contribution to diagnosis and is of special value as it is not an invasive technique.

More elaborate methods such as cardiac catheterisation, angiocardiography and coronary angiography all have important parts to play, particularly when cardiac or coronary surgery is contemplated.

## THE METHODS IN PRACTICE

In order to illustrate the practical application and integration of the various findings from the clinical examination of the cardiovascular system certain important problems have been selected, namely, acute circulatory failure, cardiac failure, myocardial and pericardial disease, massive pulmonary embolism, hypertension, the arrythmias and infective endocarditis.

### Acute Circulatory Failure

Acute circulatory failure may be transient or prolonged. The former is seen most frequently in an attack of simple syncope, i.e. the common faint (p. 37). Transient loss of consciousness also occurs in cough syncope (p. 38) and in micturition syncope (p. 38). Obstruction of venous return by a gravid uterus, or paralysis of the vasomotor reflexes by drugs or by diseases such as diabetes affecting the autonomic nervous system, may also lead to temporary syncope (p. 118).

Intermittent syncope, particularly on exertion, occurs in some patients whose cardiac output is severely restricted. Obstruction to blood flow from aortic and pulmonary stenosis, and from pulmonary vascular obstruction, provide examples of this. Mitral stenosis limits exertion by breathlessness and does not produce syncope except on the rare occasions when there is severe pulmonary arterial obstruction. Adams-Stokes attacks (p. 39) may occur at any time in patients with complete heart block.

The physician is often faced with the problem of determining the cause of a transient attack of acute circulatory failure and of its differentiation from an epileptic fit. This is dealt with when the analysis of 'blackouts' or fits and faints is discussed on page 37

More prolonged acute circulatory failure occurs when the blood volume is reduced by haemorrhage, severe injury or burns, or when there is a marked fall in cardiac output after a severe myocardial infarction or pulmonary embolism. Then there is a rapid pulse of poor volume ('thready'), low blood pressure, pale clammy skin and slow deep respiration—the so-called picture of *shock*. This clinical state is sometimes, less satisfactorily, called *peripheral circulatory failure*.

## Cardiac Failure

This may be a complication of all forms of heart disease. It is customary to divide cardiac failure into left and right heart failure depending on whether the clinical manifestations affect mainly the pulmonary or systemic circulations respectively. Right heart failure is also called congestive cardiac failure. The clinical manifestations of cardiac failure are as follows:

**Acute Pulmonary Oedema.** This is most often due to left ventricular failure as a result of myocardial infarction, hypertension or aortic valve disease. The history of being suddenly awakened at night by extreme breathlessness is characteristic (p. 44). During an attack there is pallor of the skin and cyanosis, inspiratory crepitations, and a cough which is unproductive in the early stages but which, in the absence of treatment, may later produce a frothy sputum with or without blood-staining, and extensive inspiratory crepitations. The blood pressure tends to be higher than usual, probably from the alarm which inevitably accompanies the attack. The diagnosis can be put beyond dispute by a chest radiograph, and this will be a permanent record of an unwelcome and important complication of the disease.

**Elevation of Jugular Venous Pressure** (p. 122). When persistent, this is the earliest and most reliable evidence of right heart failure; for example a rise in J.V.P. during infusion or transfusion can be overlooked only at the patient's peril.

**Subcutaneous Oedema.** Fluid retention in cardiac failure depends on numerous factors (p. 55); however, fluid tends to accumulate where the pressure across the capillary wall is greatest. In the upright position the ankles are therefore the usual site for oedema, and firm pressure by the examiner's thumb on the skin posterior to the internal malleoli will leave a significant indentation if oedema is present. When the patient is in bed, oedema accumulates over the sacrum and lumbar region, and also commonly at the backs of the thighs. In those patients with cardiac failure who are not breathless at rest and who are therefore able to lie flat in bed, oedema may be found in the arms and hands and even, rarely, in the face and neck. This may occur with chronic constrictive pericarditis, tricuspid valve lesions and occasionally with chronic cor pulmonale.

**Pleural Effusions.** Hydrothorax may occur in congestive cardiac failure from any cause, or a pleural exudate may be a sequel to pulmonary infarction which so frequently complicates congestive cardiac failure. The physical signs of a pleural effusion are described in Table 3 (p. 192).

**Hepatomegaly.** The criteria required for the diagnosis of hepatic enlargement are dealt with on page 214. Hepatomegaly is a usual complication of congestive cardiac failure. However, in the untreated patient it cannot be attributed to this cause unless accompanied by elevation of jugular venous pressure. Although usually hepatic enlargement is a crude index of cardiac failure compared to the jugular venous hypertension, in infants, where elevation of venous pressure may be impossible to detect, hepatomegaly is a particularly valuable sign. *Systolic expansion* of the liver may be appreciated if the left hand is placed under the patient's lower right ribs posteriorly, with the right hand below the right costal margin; separation of the hands by outward movement of each is characteristic of expansile hepatic pulsation found in gross tricuspid incompetence. Systolic epigastric pulsation from the aorta is not felt by the left hand. *Presystolic expansion* of the liver may be found in tricuspid stenosis.

**Ascites.** The methods for the detection of ascites are described on page 218. Although commonly found at post mortem in patients dying of congestive cardiac failure it is much less often discovered in life. Shifting dullness can be detected only when there is a considerable collection of liquid. Gross ascites is often a feature of those forms of cardiac failure in which the venous pressure is particularly high, e.g. constrictive pericarditis, tricuspid stenosis and tricuspid incompetence; in the first of these cirrhosis is commonly misdiagnosed if the jugular venous hypertension is not detected.

**Miscellaneous Findings.** There are other disturbances of function which, although not diagnostic of cardiac failure, are common accompaniments. These include *disturbance of renal function*, e.g. a concentrated urine of high specific gravity, which often contains protein. *Impairment of nutrition* may result from loss of appetite, which is a feature of severe cardiac failure, and which is often made worse by digitalis, potassium salts and other drugs; in addition there may be *impairment of hepatic function* with or without jaundice, or a protein-losing *enteropathy*. All these factors may lead to wasting. *Cerebral hypoxia* can result from ischaemia when there is hypotension, as with a severe myocardial infarction or pulmonary embolism, or from hypoxaemia, as with pulmonary oedema or chronic cor pulmonale. Alteration in behaviour, restlessness and aggressiveness, disturbance of sleep rhythm and Cheyne-Stokes respiration are the manifestations which result.

## Myocardial and Pericardial Disease

The diagnosis of myocardial or pericardial disease as the cause of heart failure is made mainly by the exclusion of other factors. The first requirement in assessing the patient with heart failure is to try and determine whether there are increased demands on the heart, such as are found in thyrotoxicosis and severe chronic anaemia, which might be the cause of, or a major contributory factor to, the heart failure. The next step is to look for evidence of increased work, such as that caused by systemic or pulmonary hypertension or by valvular disease. If these are absent, then disease of the myocardium or pericardium is likely to be the cause of the heart failure.

**Myocardial Disease.** The most common cause of myocardial disease is ischaemia as a result of coronary atheroma, and in many of these patients there will be a history of cardiac pain to point to this aetiology. There are no specific physical signs although there may be evidence of cardiac enlargement, a third heart sound at the apex, and mitral or tricuspid valvular incompetence. The ECG, however, has a special place because of its ability to throw light on abnormalities at cellular level.

**Pericardial Disease.** Many supposed signs of *pericardial effusion* are to be found in the literature, and many of them are now only of historical interest. Much the most important step towards the diagnosis is to suspect the presence of an effusion, and much the most reliable evidence is enlargement of the cardiac shadow on radiological examination, particularly when the heart is known to have been recently of normal size. Extension of the area of cardiac dullness and reduction in the intensity of the heart sounds and of the voltage of the electrocardiogram provide similar evidence in less precise ways. With the development of *cardiac tamponade*, i.e. compression of the heart by a pericardial sac distended with liquid, the venous pressure rises and pulsus paradoxus (p. 113) may be noted. The presence of a significant pericardial effusion may be difficult to disprove, for pericardial friction, normal heart sounds and even a normal ECG are not sufficient to exclude effusion. Pericardial aspiration, cardiac catheterisation or angio- or echocardiography may be necessary when a decision is important.

CHRONIC CONSTRICTIVE PERICARDITIS. Adhesion of the otherwise normal pericardium is an unimportant post-mortem finding, but when the peri-

F

cardium is thick and adherent, elevation of venous pressure and cardiac failure may occur. Interference with filling of the ventricle shows itself by a characteristic venous pulse and a right ventricular filling sound (third heart sound). When congestive cardiac failure and a normal sized heart are found together evidence of constrictive pericarditis must be carefully sought. A radiograph, particularly a lateral film, may show pericardial calcification.

## Cor Pulmonale

This merits a small section on its own, as the diagnosis is so frequently missed. These patients develop congestive cardiac failure usually for the first time during an episode of respiratory infection complicating chronic respiratory failure which in turn is most commonly due to emphysema. The distended lungs may conceal the clinical evidence of right ventricular hypertrophy and pulmonary hypertension. Paradoxically, these patients are sometimes not dyspnoeic because they have severe respiratory depression. Arterial undersaturation is the rule, and central cyanosis (p. 110) is usually detectable clinically. There is peripheral vasodilatation due to the effects of a high $Pco_2$ (i.e. partial pressure of carbon dioxide in arterial blood); the hands, nose and ears are often unusually warm, or at least lack the chill which is a feature in most patients with heart failure secondary to cardiac disease. The volume of the radial pulse is often greater than normal. The conjunctival vessels may be congested, sometimes with chemosis, the retinal veins are engorged and rarely papilloedema and retinal haemorrhages may develop. In addition, flapping tremor of the outstretched arms, mental confusion and even coma may occur.

## Massive Pulmonary Embolism

The patients most liable to pulmonary embolism are those confined to bed, particularly after a surgical operation or child-birth. The symptoms may include sudden dyspnoea, shock, or, particularly in the elderly, cardiac ischaemic pain. Pleural pain is a symptom of pulmonary infarction not of embolism. The signs of massive embolism are cyanosis, shock, a right ventricular impulse, a loud second heart sound in the pulmonary area and, occasionally, a pulmonary diastolic murmur. The jugular venous pressure is often elevated. The legs should be examined for evidence of a deep venous thrombosis (p. 143). However, a major pulmonary embolism can occur without producing any of these signs, and without a source for the embolus being demonstrable.

## Hypertension

### SYSTEMIC HYPERTENSION

In the clinical assessment of this condition the following points have especially to be borne in mind.

The important symptoms are those of the complications, i.e. left ventricular failure, cerebrovascular accidents, ischaemic heart disease and renal failure. Symptoms, such as headache, malaise and tiredness which are found in many other conditions, are of little value in assessment and in decisions as to the need for treatment. Clinical evidence of left ventricular hypertrophy should be sought by palpation, and of left atrial hypertrophy from an apical fourth heart sound. The retina must be examined for evidence of hypertensive changes. Left ventricular failure may be inferred from fine basal crepitations which persist after coughing but a radiograph showing pulmonary oedema is better evidence. The peripheral arteries must be palpated for evidence of occlusion. The urine must be examined by microscopy for casts, polymorphonuclear leucocytes and protein.

In searching for a cause for the hypertension, particularly careful scrutiny of patients aged less than 40 and who have no family history of hypertensive disease may well be rewarding. When hypertension is due to a phaeochromocytoma there may be symptoms of increased adrenaline production (sweating, dyspnoea, palpitations and apprehension). Very rarely such a tumour is palpable. Coarctation of the aorta is easily overlooked unless a search is always made for the femoral pulse in the presence of hypertension; even with a coarctation it is almost always palpable, but usually only with great difficulty. The delay in arrival of the pulse wave at the femoral pulse when compared with the simultaneously palpated radial artery is characteristic. Renal artery stenosis may cause hypertension, and may be suspected if a systolic murmur is audible over the kidney either anteriorly or posteriorly. Hypertension is also a feature of Cushing's syndrome.

### PULMONARY HYPERTENSION

Pulmonary hypertension occurs in some cases of severe mitral stenosis and congenital heart disease (e.g. in some cases of atrial septal defect, ventricular septal defect, patent ductus arteriosus and Eisenmenger's syndrome), from repeated pulmonary embolism, and sometimes without recognisable cause. The physical signs can be grouped as follows: firstly, those of high pressure in the pulmonary artery, namely a pulsation to the left of the sternum in the second intercostal space, a loud pulmonary second sound and a Graham-Steell murmur (p. 137); secondly, those of right ventricular hypertrophy, i.e. a forceful systolic impulse to the left of the sternum; and thirdly, those of right atrial hypertrophy, namely a large 'a' wave, and a right atrial fourth heart sound over the right ventricle.

## Elucidation of an Attack of Tachycardia

This is a common problem with which the medical practitioner is faced, and it has to be tackled by a logical system of analysis. Complications such as breathlessness or hypotension develop during a paroxysm only if there is some other abnormality of the heart which makes it unable to tolerate a tachycardia and to maintain the cardiac output, or if the patient is an infant or is elderly. The first step is to reassure the patient if he appears to be alarmed, and then to proceed with the history and examination. The following questions have to be asked:

1. *Have there been other attacks?* This is probable in supraventricular tachycardia and paroxysmal atrial fibrillation.

2. *Has heart disease been previously suspected?* If so what was the reason for this? In rheumatic heart disease atrial fibrillation and flutter are likely to be the cause of the arrhythmia.

3. *Are there other signs or symptoms?* These might suggest that the tachycardia is symptomatic of some sudden circulatory crisis, such as major haemorrhage, pulmonary embolism or myocardial infarction. Is there evidence of possible causative disease such as thyrotoxicosis?

4. *Is the patient under treatment?* Any arrhythmia may be provoked by digitalis, and some, e.g. ventricular tachycardia and paroxysmal atrial tachycardia with atrioventricular block (P.A.T. with block) may prove fatal if more digitalis is given.

5. *Is the pulse regular or irregular?* If the pulse is regular and fast the main possibilities are *sinus tachycardia, paroxysmal tachycardia, atrial flutter* and *P.A.T. with block.* In *sinus tachycardia* the rate usually varies from minute to minute, and slows with carotid sinus pressure. In *paroxysmal tachycardia* the signs depend on whether it is of supraventricular (i.e. atrial or nodal) or of ventricular origin. In both the heart rate is absolutely regular between 130 and 180 per minute. Youth, and the absence of other evidence of heart disease suggest supraventricular origin; it is proved if sinus rhythm can be restored by carotid sinus pressure. Ischaemic heart disease and digitalis intoxication are common causes of ventricular tachycardia. The dissociated waves in the jugular venous pulse resulting from atrial contraction may be seen, and the intensity of the first heart sound at the apex and the pulse volume often vary from beat to beat. These last two signs depend on variations from beat to beat in ventricular filling due to dissociation of atrial and ventricular contractions. In *atrial flutter* the rapid five per second venous pulse may be seen. Carotid sinus pressure may increase the A.V. block and result in a regular and slower ventricular beat while the pressure is maintained; the new heart rate is mathematically related to the one before carotid sinus pressure was used. If carotid sinus pressure fails, or the other signs are inconclusive, it is better to record ECGs than to guess at the cause of the tachycardia.

If the pulse is *irregular and fast* the most likely arrhythmia is *atrial fibrillation* and the signs of mitral stenosis or of thyrotoxicosis should be sought. When the ventricular rate is very fast with this arrhythmia the irregularity is easily overlooked. *Atrial flutter with varying block,* and *P.A.T. with block* are rarer possibilities. Nowadays these attempts at bedside diagnosis are seldom sustained for long when an ECG can give precise information so readily.

## Infective Endocarditis

This disease does not usually present itself primarily as a cardiological problem; its detection is an important responsibility of all physicians as it is remediable and yet readily overlooked, particularly in the elderly. A prolonged fever, malaise, tiredness, embolism, an obscure anaemia, premature cardiac failure, generalised aches and pains—any of these may be the main feature. The diagnosis may be straightforward, provided the possibility is considered when the patient is known to have congenital heart disease (particularly a ventricular septal defect, a patent ductus arteriosus or a coarctation of the aorta) or rheumatic heart disease (particularly mitral incompetence and aortic valve disease). The diagnosis is difficult when the disease affects a bicuspid aortic valve as there may be, initially at least, only a soft aortic systolic murmur. However, the development of a soft early diastolic murmur of aortic incompetence in a patient under investigation for symptoms such as those already described, and who is known not to have had such a murmur on previous careful examination, is highly suggestive, and is almost the only occasion when the skilled use of a good stethoscope in detecting this particular murmur may make a crucial difference to the patient's welfare. Its recognition enables prompt and effective treatment to be started before severe damage to the valve has taken place. The following physical signs should be sought.

*Clubbing of the fingers* (p. 167) is usually a fairly late manifestation of the disease, but not invariably so, and rarely it may be the only extracardiac abnormality. *Splinter haemorrhages* under the nails, too far from the free margin to be due to a splinter beneath the nail—of which patients are usually aware—are seen occasionally in normal subjects. They occur more frequently in patients with rheumatic heart disease, and in greatest numbers in those with infective endocarditis. When found in large numbers they are highly suggestive of infective endocarditis, but their absence does not exclude the disease. *Petechial haemorrhages* may occur in skin, mucous membranes and conjunctivae, and there may be retinal haemorrhages and exudates. Exquisitely tender spots appearing in the pulp of a finger, sometimes accompanied by swelling or redness, are called *Osler's nodes*. *Palpable enlargement of the spleen* is usually slight and detected only with careful examination. *Microscopic haematuria* is often found and proteinuria may also occur.

# CHAPTER 6
# The Respiratory System

'Take care of the sense, and the sounds will take care of themselves.'
LEWIS CARROLL

Many of the methods of physical examination we use today for the investigation of respiratory disease differ remarkably little from those described by Laënnec in his *Treatise on the Diseases of the Chest*, published in 1819. We still seek by means of inspection, palpation, percussion and auscultation to detect abnormalities in the bronchi, lungs and pleura and by analysis of the various physical signs to determine the gross pathology of the lesions. Advances in radiology, bacteriology, physiology, endoscopy and thoracic surgery have, however, enabled us not only to diagnose respiratory disease with more precision but also to reappraise the value of clinical investigation in its various forms. Nowadays, for example, we place more weight on careful history-taking than on the elicitation of elegant, but possibly misleading, physical signs. We also realise that in many disorders the disease process may reach an advanced stage before any abnormal signs can be detected and that unless symptoms are promptly investigated by special techniques, such as radiology, serious delays in diagnosis and treatment may result. More is known, too, of the relationship between clinical findings and disturbances of respiratory function, and there is a better understanding of the significance of features such as dyspnoea and cyanosis.

The principal effects of these advances are threefold. Firstly, the technique of physical examination of the chest has been greatly simplified by the omission of tedious procedures which are now known to have little, if any, practical application, by discarding elaborate and meaningless terms previously in common use for the description of physical signs and by emphasising the importance of those items of clinical examination which provide information of genuine diagnostic value. Secondly, the limitations of physical examination have been recognised and defined in relation to the diagnosis of conditions such as pulmonary tuberculosis and bronchial carcinoma, in which physical signs are notoriously unreliable. Thirdly, the modern approach to clinical examination reflects the importance accorded to respiratory physiology and embodies acceptance of the principle that a morbid anatomical diagnosis can no longer be regarded as an end in itself. If, for example, a diagnosis of emphysema is made, the patient's investigation is considered incomplete until the effects of the disease on respiratory function have been assessed.

# THE HISTORY

The approach to history-taking in patients thought to have respiratory disease differs according to the nature of the illness, the main distinction being that between an acute or subacute illness and a chronic respiratory disorder. The methods used to obtain a coherent account of the patient's symptoms are, however, the same in the two types of case. Firstly, a narrative history is taken, the patient being encouraged to describe his symptoms in his own way, curbed only by restrictions on verbosity and irrelevance as outlined in Chapter 1. Specific enquiry is then made about any of the six cardinal respiratory symptoms (cough, sputum, haemoptysis, chest pain, dyspnoea and wheeze) not mentioned in the narrative history. At this stage the doctor may find it convenient to review the data so far obtained and make a mental note of all the conditions which might conceivably be responsible for the patient's symptoms. This will seldom be a formidable list, perhaps three or four items in the average case. He should then ask a series of supplementary questions designed to provide evidence for and against each possible diagnosis. In the course of this interrogation he may have to ask the patient to confirm or expand some of the information previously given. This method of integrating and rationalising the history has an important place in the diagnosis of respiratory disease because it facilitates the recognition of certain character-istic symptom-patterns, such as those presented by chronic bronchitis and bronchial asthma, in which physical signs and even specialised investigations may be of limited diagnostic value.

In an *acute respiratory illness* history-taking usually presents no special difficulties, but one or two points are worthy of mention. It is always important to enquire carefully about the onset of the illness, which may provide a valuable clue to its nature. In pneumococcal pneumonia, for example, systemic disturbance (rigor, pyrexia, malaise) seldom precedes the first respiratory symptom (usually pleural pain) by more than a few hours, while in virus pneumonia the patient may be pyrexial and generally unwell for several days before there are any symptoms or signs to suggest pulmonary involvement. Acute dyspnoea is a presenting symptom of particular import-ance since it often demands urgent treatment, and an error in diagnosis between, say, tension pneumothorax, status asthmaticus and left heart failure may have catastrophic consequences. There, too, a carefully taken history, from a relative if the patient is too breathless to give a coherent account of his illness, may enable such a mistake to be avoided. The nature and effect of treatment prescribed before the patient is seen should also be carefully noted. If, for example, the symptoms are suggestive of an acute pulmonary infection but there had been no improvement after a few days of treatment with an antibiotic, consideration must be given to the possibility of the patient having a drug-resistant bacterial infection, a tuberculous or viral infection, an empyema or even a pulmonary infarct.

In *chronic respiratory disorders* history-taking is always a complex and time-consuming procedure. Care must be taken to record not only major incidents in the course of the illness but also to describe and assess the 'interval' or 'background' symptoms. In the case of acute episodes, such as exacerbations of chronic bronchitis, an enquiry should be made into the events which preceded them and the effects which they appeared to have on the course of the disease. Most chronic respiratory disorders pursue a fairly predictable course, and if a patient exhibits symptoms out of line with the established pattern of his illness, the development of another disease should be suspected. The influence of environmental factors, such as weather and time of year, changes of room temperature and exposure to smoke and dust, should always be recorded. Such information, in addition to its diagnostic relevance, may prove of value from the therapeutic aspect. A clinical assessment of respiratory function is an essential item in the history of every patient with chronic respiratory disease.

## The Cardinal Symptoms of Respiratory Disease

The six cardinal symptoms of respiratory disease are *cough, sputum, haemoptysis, chest pain, dyspnoea* and *wheeze*. It is important to remember that some of these symptoms may occur in the absence of primary respiratory disease. Certain types of chest pain, for example, may be of cardiac or oesophageal origin, dyspnoea may be due to pulmonary oedema secondary to heart disease, and haemoptysis may occasionally be the presenting symptom in disorders of the blood clotting mechanism. Nevertheless, all six symptoms in the vast majority of cases are indicative of respiratory disease, and will be discussed in that context.

**Cough.** Cough, the most frequent symptom of respiratory disease, may be excited by stimuli arising in the mucosa of any part of the respiratory tract from the pharynx to the smaller bronchi. Stimuli arising in the parietal pleura may, on rare occasions, also produce cough, for example in dry pleurisy or during pleural paracentesis. The frequency, severity and character of cough are dependent on several factors including (*a*) the situation and nature of the lesion responsible for the cough, (*b*) the presence or absence of sputum and (*c*) coexisting abnormalities such as vocal cord paralysis, impairment of ventilatory function and pleural pain.

### TYPES OF COUGH

1. Cough produced by stimuli arising in the *pharyngeal mucosa* occurs in pharyngitis or may be caused by secretions trickling down the posterior pharyngeal wall from the nasal sinuses. It is typically a dry, persistent cough, but may be paroxysmal and explosive at times when the pharynx is coated with tenacious mucus or mucopus.

2. Cough arising in the *larynx* has a harsh, barking quality and may be painful, especially when it is a manifestation of acute laryngitis. If a vocal

cord is paralysed, a cough, whatever its site of origin, will lose its normal explosive force (p. 274) and will cease to be effective in clearing the respiratory tract of secretion. Cough in patients with whooping-cough occurs in prolonged, severe paroxysms culminating in the characteristic long inspiratory 'whoop'. This is produced by the passage of air between vocal cords approximated by spasm of the laryngeal muscles.

3. Cough arising in the *trachea* is usually caused by tracheitis, in which it is harsh, 'dry' and painful at first, becoming 'loose', productive and less painful later. Cough caused by a malignant tumour partially obstructing the trachea is persistent and at times severe and suffocating. Such patients may become deeply cyanosed and even unconscious during paroxysms of coughing.

4. Cough of several different types may be produced by stimulation of nerve endings in the *bronchial mucosa*.

Cough in *acute bronchitis* is similar in character to that which occurs in tracheitis but is often preceded or accompanied by transient wheeze and a feeling of diffuse 'tightness' in the chest. In the early stages it is 'dry'; when it later becomes productive it assumes a 'loose' and painless quality.

Cough in *chronic bronchitis* tends to occur in prolonged paroxysms, which usually culminate in the production of sputum. When the sputum is very tenacious, however, or if there is serious impairment of ventilatory function, the patient, exhausted by the effort of coughing, may abandon the attempt to clear his bronchi of secretions and the bout of coughing comes to an indecisive stop. This 'unfinished cough', as some patients describe it, is typical of chronic bronchitis and emphysema. Bouts of coughing in these patients often produce severe dyspnoea, frequently accompanied by wheezing, and may be very distressing. Cough in chronic bronchitis has other typical characteristics. It is particularly frequent and severe when the patient retires to bed at night and, even more so, when he gets up in the morning, possibly because of the sudden changes in the temperature of the inspired air to which he is exposed at these times. Sleep is seldom disturbed by coughing, but most patients with chronic bronchitis waken in the morning with a slight wheeze and a sensation of tightness in the chest. These symptoms do not improve until sputum is brought up by a violent bout of coughing which may continue for several minutes. Cough in chronic bronchitis is stimulated not only by changes in atmospheric temperature but also by bronchial irritants such as smoke, fumes or dust, and by the sudden increase in the depth of ventilation which occurs with exertion and laughter. Some patients may experience 'cough syncope' (p. 38) during bouts of violent coughing. When patients with chronic bronchitis develop ventilatory failure, cough becomes progressively more feeble and ineffective, and eventually the accumulation of secretions in the larynx and trachea gives rise to a so-called 'death rattle'.

Prolonged paroxysms of coughing may also occur in patients with *chronic asthma*. The cough, which invariably aggravates the dyspnoea and wheeze, is less directly related to atmospheric conditions than the cough of chronic bronchitis and often wakens the patient in the middle of the night. The dyspnoea and wheeze which follow may be confused with cardiac asthma (p. 44).

In *bronchial carcinoma* cough may be and often is an early and persistent symptom. At first it is a frequent short 'dry' cough, but later, when the tumour has caused bronchial obstruction with distal pulmonary infection, it becomes more severe and distressing. If the bronchus is not completely occluded, pus may be coughed up. The type of cough associated with interruption of the left recurrent laryngeal nerve, a common complication of tumour at the left pulmonary hilum, is described on page 274.

Cough in *bronchiectasis*, uncomplicated by chronic bronchitis or asthma, is characteristically a 'loose' cough, readily productive of sputum. It may be brought on by changes in posture, e.g. by stooping if the bronchiectasis affects the lower lobes. Patients with severe unilateral bronchiectasis prefer to sleep on the affected side in order to prevent cough being stimulated by the dislodgement of sputum. Cough in *pneumonia* and *lung abscess* is 'dry' and irritable at first, later becoming loose and productive. When pleural pain is present, cough is typically short and half-suppressed. Cough in *acute pulmonary oedema* secondary to left heart failure is generally short, persistent and exhausting. A similar type of cough may occur in *allergic* and *fibrosing alveolitis*.

**Sputum.** When a patient has sputum, information should be obtained as to *amount, character, viscosity* and *taste or odour*.

AMOUNT. This can seldom be accurately estimated by the patient although statements that it is very large (e.g. a teacupful per day) or very small (one or two spits per day) are usually reliable. If it is important to obtain precise information about the amount of sputum, the patient should be given a graduated container and a 24-hour collection should be measured. It should be appreciated that some patients deny cough while admitting to the presence of sputum, saying that they bring it up merely by 'clearing the throat'. A specific enquiry about sputum should, therefore, be made in every case. Most children and some women swallow their sputum, even when it is being produced in large amounts. The character of the cough, if it is loose or moist, will, however, indicate that sputum is present.

CHARACTER. This is seldom described accurately by the patient and, wherever possible, a specimen should be inspected by the doctor. Apart from haemoptysis, there are four types of sputum—serous, mucoid, purulent and mucopurulent. Serous sputum, which is usually described by patients as clear and/or frothy, is seen in acute pulmonary oedema, in which it may acquire a pink colour through admixture with red blood cells, and in the rare condition of alveolar-cell carcinoma. Mucoid sputum, which is a characteristic feature of chronic bronchitis, is usually described by patients as 'grey', 'white', 'clear' or sometimes 'black' (when it contains soot particles). Purulent and mucopurulent sputum is usually described as 'yellow' or 'green', but occasionally 'white' sputum proves on inspection to be purulent. The term 'dirty spit' used by many patients is a misleading one, as it may refer either to purulent sputum or to mucoid sputum containing soot particles. Mucoid sputum may be copious and frothy in some cases of chronic bronchitis and asthma. Hysterical patients may spit out large amounts of saliva which they claim to be sputum.

VISCOSITY. Mucoid sputum is more viscous than purulent sputum and for that reason is often more difficult to cough up. Sputum is particularly viscous in the early stages of pneumococcal pneumonia and in status asthmaticus.

TASTE OR ODOUR. When this is described as 'nasty' the patient may merely be referring to the normal taste of purulent sputum. Only when terms such as 'horrible', 'like rotten eggs' or 'like a sewer' are used can it be assumed that the sputum is foetid (as in bronchiectasis or lung abscess with anaerobic bacterial infection). The doctor must always use his own sense of smell to confirm this.

**Haemoptysis.** Haemoptysis occurs in many respiratory diseases (e.g. bronchial carcinoma and adenoma, pulmonary tuberculosis, bronchiectasis, pulmonary infarction), in certain cardiovascular diseases (e.g. mitral stenosis) and occasionally in the absence of any demonstrable lesion in bronchi, lungs or heart. The blood in haemoptysis is bright red at first but may later become dark red. It is often frothy and may be mixed with sputum. Although most patients readily appreciate whether blood has been coughed up or vomited, haemoptysis is occasionally confused with haematemesis. Blood from the stomach can, however, usually be recognised by its consistently dark colour, by the absence of froth and sometimes by its admixture with food.

Whenever a history of haemoptysis is obtained, questions must be asked about its type, degree, frequency and duration. In some cases the events preceding it may be of importance in diagnosis, e.g. deep venous thrombosis in a lower limb or a respiratory infection.

TYPE AND DEGREE OF HAEMOPTYSIS

1. *Frank haemoptysis*, in which the material coughed up consists wholly of blood, occurs most commonly in bronchiectasis, pulmonary infarction, tuberculosis and mitral stenosis. A rough estimate should be made of the amount of blood lost, bearing in mind that most patients tend to exaggerate this.

2. *Blood-stained sputum*, in which the blood and sputum are intimately mixed in various proportions, occurs most commonly in bronchial carcinoma and lung abscess.

3. *Blood-streaked sputum*, in which streaks of blood are present in mucoid or purulent sputum, is a fairly frequent symptom in chronic bronchitis but may also occur in bronchial carcinoma.

4. *'Rusty' sputum*, in which degradation products of haemoglobin give the sputum a colour varying between rust and golden-yellow, is a common feature of pneumococcal pneumonia and occurs in few other conditions.

FREQUENCY AND DURATION OF HAEMOPTYSIS. With frank haemoptysis it is usual for the blood in the sputum to become progressively darker in colour for

24 to 48 hours at least after the bleeding ceases. Such prolongation of haemoptysis, which is common in, for example, pulmonary infarction, has no diagnostic importance. When, however, small amounts of fresh blood are coughed up frequently either as frank haemoptysis or blood-stained sputum, for example daily for a week, the symptom strongly suggests a diagnosis of bronchial carcinoma.

**Chest Pain.** Three types of chest pain are directly due to respiratory disease:

1. *Upper retrosternal pain* of the type experienced in acute tracheitis (p. 162).

2. *Retrosternal pain associated with lesions of the mediastinum*, e.g. tumours, acute mediastinitis and mediastinal emphysema. This type of pain, which is an uncommon but important symptom, has a constrictive or oppressive character similar to that of cardiac pain and may radiate into the arms or neck, but is seldom severe and is not related to exertion.

3. *Pleural pain*, caused by stretching of an inflamed parietal pleura, occurs in all forms of fibrinous ('dry') pleurisy. Identical pain is produced by fractures of ribs. Pleural pain is recognised by its sharp, 'knife-like' character and by its relationship to breathing and coughing. It may be present only at the end of a deep inspiration or during a cough; with more severe degrees even shallow breathing may produce intense pain. Occasionally the pain is aggravated by exertion (which causes an increase in the depth of breathing) or by movements of the thoracic spine. Pleural pain often, but not invariably, subsides when an effusion develops, probably because the fluid limits expansion of the lung and thus reduces the range of movement of the chest wall.

In spontaneous pneumothorax typical pleural pain may be present, particularly if the amount of air in the pleural space is small. More often, however, after a brief initial episode of severe unilateral pain the patient complains mainly of tightness across the front of the chest, which may later become localised to the affected side. Rarely, there may be central retrosternal pain resembling that of cardiac infarction, with radiation into the neck and upper limbs. This type of pain may be due to mediastinal emphysema, with which spontaneous pneumothorax is occasionally associated.

Chest pain may also be caused by lesions of the heart and great vessels (p. 105, 106) or of the oesophagus (p. 202), or it may be due to irritation of a spinal nerve root. The pain of herpes zoster may also be referred to the chest wall (p. 97). Pain caused by invasion of the chest wall by a malignant pulmonary tumour or by a metastatic deposit in a rib is due to involvement of intercostal nerves. It is a constant, severe, aching pain, usually unrelated to respiration. Chest pain in the absence of organic disease may be a manifestation of anxiety (p. 28).

When a patient complains of chest pain the following information should be obtained about it:

(1) Situation, (2) severity, (3) duration, (4) whether constant or intermittent, (5) nature and circumstances of onset, e.g. whether sudden or gradual; whether accompanied by other respiratory symptoms such as cough or dyspnoea, and (6) whether related to breathing, coughing, sneezing, spinal movements or exertion.

**Dyspnoea** (p. 41).

**Wheeze.** When a patient complains of 'wheeze' it is important first to discover what he means by the term. Some patients use it merely to describe noisy and laboured breathing while others apply it to the rattling or rustling of secretions in the upper air passages. Wheeze is, however, usually applied to the musical sounds produced by the passage of air through narrowed bronchi. It is invariably louder during expiration and is often confined to that phase of the respiratory cycle. It is always more conspicuous during deep breathing and sometimes may become audible only when the depth of respiration is increased. Many patients become so accustomed to wheeze that they cease to be aware of its presence until a relative or friend draws attention to it. When making enquiries about wheeze the doctor should listen carefully to the patient's breathing and from his own and the patient's observations find out when wheeze is present and whether it is aggravated by factors such as exertion, inhalation of dust or a respiratory infection.

## Symptoms indicative of Disease of the Upper Respiratory Tract

**Nose and Nasopharynx.** The most frequent symptoms of disease in the nose and nasopharynx are *obstruction of the nasal airway*, often described by patient's as 'catarrh', and *nasal discharge*. Not uncommonly, these two symptoms co-exist.

It is important to enquire whether the nasal obstruction consistently affects the right or left nasal airway (or both), or whether it changes from one side to the other, according to the position of the head. This may be a relevant point since persistent nasal obstruction is usually due to adenoids, to a deflected nasal septum or to a collection of polypi, whereas intermittent obstruction is more often caused by mucosal oedema and excessive secretions. Bilateral nasal obstruction may lead to chronic mouth breathing, which, in children particularly, is often the reason for seeking medical advice.

The amount, nature and colour of any nasal discharge should normally be recorded in lay terms, e.g. 'profuse and watery', 'scanty', 'tenacious' or 'green', unless a specimen is inspected by the doctor, in which case technical terms, such as serous, mucoid or purulent, may be used. An attempt should be made to discover whether the discharge comes entirely from the nostrils or whether it drips into the back of the throat.

Factors which precipitate recurrent nasal obstruction and discharge, e.g. the inhalation of dust or grass pollens, should be identified whenever possible. An enquiry should also be made about excessive *sneezing*, a common feature of allergic rhinitis, and *frontal headache* which may accompany an acute sinus infection.

*Epistaxis* may give rise to haemoptysis if blood in the posterior nares is inhaled and then coughed up. This possibility should always be kept in mind when a history is being taken from a patient with a complaint of haemoptysis.

**Larynx.** The two chief symptoms of laryngeal disease are hoarseness and stridor, but lesions of the larynx may also produce cough and pain.

*Hoarseness* may vary in degree from a slight harshness of the voice to aphonia. Enquiries should be made about the duration of hoarseness and about events which may have preceded its onset, such as a head cold, abuse of the voice, chronic cough or an operation on the neck or throat. The patient should also be asked whether it is improving, worsening or remaining static.

*Cough* of a short, dry, 'barking' character almost invariably accompanies hoarseness caused by an organic lesion within the larynx. The 'bovine' cough of laryngeal paralysis is described on page 274.

*Laryngeal stridor* is recognised by a high-pitched crowing sound with each inspiration, and may be produced by a foreign body lodged between the cords, laryngeal spasm, exudate or oedema and bilateral vocal cord paralysis.

*Laryngeal pain* of mild degree occurs transiently in acute laryngitis, constant severe pain in advanced tuberculous laryngitis and laryngeal carcinoma.

All patients with stridor and those in whom a marked degree of hoarseness persists for more than a fortnight should have laryngoscopy (p. 170) carried out.

**Trachea.** Disease of the trachea may produce pain, cough, stridor and dyspnoea.

*Tracheal pain* is referred to behind the manubrium sterni. In the early stages of acute tracheitis there may be quite severe pain in this situation, which may become momentarily intense on coughing but which subsides as soon as the cough becomes productive.

*Tracheal stridor* is usually due to obstruction of the tracheal lumen by a malignant tumour and is always accompanied by dyspnoea. It is lower in pitch than laryngeal stridor, is heard best during inspiration and is accentuated by coughing.

## History of Previous Illness

When the present illness appears to be involving the respiratory system, information of considerable value in diagnosis, prognosis, and treatment may be obtained from the past medical history. The following conditions are of particular importance in this respect:

**Tuberculosis.** Primary tuberculous infection in childhood may be responsible for lobar or segmental bronchiectasis in later life. Post-primary tuberculosis, if inadequately treated, may relapse. Extensive bilateral tuberculosis, although no longer active, produces severe pulmonary fibrosis which may ultimately cause respiratory failure and pulmonary heart disease. Bronchiectasis at the site of a healed tuberculous lesion may give rise to severe haemoptysis.

Enquiries about a past history of tuberculosis should always be made tactfully since some patients still have an irrational fear of the disease and take fright at the merest suggestion that the diagnosis is being considered. If a history of tuberculosis is given, full details of the nature and duration of treatment should be obtained, if necessary from the hospital or chest clinic which the patient attended.

Another point worthy of enquiry is a history of B.C.G. vaccination which for the past 20 years has been offered to all tuberculin-negative British children at the age of 13. Successful vaccination affords considerable protection against tuberculosis and this information may be of value in differential diagnosis.

**Pneumonia and Pleurisy.** Some chronic respiratory disorders, e.g. chronic bronchitis and bronchiectasis, appear to date from an attack of pneumonia, sometimes described by patients as 'pleurisy' or 'congestion'. A history of recurrent pneumonia, particularly if it occurs on the same side each time, is suggestive of bronchiectasis, or, if the history is short (e.g. less than a year), of bronchial carcinoma. Rarely, recurrent pneumonia may be a feature of myelomatosis or hypogammaglobulinaemia, or in children of mucoviscidosis.

**Severe Measles or Whooping-cough in Childhood.** Such illnesses, particularly if complicated by pneumonia, are a frequent cause of bronchiectasis and an enquiry should always be made about them whenever that diagnosis is suspected.

**Chest Injuries and Operations.** It is important to enquire into the circumstances and nature of any chest injury or operation and to consider whether it might be related to the patient's current illness. For example, surgical or accidental trauma may produce deformities of the chest wall. A traumatic haemothorax, particularly if complicated by infection, may result in gross pleural thickening. A metallic foreign body lodged in the lung may cause recurrent haemoptysis or be responsible for the development of a chronic pulmonary abscess or bronchiectasis.

**Other Surgical Procedures.** The inhalation of septic material from the mouth or throat during dental extractions or tonsillectomy under general anaesthesia may result in the development of a pulmonary abscess. Any abdominal or thoracic operation, particularly an operation on the upper abdomen, may give rise to atelectasis and subsequent pulmonary infection which, if severe, may lead to the development of a pulmonary abscess or, at a later date, to bronchiectasis. Any major operation may also be complicated by pulmonary embolism and infarction. Certain surgical conditions in the abdomen, notably a perforated gastric or duodenal ulcer may mimic pulmonary disease or even produce secondary lesions in pleura and lungs.

**Allergic Disorders.** Patients who are believed to have an allergic disorder, such as bronchial asthma or allergic rhinitis, should be asked about previous manifestations of allergy, e.g. eczema, urticaria, and angio-oedema. A detailed enquiry should also be made regarding the effects of exposure to substances capable of producing allergic reactions, such as grass pollen, house dust, animal dander and certain foods and drugs.

**Previous Radiological Examination.** Often of considerable relevance to the diagnosis and management of the current illness is a history of previous radiological examination of the chest. If a radiographic abnormality is present, vital information as to its nature and significance may be obtained by reviewing the previous films and reports, if they can be obtained. This information may be of great value in the diagnosis of bronchial carcinoma and in assessing the activity of a tuberculous lesion. All patients should, therefore, be asked about previous radiological examination of the chest and a note made of the date and place of the examination.

## Family and Social History

The *family history* of patients with respiratory disease may be important in three ways:

1. *Certain infections*, notably tuberculosis, may be transferred from one person to another. In such cases a history of contact with an infected person is, of course, more important than the family relationship.

2. In *allergic disorders*, such as bronchial asthma, there may be an inherited predisposition, and a family history is not uncommon. Routine enquiries into family circumstances may, however, reveal potential causes of anxiety, stress and domestic conflict, which may prove to be much more important aetiological factors than heredity.

3. In *chronic bronchitis*, although an inherited predisposition cannot be excluded, the liability of several members of one family to develop the disease is more likely to be related to the conditions under which they all live, e.g. an overcrowded house situated in a district with a high level of atmospheric pollution.

From the diagnostic point of view, only enquiries regarding tuberculosis are likely to be rewarding, but a detailed knowledge of the family history will often highlight the social and economic consequences of chronic bronchitis and reveal psychological maladjustments which may be influencing the course of bronchial asthma.

*Social problems*, such as those of housing, finance and employment, loom large in the management of patients with all types of chronic respiratory disease and should be investigated fully in every case. The type of information which should be obtained from a patient with chronic bronchitis, for example, is the nature of his employment and, in more advanced cases, the number of stairs he has to climb to reach his house. Should he be advised to give up a well-paid job as an underground miner in favour of relatively poorly paid work in a less harmful atmospheric environment? Can anything be done to persuade the local authority or the landlord to exchange a top-floor flat without a lift for ground-level accommodation?

*Cigarette smoking* is now accepted as the most important cause of bronchial carcinoma and chronic bronchitis. In the case of bronchial carcinoma this fact is of some diagnostic relevance as the condition is rare in non-smokers. Tobacco smoking, especially of cigarettes, aggravates the symptoms of chronic bronchitis. A smoking history should include details such as the age when regular smoking started, the age when smoking was given up (where applicable), and the average consumption of tobacco (number of cigarettes or cigars per day, amount of pipe tobacco per week).

*Overeating and overindulgence in alcohol* may contribute to the development of obesity, which invariably causes an increase in exertional dyspnoea, whatever the basic pulmonary pathology. Extreme obesity may be directly responsible for respiratory and cardiac failure.

### Occupational History

Since both acute and chronic respiratory disease may be caused by the inhalation of certain types of dust encountered at work, it is important to record a complete occupational history, covering both present and previous employment. Industrial dust hazards may be responsible for respiratory disease in coal miners, iron and steel foundry workers, stonemasons, arc welders, pottery workers, asbestos workers, farmworkers and cotton operatives. Whenever an occupational history of this type is obtained, detailed information should be sought regarding the degree and duration of exposure to dust, and the time relationship of such exposure to the onset of symptoms.

In a separate but equally important category are dust hazards encountered in the patient's environment, but not necessarily at his place of work. Persons in close contact with pigeons, parrots, budgerigars or canaries may develop extrinsic allergic alveolitis or psittacosis, while atopic subjects may develop allergic rhinitis or bronchial asthma when exposed to allergens such as pollen, house dust, feathers, animal dander or certain types of fungal spore. An enquiry should always be made about these and other environmental hazards when an occupational history is being taken.

## THE PHYSICAL EXAMINATION

### The External Features of Respiratory Disease

**Initial Impression.** There are a number of features which may have become evident during the course of history-taking and should immediately cause the observer to suspect respiratory disease. These are (1) cough, (2) wheeze or stridor, and (3) respiratory discomfort.

The frequency, severity and type of cough (p. 156) should be noted. The character of wheeze and the degree of respiratory distress should also be observed. The speed with which a patient can dress or undress is often a useful index of his respiratory disability. Attention should be paid to any abnormality of the voice and to foetor of the breath, for which an anaerobic infection of the lung may be responsible if a local cause in the mouth has been excluded (p. 62). The state of nutrition should be roughly assessed (overweight, underweight, normal) pending precise measurements of height and weight. Finally, any suggestion of anaemia or polycythaemia should be noted either of which may be a relevant finding in certain types of respiratory disease.

**Cyanosis.** The presence of cyanosis should be noted, and the mechanism of its production determined. Central cyanosis of respiratory origin is most frequently seen in chronic bronchitis, emphysema and fibrosing alveolitis. In these conditions, especially if they are sufficiently advanced to cause pulmonary heart disease, peripheral vasodilatation is often a prominent feature and the warm, blue hands in such cases afford a striking demonstration of severe central cyanosis. Central cyanosis may also develop in pneumonia, bronchial asthma and tension pneumothorax. The cardiac causes of central cyanosis are described on page 110.

Peripheral cyanosis affecting the face and neck, and in some cases the upper limbs also, occurs in superior vena caval obstruction (see below).

In polycythaemia increased viscosity of the blood produces peripheral cyanosis by reducing the rate of blood flow through skin capillaries. Severe chronic hypoxia of either pulmonary or cardiac origin is often associated with polycythaemia, and an extreme degree of cyanosis, partly central and partly peripheral, may be seen in these conditions.

**Oedema.** The detection of peripheral oedema, which has been fully described on page 52, is an essential part of the investigation of respiratory disease and is especially important in patients with conditions such as chronic bronchitis, emphysema and diffuse pulmonary fibrosis, which are often complicated by right ventricular failure. Oedema of a different distribution is seen when the *superior vena cava is obstructed*. In this condition, which is a fairly common complication of bronchial carcinoma but may also be caused by a very large benign tumour or by chronic mediastinal fibrosis, the face and neck appear swollen and 'puffy'—although the tissues seldom 'pit' on pressure—and conjunctival oedema (chemosis) is often present. Because of more efficient collateral venous drainage the upper limbs are less frequently affected, but in some cases there is pitting oedema of the hands and forearms. When the superior vena cava is obstructed the external jugular veins become grossly distended but no venous pulsation is visible in these veins or in the internal jugular veins. After a week or two, dilated superficial veins and venules appear on the anterior and lateral aspects of the chest wall from the clavicles to below the costal margins. These veins convey blood from the tributaries of the subclavian and axillary veins to the drainage area of the inferior vena cava. The downward direction of blood flow can be demonstrated by the method described on page 143.

**Hands.** Examination of the hands in patients with suspected respiratory disease, apart from the observation of cyanosis (p. 166), is chiefly concerned with the recognition of *clubbing of the fingers*. This phenomenon occurs in a variety of respiratory, cardiovascular and alimentary diseases, including: (*a*) bronchial carcinoma and certain other intrathoracic tumours, some forms of pulmonary and pleural suppuration, e.g. bronchiectasis, pulmonary abscess and empyema, and some cases of fibrosing alveolitis (*b*) cyanotic congenital heart disease and infective endocarditis; and (*c*) the malabsorption syndrome, Crohn's disease, ulcerative colitis and hepatic cirrhosis. It has also been observed as a familial trait and may occur unilaterally in association with an

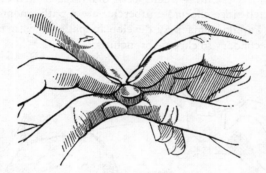

FIG. 26    Testing for Fluctuation at the Base of the Nail.

aneurysm of the subclavian artery. The swelling of the terminal phalanges in clubbing, which usually, but less obviously, affects the toes also, is due to interstitial oedema and dilatation of the arterioles and capillaries. In the earlier stages there may be little or no visible swelling, but the test of abnormal fluctuation at the nail bases will be positive (Fig. 26).

The finger is placed on the pulp of the examiner's two thumbs and the dorsum of the finger is palpated immediately proximal to the base of the nail by the tips of the examiner's two index or middle fingers. If a sensation of fluctuation is elicited, the test is said to be positive, provided that this is greater than the very slight degree of fluctuation which can be detected in normal fingers. When fluctuation is marked, palpation of the nail itself may give the impression that it is floating free on its bed. The difference between normal and abnormal fluctuation is, with practice, fairly easily recognised.

With more advanced degrees of clubbing, various visible changes develop progressively:

1. Swelling of the subcutaneous tissues at the base of the nail causes the overlying skin to become tense, shiny and red, with obliteration of the skin creases and loss of the angle between the nail and the nail base.

2. Later, as the swelling involves the nail bed, the curvature of the nail, especially in its long axis, increases.

3. Finally, swelling of the pulp of the finger in all its dimensions occurs in fully developed clubbing. In a few cases there may also be hypertrophic pulmonary osteoarthropathy causing pain in the forearms.

Increased curvature of the finger nails is commonly seen in normal subjects and, as an isolated phenomenon without other evidence of clubbing, is of no significance.

**Eyes.** The importance of examining the eyes in patients suspected of having respiratory disease is to recognise conditions such as phlyctenular keratoconjunctivitis, which may be a manifestation of primary tuberculosis, and iridocyclitis, which may be seen in tuberculosis or sarcoidosis. Opthalmoscopy (p. 412) is essential whenever a diagnosis of acute miliary tuberculosis is suspected since choroidal tubercles are a pathognomonic feature of that condition. Papilloedema may develop in patients with hypercapnia of long duration, secondary to chronic bronchitis.

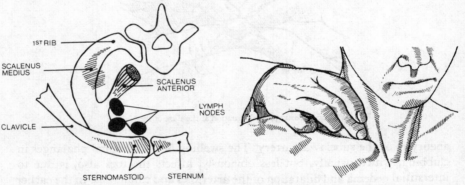

FIG. 27   Relation of Lymph Nodes to Scalenus Anterior.

FIG. 28   Palpation of Lymph Nodes on Scalenus Anterior.

**Neck.** A systematic method of examining the neck has already been described (p. 82). The part of the examination which is of particular importance in patients believed to have respiratory disease is that concerned with the detection of enlarged supraclavicular lymph nodes. These nodes are often involved when a pathological process, such as carcinoma, sarcoidosis, reticulosis or tuberculosis, affects the mediastinal nodes, and biopsy of an enlarged supraclavicular node may yield information of conclusive diagnostic value. The group of nodes most frequently implicated lies in a pad of fat on the surface of the scalenus anterior muscle, just above its insertion into the scalene tubercle of the first rib (Fig. 27). To reach this situation the palpating finger must dip behind the clavicle through the clavicular origin of sterno-mastoid and for the examination to be adequate all the anterior cervical muscles must be completely relaxed. This is best achieved by having the patient sitting in a chair with his elbows hanging loosely at his sides and his cervical spine partially flexed. The examination should be carried out from behind, one side at a time, and the whole of the supraclavicular and retroclavicular regions of the neck from the trachea to the anterior border of trapezius should be carefully palpated for enlarged nodes, special attention being devoted to the vicinity of the scalene tubercle (Fig. 28). When a node is found it should be described in the terms recommended on page 48. Nodes which are greater than 0.5 cm in diameter, firm in consistence and round in shape are usually of pathological significance, many of them containing metastatic deposits from a bronchial carcinoma. Large, fixed masses are present in some of these cases. Hard, craggy nodes may, however, signify healed and calcified tuberculosis, the calcification generally being demon-strable radiographically.

**Skin.** Examination of the skin may, on occasion, yield information of considerable value in the diagnosis of respiratory disease. Some of the cutaneous and subcutaneous lesions which may be relevant in this connection are:

1. Erythema nodosum (p. 99), which may be the initial clinical mani-festation of a primary tuberculous infection or of sarcoidosis.

2. Metastastic tumour nodules, which may be derived from a primary bronchial carcinoma.

3. Cutaneous sarcoids and lupus pernio, which may occur in association with sarcoidosis involving the intrathoracic lymph nodes or the lungs.

4. The rash of lupus erythematosus (p. 99), which may accompany systemic, including pulmonary or pleural, manifestations of this connective tissue disorder.

5. Lupus vulgaris and erythema induratum which, although manifesta-tions of tuberculosis, are seldom associated with pulmonary lesions.

### The Upper Respiratory Tract

The upper respiratory tract extends from external nares to the junction of the larynx with the trachea at the vocal cords. It includes the nasal cavity, the nasopharynx, the nasal sinuses, the oropharynx and the larynx. Infective and allergic disorders of the upper respiratory tract are amongst the most common afflictions of mankind and infection in any part of it may produce or aggravate disease of the bronchi and lungs. Clinical examination of the nose and throat is therefore an essential part of the investigation of all patients with respiratory disease. Since oral sepsis, particularly suppurative gingivitis, may also cause pulmonary disease, such as lung abscess, the buccal cavity, the teeth and the gums should also be included in the examination. The procedure recommended for examination of the nose, mouth and throat is described on pages 77 to 82.

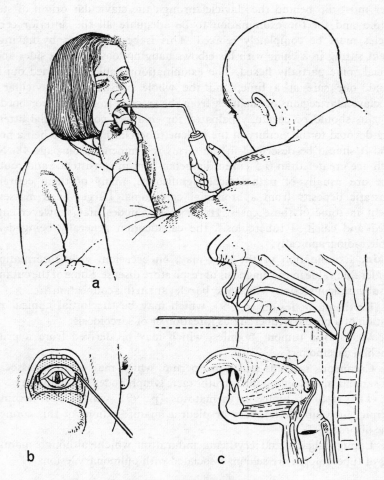

FIG. 29   INDIRECT LARYNGOSCOPY

(*a*) Positions of the patient and doctor.    (*b*) View of larynx in mirror.    (*c*) Position of mirror in relation to
soft palate and larynx.

## THE LARYNX

External examination of the larynx seldom yields any useful information, but swelling on the front of the neck caused, for example, by a hypersensitivity reaction (angio-oedema) should be noted, since the oedema may involve the glottis and give rise to dyspnoea and stridor, which may be followed by complete respiratory obstruction.

Examination of the interior of the larynx by indirect or direct laryngoscopy is an essential step in the investigation of hoarseness (p. 162). In indirect laryngoscopy, a small (warmed) mirror reflecting light from a head lamp, from a head mirror, or from the small electric bulb on the laryngoscopic attachment of a diagnostic set is placed just in front of the uvula and with a co-operative patient a clear view can be obtained of the epiglottis, the arytenoid region and the vocal cords (Fig. 29). The examination can often be facilitated by the use of an anaesthetic lozenge (benzocaine). Direct laryngo-scopy, using a laryngoscope, is necessary in some cases, particularly if a biopsy has to be taken, but is an uncomfortable procedure which requires more extensive local anaesthesia. Lesions which can be detected by laryngo-scopy include laryngeal tuberculosis, laryngeal tumours and vocal cord paralysis (p. 274).

A paralysed vocal cord adopts a position midway between abduction and adduction and fails to adduct on phonation. Paralysis of abduction may precede complete paralysis of the cord.

## THE TRACHEA

In normal subjects the upper 4 to 5 cm of the trachea can be felt in the neck between the cricoid cartilage and the suprasternal notch, but in thick-set or obese subjects it may be so deeply placed that it is difficult or impossible to reach with the palpating finger.

The trachea should be examined with the thumb and index finger, and identified by the presence of cartilaginous rings. The position of the trachea is determined by gently thrusting the tip of the index finger into the sup-rasternal notch, exactly in the midline (Fig. 30). By this manœuvre any deviation of the trachea to either side can readily be detected. Thyroid enlargement may displace the trachea, and the thyroid gland should always be examined before tracheal deviation is attributed to intrathoracic disease. In patients with chronic airways obstruction there is a downward movement of the trachea during inspiration. This can be detected by placing a finger on the thyroid cartilage.

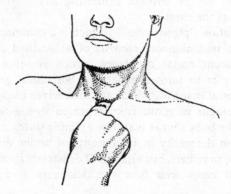

FIG. 30   Determining the Position of the Trachea.

## THE CHEST

Physical examination of the chest comprises three procedures:

1. Examination of the chest wall.
2. Observation of respiratory movements.
3. The elicitation of specific 'physical signs' by means of which abnormalities in the structure and function of the bronchi, lungs and pleura can be recognised.

### 1. Examination of the Chest Wall

With the patient sitting erect in a good light and preferably stripped to the waist, the chest is inspected from the front, from the back and from each side. Abnormalities in the shape of the chest are observed, and by means of combined inspection and palpation a careful search is made for lesions of the chest wall.

**Abnormalities in the Shape of the Chest.** Those of clinical importance are as follows:

1. *The anteroposterior diameter may be increased* relative to the lateral diameter. In normal subjects the ratio is usually about 5 : 7, and in 'flat-chested' patients without respiratory disease, it may be as low as 1 : 2. In some patients with emphysema, however, the two measurements may approximate ('barrel-chest'). It is important to note whether the increase in the antero-posterior diameter is due chiefly to thoracic kyphosis (which may be unrelated to respiratory disease), to displacement forwards of the anterior chest wall or to a combination of both factors. Chest deformity in emphysema is not a reliable guide to the severity of the functional defect. It is seen most frequently in patients who have developed chronic respiratory disease (bronchitis or asthma) relatively early in life, i.e. before the age of 30 years. Those in whom the onset is delayed until after the age of 40 years may progress even to the stage of respiratory failure without exhibiting any increase in the antero-posterior diameter of the chest.

2. *Pectus carinatum* ('pigeon chest'), which is a common sequel to chronic respiratory disease in childhood, consists of a localised prominence of the sternum and adjacent costal cartilages, which is often accompanied by indrawing of the ribs to form symmetrical horizontal grooves (Harrison's sulci) above the costal margins, which are themselves usually everted. These deformities are thought to result from repeated strong contractions of the diaphragm while the bony thorax is still in a pliable state.

Pectus carinatum deformity in inhabitants of under developed countries may be entirely due to rickets, but vitamin D deficiency is now rare in Britain, and in almost all cases seen here the deformity is a manifestation of respiratory disease.

3. *Pectus excavatum* ('funnel-chest') is a developmental defect in which there is either a localised depression of the lower end of the sternum, or, less commonly, depression of the whole length of the sternum and of the costal

cartilages attached to it. Pectus excavatum is usually asymptomatic, but when there is a very marked degree of depression of the sternum the heart may be compressed between it and the vertebral bodies. This may produce displacement of the apex beat to the left, murmurs and disturbances in cardiac function, e.g. paroxysmal tachycardia and, rarely, a clinical picture akin to constrictive pericarditis. The ventilatory capacity of the lungs may also be restricted in severe cases.

4. *Thoracic kyphoscoliosis* (p. 344) ranges in degree from the minor variations in spinal curvature seen in many otherwise healthy subjects to grossly disfiguring and disabling deformities. Thoracic scoliosis may alter the position of the mediastinum in relation to the anterior chest wall, with the result that abnormalities in the position of the trachea and the cardiac apex beat may be mistakenly attributed to cardiac or pulmonary disease. Severe kyphoscoliosis may have profound effects on pulmonary function, as the chest deformity reduces the ventilatory capacity of the lungs and increases the work of breathing. Many such patients eventually develop hypoxia, hypercapnia and pulmonary heart failure.

5. *Thoracic operations*, particularly thoracoplasty, may result in a considerable degree of chest deformity, of which scoliosis may be an important secondary feature.

**Lesions of the Chest Wall.** Combined inspection and palpation of the whole chest wall is essential for the detection of these lesions. The abnormalities which may be found include:

1. *Cutaneous lesions*, e.g. skin eruptions, sarcoid or other nodules, purpuric spots, bruises, scars (accidental or surgical), sinuses.

2. *Subcutaneous lesions*, e.g. inflammatory swellings, metastatic tumour nodules, neurofibromas, lipomas. (The nature of certain cutaneous and subcutaneous lesions, e.g. sarcoid nodules and tumours, may require to be determined by biopsy.)

3. *Subcutaneous emphysema* (air in the subcutaneous tissues) may cause diffuse swelling of the chest wall, the neck and, in some cases, the face. The condition is recognised by the characteristic 'crackling' sensation elicited by palpation of the air-containing tissues. When subcutaneous emphysema is localised to the chest wall, it is usually derived from a tension pneumothorax from which it has escaped along the track of a needle or intercostal catheter used to decompress the pleural space. In most other cases air extruded from the lungs as a result of interstitial rupture of the alveoli tracks into the mediastinum (*mediastinal emphysema*). Rarely a large collection of air under pressure in this situation may interfere with the venous return to the heart and cause cardiac arrest, but the air usually escapes innocuously into the neck and produces subcutaneous emphysema of the neck, face and chest wall which in severe cases may be very gross but is not in itself dangerous. When air is present in the mediastinum the heart sounds may be replaced by a 'churning' noise, accentuated during systole.

4. *Vascular anomalies*, e.g. spider naevi (p. 96), enlarged vascular channels (arterial in coarctation of aorta; venous in superior vena caval obstruction).

5. *Localised prominences and deformities of the bony thorax*, involving clavicles, scapulae, sternum, ribs, costochondral junctions and spinous processes.

6. *Localised tenderness on palpation of chest wall*, e.g. from a fractured rib, from tumour invading chest wall, from spinal injury or disease, or in association with pleural or nerve root pain.

7. At the same stage in the examination the *breasts* (p. 87) and the *axillary lymph nodes* (p. 86) should be palpated, and the presence of *lumbar or sacral oedema* should be noted.

## 2. Observation of Respiratory Movements

(a) **Respiratory Frequency.** The number of breaths in a full minute is countered by surreptitiously observing the movements of the chest wall, with the fingers held on the pulse to avoid drawing the patient's attention to his breathing. The normal frequency at rest in a healthy adult is about 14 respirations per minute. The rate is increased in a variety of pathological states, including pyrexia from any cause, acute pulmonary infections, particularly those accompanied by pleural pain, and conditions in which there is a sudden increase in the work of breathing, e.g. bronchial asthma and acute pulmonary oedema.

(b) **Respiratory Depth.** This is difficult to estimate clinically as the movements of the chest and diaphragm, on which it is dependent, cannot be accurately measured. Furthermore, it is only too easy to confuse a dyspnoeic patient's strenuous but unavailing efforts to achieve an adequate tidal volume with a genuine increase in the depth of breathing. It is usually possible with practice, however, to recognise marked degrees of overventilation and underventilation. The latter may be of considerable clinical importance in the diagnosis of respiratory failure, while hyperventilation may give rise to tetany or epilepsy.

In states of metabolic acidosis, such as those produced by diabetic ketosis and uraemia, pulmonary ventilation at rest may be considerably raised. This can be recognised clinically by a marked increase in the depth of respiration ('*air hunger*') which may on occasion give rise to the subjective sensation of dyspnoea. In *periodic* or *Cheyne-Stokes breathing* there is a cyclical variation in the depth of respiration believed to be caused by a decrease in the sensitivity of the respiratory centre to carbon dioxide. This occurs in left ventricular failure and in certain neurological conditions, particularly those associated with increased intracranial pressure. The cycle usually takes two to three minutes to complete and during the phase of hyperventilation the patient may experience respiratory distress.

Hyperventilation may also occur in patients who are unconscious as a result of severe brain damage caused by trauma, haemorrhage or infarction.

In such patients laxity of the soft palate may give rise to the phenomenon of 'stertorous breathing'.

(c) **Maximum Chest Expansion.** This is estimated by placing a tape measure round the chest at nipple level and recording the maximum inspiratory/expiratory difference in the chest circumference. There is a considerable degree of observer variation with this measurement and it does not correlate well with vital capacity, probably because in some subjects breathing is predominantly diaphragmatic. A figure of above 5 cm can, however, be regarded as normal and one of 2 cm or less as definitely abnormal. Chest expansion is diminished in all conditions which reduce or restrict the movement of ribs and in almost every type of diffuse bronchopulmonary disease, e.g. bronchial asthma, emphysema and pulmonary fibrosis.

(d) **Mode of Breathing.** In normal subjects inspiration is effected by contraction of the intercostal muscles and the diaphragm while expiration is a passive process dependent upon the elastic recoil of the lungs towards the hila. Women make more use of the intercostal muscles than of the diaphragm and their respiratory movements are predominantly thoracic. Men, on the other hand rely more on the diaphragm and their respiratory movements at rest are mainly abdominal. Babies of both sexes are also diaphragmatic breathers. Any departure from the normal mode of breathing should receive close attention. If respiratory movements are exclusively thoracic this may indicate that diaphragmatic movement is inhibited by pain caused, for example, by peritoneal irritation, or prevented by severe abdominal distension resulting from conditions such as ascites, gaseous distension of the bowel, a large ovarian cyst or pregnancy. If respiratory movements are exclusively abdominal, ankylosing spondylitis, intercostal paralysis or pleural pain may be responsible for the lack of chest expansion.

Although dyspnoea (p. 41) is a subjective phenomenon it is often accompanied by objective evidence of respiratory difficulty or distress. There is often an increase in respiratory frequency, which may be accompanied by dilatation of the alae nasi during inspiration, but as these features may be observed in the absence of dyspnoea they are not reliable indices of respiratory distress. A much more useful criterion is the presence of abnormal respiratory movements of the following types:

(i) *Abnormal inspiratory movements* produced by contraction of the cervical muscles (principally the sternomastoids, scaleni and trapezii), by which the whole thoracic cage is, in effect, lifted off the diaphragm with every inspiration. Patients breathe in this way if adequate pulmonary ventilation cannot be achieved by normal inspiratory efforts, as, for example, when there is gross overdistension of the lungs in conditions such as advanced emphysema and severe bronchial asthma. More violent inspiratory movements of a similar character are observed in patients with obstruction of the larynx or trachea. Indrawing of the suprasternal and supraclavicular fossae, the intercostal spaces and the epigastrium with each inspiration invariably accompanies airways obstruction of this type and may also be seen, although it is usually less conspicuous, in emphysema and asthma.

A much more striking degree of indrawing of the chest wall is seen in patients who have sustained double fractures of a series of ribs or of the sternum. The portion of the thoracic cage between the fractures becomes mobile and, with the overlying soft tissues, is sucked in with every inspiration. 'Paradoxical movement' of this type interferes seriously with pulmonary ventilation and may cause grave respiratory distress.

(ii) *Abnormal expiratory movements* produced by powerful contractions of the abdominal muscles and latissimus dorsi. These are observed when the elastic recoil of the lungs is insufficient to complete the expulsion of air from the alveoli, as in some types of emphysema, or when expiratory airway obstruction is present, as in bronchial asthma and some cases of chronic bronchitis. Patients with a severe degree of expiratory obstruction prefer to sit upright, grasping a bed table or the back of a chair. This enables them to fix the shoulder girdle so that the latissimus dorsi can be used exclusively for approximating the ribs and augmenting the expiratory efforts. Many patients who breathe in this way can be seen to purse their lips with every expiration. This manoeuvre keeps the intrabronchial pressure above that of the surrounding alveoli and prevents the collapse of the bronchial walls which would otherwise result from the unopposed effect of air trapped in the alveoli.

(iii) *Localised impairment of respiratory movement* is usually caused by disease in the underlying lung or pleura, and is almost invariably associated with abnormal findings on percussion and auscultation. The methods used for detecting differences in the range of respiratory movement on the two sides of the chest are described in the section on physical signs (p. 77). Testing the strength of the respiratory muscles is discussed on page 283.

### 3. The Elicitation of Physical Signs

In health the two sides of the chest are seen to move to an equal extent with respiration. The trachea is central and the apex beat is in the normal position (p. 125). Percussion of the chest wall produces a resonant note over both lungs. The breath sounds heard on auscultation are 'vesicular' in type (p. 185). In diseases of the bronchi, lungs and pleura, various changes in these physical signs may be observed. For example, movement of one side of the chest may be reduced, the percussion note may lose its normal resonance, the breath sounds may alter in type and may be accompanied by 'added sounds', and there may be displacement of the trachea and apex beat to one or other side.

Certain groups of physical signs are typically associated with certain pathological changes in the lungs and pleura. Such changes are not necessarily specific for one particular disease. For example, the physical signs of consolidation may occur in pneumonia or tuberculosis and those of pleural effusion may be present in tuberculous pleurisy, empyema or congestive cardiac failure. Each group of physical signs therefore gives an indication only of the gross pathology of the lesion, and not of its precise nature, the diagnosis of which depends on an analysis of all the clinical and other evidence. The characteristic physical signs of the more common lesions are summarised in Table 3 (p. 192).

The most convenient method of eliciting physical signs is to examine the front and sides of the chest and then the back. When the anterior and lateral aspects are being examined the patient should lie in a supine or semi-recumbent position on a bed or couch, with the chest and upper abdomen fully exposed and evenly illuminated down to the level of the umbilicus, and with the arms sufficiently abducted to allow access to the axillary regions. When the posterior aspect of the chest is being examined the patient should sit upright with arms folded across the chest. Some patients are unable to maintain this position and have to be held forward by a third person standing at the foot of the bed and grasping the patient's outstretched hands. At this stage all pillows should be removed to allow unimpeded access to the whole length of the back.

Examination of the anterior and lateral aspects of the chest should begin with a comparison of the range of respiratory movement on the two sides during both normal and deep breathing. The position of the trachea (p. 171) and the cardiac apex beat (p. 125) should then be determined and vocal fremitus (p. 179) tested over equivalent areas of the right and left lung. Next, the percussion note on the two sides should be compared and any areas of dullness carefully delineated, including cardiac and hepatic dullness (pp. 126, 219). Finally, by means of auscultation, the quality and intensity of the breath sounds and voice sounds should be assessed and the nature of any added sounds identified.

A similar procedure is adopted for examination of the back of the chest, omitting those items concerned with anteriorly situated structures. A crude estimate of diaphragmatic movement may be obtained by the technique of tidal percussion (p. 185).

### Inspection and Palpation

The object of these procedures is to detect differences in the range of movement on the two sides of the chest. Palpation is also used to elicit vocal fremitus and palpable accompaniments.

METHODS OF COMPARING RANGE OF MOVEMENT OF THE
CHEST WALL

(a) Respiratory movement in the *infraclavicular* regions is best gauged by inspection, palpation being almost valueless in this situation. The patient lies supine with his head on a single low pillow. Care must be taken to ensure that the head and trunk are in a straight line and that the shoulders are relaxed and in a symmetrical position. The doctor crouches at the foot of the bed, views the infraclavicular regions tangentially (Fig. 31) and asks the patient to take steady deep breaths. By this technique very slight unilateral impairment of chest wall movements can be readily and reliably detected.

(*b*) *Respiratory movement at the costal margins* can also be accurately gauged by inspection if the patient is thin. In most cases, however, this cannot be done and reliance has to be placed on palpation. The sides of the chest are grasped firmly with the fingers in such a way as to approximate the tips of the outstretched thumbs in the region of the xiphoid process. The grip should be adjusted to ensure that there is a loose fold of skin between the two thumbs so that they can move apart as the chest expands. The movement of the two thumbs with deep breathing can then be used to estimate the relative degree of movement on the two sides.

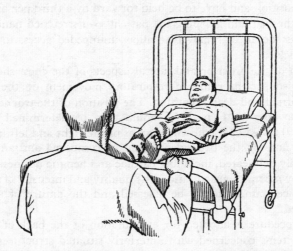

FIG. 31   Inspection of Respiratory Movement in the Infraclavicular Regions.

(*c*) *Respiratory movements of the lower ribs posteriorly* is estimated by a similar technique (Fig. 32). With the patient sitting erect, the chest is grasped from behind with the two hands and the tips of the outstretched thumbs are brought together in the region of the tenth thoracic spine. It is again important to ensure that there is a loose fold of skin between the thumbs, the movement of which can then be used to estimate the relative degree of chest expansion on the two sides.

THE SIGNIFICANCE OF RESTRICTED MOVEMENT. Unilateral restriction of chest wall movement occurs in many types of respiratory disease. In pleural effusion and empyema, movement may be absent, and if the lesion has persisted for some weeks retraction of the ribs and intercostal spaces may produce flattening of the affected side of the chest, which is most marked in the pectoral region. The term 'frozen chest' is sometimes applied to this condition. Restriction of movement of a less severe but easily discernible degree occurs in pneumonia and atelectasis, particularly if these conditions are accompanied by pleurisy. In pneumothorax the limitation of movement is related to the amount of air in the pleural space and thus to the degree of pulmonary collapse; in tension pneumothorax the affected side of the chest may be immobilised in a position of almost full inspiration. In pulmonary tuberculosis even extensive lesions may have little effect on chest wall movement during the early stages of the disease, but later, when fibrosis becomes a predominant feature of the pathology, there may be severe restriction of movement with flattening of the affected side of the chest.

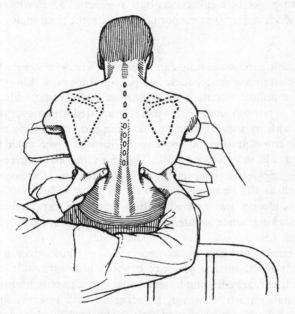

FIG. 32    Estimation of Respiratory Movements of the Lower Ribs Posteriorly.

In bronchial asthma, emphysema and diffuse pulmonary fibrosis movements of the chest wall are symmetrically reduced. In the first two conditions the restriction is chiefly of expiratory movement, which is hindered by airways obstruction. In diffuse pulmonary fibrosis, on the other hand, inspiratory movement is restricted by the reduced distensibility of the lungs. In severe cases this may bring each inspiration to an abrupt halt and produce the phenomenon of 'door stop' breathing.

**Vocal Fremitus.** This is tested by placing the palm of the hand on equivalent areas of the chest wall on each side in turn and asking the patient to say 'one, one, one'. This should be done at three levels anteriorly, at three levels posteriorly and at one level laterally. Vocal fremitus is a crude test and only when it is absent, e.g. over a large pleural effusion, is the test likely to provide useful informatior

**Palpable Accompaniments.** The low-frequency vibrations from a low-pitched rhonchus or a coarse pleural rub can occasionally be detected by a hand placed on the chest wall. In such cases an unusually loud rhonchus or rub is invariably present on auscultation and there is seldom any difficulty in distinguishing between the two (p. 190). A palpable rhonchus generally has its origin in a large bronchus and, if persistent and unilateral, may be due to partial bronchial obstruction by a tumour or foreign body. A palpable pleural rub, which may be recognised by the patient as a grating sensation within the chest, has no specific significance, but, in general, a rub which can be detected by palpation is more often encountered in chronic than in acute pleurisy.

## Percussion

A resonant percussion note can be elicited wherever aerated lung tissue or a large air-containing space, such as a pneumothorax, a thin-walled pulmonary cavity or a hollow viscus, is in apposition to the chest wall. The percussion note loses its normal resonance whenever aerated lung tissue is separated from the chest wall by pleural fluid or thickening, or when lung tissue is rendered airless by consolidation, atelectasis or fibrosis. Over such lesions the percussion note is impaired or dull. The most marked degrees of dullness on percussion are found over large pleural effusions. Percussion over a solid viscus such as the heart or the liver may elicit a dull note, but the area of dullness is always less extensive than would be expected from anatomical surface marking, since aerated lung is interposed between part of the viscus and the chest wall.

A hyperresonant percussion note may be found over a pneumothorax, particularly if the pleural pressure is above atmospheric level, and also over lung which is markedly emphysematous. An apparent finding of generalised hyperresonance must, however, be accepted with reserve, since a change in the absolute pitch of a percussion note is always difficult to recognise and may depend merely upon the thickness of the chest wall. For that reason it is not usually advisable to attempt to distinguish between normal resonance and hyperresonance when the percussion note is resonant on both sides.

**Anatomical Considerations.** The regions of the thorax over which a resonant percussion note is normally found correspond approximately with the surface marking of the lungs (Fig. 33).

When an abnormality of the percussion note is due to pulmonary consolidation or atelectasis it is usually possible to identify the lobe or lobes involved by reference to the surface marking of the fissures but it must be emphasised that, unless a lobe is totally consolidated, the area over which the percussion note is impaired is often much smaller than would be expected from its surface marking. This is also the case when a lobe is collapsed. With a pleural

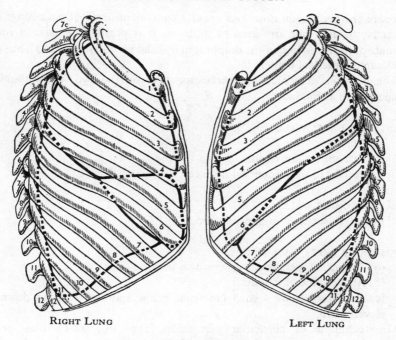

RIGHT LUNG    LEFT LUNG

FIG. 33    Surface Markings of the Lungs.

effusion the area of dullness on percussion is, of course, unrelated to the surface anatomy of the lobes. Except with localised effusions, it is situated over the lower part of the hemithorax and usually extends to a higher level posteriorly and laterally than at the front of the chest.

In localising the position of a pulmonary or pleural lesion the observer should make use of the breath sounds and voice sounds in addition to the percussion note. It should, however, always be borne in mind that small lesions, such as areas of segmental consolidation or collapse, may not produce any abnormal physical signs. Even with larger lesions the signs may be partly or completely obscured if the lungs are emphysematous.

**Technique of Percussion.** The basic technique of percussion is as follows:

1. The left hand is placed on the chest wall, palm downwards and with the fingers slightly separated, so that the second phalanx of the middle finger is precisely over the area to be percussed.

2. The middle finger of the left hand is then pressed firmly against the chest wall and the centre of its second phalanx is struck sharply with the pad of the right middle finger. In order to produce a satisfactory percussion note the right middle finger must be held in a position of partial flexion (to produce a 'hammer' effect) and the entire movement must come from the wrist joint.

The terms used to describe different types of percussion note are shown on page 184. The procedure recommended for percussion of the chest is, firstly, to

G

compare the percussion note over exactly equivalent areas of both lungs and secondly, to map out any area of dullness. It is possible to make a rough estimate of the excursion of the diaphragm by tidal percussion (p. 185), but this is seldom of practical value.

The positions in which the percussion note on the two sides should be compared are as follows:

ANTERIOR CHEST WALL (Fig. 34)
    (*a*) Clavicle.
    (*b*) Infraclavicular region.
    (*c*) Second to sixth intercostal spaces.

LATERAL CHEST WALL
    Fourth to seventh intercostal spaces.

POSTERIOR CHEST WALL (Fig. 35).
    (*a*) Trapezius (percussing downwards on lung apex).
    (*b*) Above spine of scapula.
    (*c*) At intervals of 4 to 5 cm from below spine of scapula down to eleventh rib.

The technique of clavicular percussion (Fig. 36), which may be of considerable value in detecting lesions of the upper lobes, particularly when they are contracted by collapse or fibrosis, differs from that used elsewhere in that the clavicles can be percussed directly with the right middle finger or, if preferred, with the right index, middle and ring fingers held closely together. The correct situation for percussion is within the medial third of the clavicle,

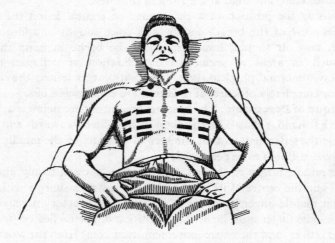

FIG. 34 ·Sites for Percussion of Anterior and Lateral Chest Wall.

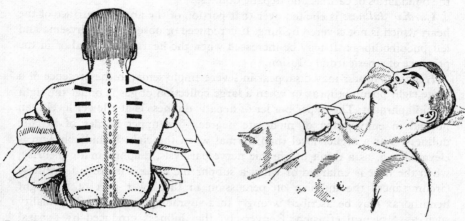

FIG. 35  Sites for Percussion of Posterior Chest Wall.

FIG. 36  Clavicular Percussion.

just lateral to its expanded medial end. Percussion more laterally will merely elicit the dullness produced by the muscle masses of the shoulder. Clavicular percussion should be directed backwards and downwards. The lung apices are percussed by placing the left middle finger across the anterior border of each trapezius muscle, 5 cm from the midline, and directing the percussion downwards (Fig. 37).

When an area of impaired resonance is discovered, its boundaries should be carefully mapped out by percussing from a zone of normal resonance towards

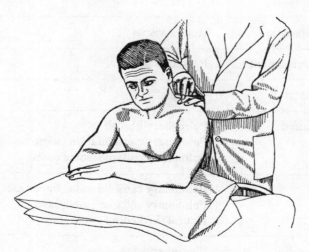

FIG. 37  Percussion of Apex of Lung.

the suspected abnormality. The same technique should be used to determine the boundaries of cardiac and hepatic dullness.

*Cardiac dullness* is elicited over that portion of the anterior surface of the heart which is not covered by lung. It is reduced or absent in emphysema and left pneumothorax. It may be increased when the heart is enlarged or in the presence of a pericardial effusion.

*Hepatic dullness* may disappear in severe emphysema, in the presence of a large right pneumothorax or when a large collection of gas is under the right hemidiaphragm. The upper border of hepatic dullness is at a lower level than normal in emphysema of moderate degree. The upper border of hepatic dullness is at a higher level than normal when the right hemidiaphragm is elevated, e.g. as a result of phrenic nerve paralysis, diaphragmatic pleurisy, when the liver is enlarged or when a subphrenic abscess is present. In these circumstances the dullness on percussion in the lower part of the right hemithorax may be ascribed wrongly to a supradiaphragmatic abnormality such as a pleural effusion. Conversely, the dullness produced by a basal pulmonary or pleural lesion may be mistaken for that caused by a high diaphragm. Obesity, pregnancy and ascites, which frequently cause elevation

TABLE 2

*Percussion Note*

| Type | Lesions by which produced |
| --- | --- |
| Tympanitic | Hollow viscus |
| Hyperresonant | Pneumothorax |
| Resonant | Normal |
| Impaired | Pulmonary fibrosis<br>Pulmonary consolidation (some cases)<br>Pulmonary collapse (some cases) |
| Dull | Pulmonary consolidation (some cases)<br>Pulmonary collapse (some cases)<br>Pleural thickening |
| Stony dull | Pleural effusion |

of both hemidiaphragms, may be responsible for raising the upper border of hepatic dullness.

Few clinicians nowadays make a routine practice of determining precisely the areas of cardiac and hepatic dullness. The extent and degree of cardiac dullness may, however, provide information of diagnostic value when a pericardial effusion is suspected, and the level of the upper border of hepatic dullness may be a useful guide to the position of the right hemidiaphragm or, in certain cases, to the size of the liver.

**Tidal Percussion.** This technique, which is of limited practical value, gives a rough indication of the range of diaphragmatic movement. The lower border of pulmonary resonance at the back of the chest on each side is carefully marked by a skin pencil (*a*) in full expiration and (*b*) in full inspiration. The distance between the two marks represents approximately the range of diaphragmatic movement and this is impaired on one side when an inflammatory lesion is present immediately above or below the diaphragm.

### Auscultation

Auscultation of the lungs has an important place in the diagnosis of certain respiratory diseases, but is of little or no value in others. In bronchial asthma and 'dry' pleurisy, for example, the stethoscope provides information of diagnostic value which cannot be obtained in any other way. In contrast, auscultation is unhelpful in the early diagnosis of pulmonary tuberculosis, which may reach an advanced stage before any abnormality can be detected with the stethoscope.

**Breath Sounds and Voice Sounds.** Breath sounds are produced by vibrations of the vocal cords caused by the rapid flow of air through the larynx during inspiration and expiration. The sounds so produced are transmitted along the trachea and bronchi and through the lungs to the chest wall. In their passage through normal lungs the intensity and frequency-pattern of the sounds are altered. When they are heard through a stethoscope on the chest wall they have a characteristic 'rustling' quality to which the name *'vesicular'* is given. The intensity of the sounds increases steadily during inspiration and then quickly fades away during the first one-third of expiration. Diseases of the bronchi, lungs and pleura may alter the breath sounds in several ways:

1. If the conduction of the breath sounds to the chest wall is attenuated by airway obstruction (either general, as in bronchial asthma, or local, as when a large bronchus is obstructed by a tumour) or by pneumothorax, pleural effusion or pleural thickening, they remain vesicular but are diminished in intensity. This change in the breath sounds is invariably accompanied by a reduction in the intensity of the conducted voice sounds.

2. If the lung tissue through which the breath sounds are transmitted from

the air passages to the chest wall has lost its normal spongy consistence and has become firm or solid, e.g. in consolidation or fibrosis, the sounds picked up by the stethoscope resemble more closely those produced at the larynx than those heard over a normal lung. They are usually louder during both inspiration and expiration, and the expiratory murmur is audible through the whole of expiration instead of only during the first one-third. The sounds also retain the 'blowing' quality derived from their origin in the larynx. The term *'bronchial'* is given to breath sounds of this type. Bronchial breath sounds, as would be expected, are similar in quality to those heard when the chest piece of a stethoscope is placed on the larynx or trachea, but they are, of course, less loud.

Voice sounds conducted through consolidated lung tissue also resemble more closely those produced at the larynx than those heard over normal lungs, in that they are louder and more distinct. In some cases the whispered voice may be transmitted almost without distortion, so that individual syllables can be clearly recognised (*'whispering pectoriloquy'*).

The pitch of bronchial breath sounds varies according to the nature of the pulmonary changes. As high-frequency sounds are selectively conducted through consolidated lung tissue, high-pitched bronchial breath sounds are heard in lobar or segmental pneumonia. Fibrotic lung tissue, on the other hand, transmits sounds of lower frequency and thus produces low-pitched bronchial breath sounds. With voice sounds, there is a similar selective conduction of certain frequencies. High-pitched bronchial breath sounds are associated with voice sounds of a 'bleating' high-pitched quality, often described as *'aegophony'*, a phenomenon which is not observed in the presence of low-pitched bronchial breath sounds.

3. When bronchial breath sounds traverse air-containing cavities in their passage to the chest wall, they may acquire a resonating *'amphoric'* quality, resembling the sound produced by blowing across the top of a bottle. Amphoric breath sounds are, however, present in only a small proportion of those cases in which an abnormality of this type is present. In lung abscess and tuberculous cavitation, for example, they are heard only when the cavity is very large and superficial, and the draining bronchus or bronchi are patent, while in spontaneous pneumothorax the production of amphoric breath sounds is confined to those cases in which the intrapleural pressure is above atmospheric level (tension pneumothorax). When amphoric breath sounds are present the voice sounds are conducted more clearly and usually more loudly than normal, and whispering pectoriloquy can always be elicited.

The main importance of identifying breath sounds as bronchial in type lies in the fact that this indicates the presence of a pulmonary lesion. The criteria for their recognition must therefore be strict and unambiguous. Three conditions must be satisfied before breath sounds can be described as bronchial.

1. Both the inspiratory and expiratory sound must be blowing in character.

2. The expiratory sound must be as long and as loud as the inspiratory sound.

3. There must be a pause between the end of the inspiratory sound and the beginning of the expiratory sound.

Breath sounds may be intermediate in type between vesicular and bronchial, for example, vesicular with prolonged expiration. This type is heard commonly in the presence of diffuse airways obstruction in conditions such as chronic bronchitis and emphysema. Other variants, such as bronchovesicular breath sounds, in which the inspiratory component is bronchial in type and the expiratory sound is vesicular, have no specific significance.

**Added Sounds.** For many years the terminology of added sounds has been confused by the ambiguity which has surrounded the use of the French word 'râle'. Translated literally from the French it means 'rattle', but Laënnec wrongly regarded it as equivalent to the Latin term 'rhonchus'. In fact, 'rhonchus' is a latinised version of the Greek 'rhonchos', meaning 'wheezing', and its use should logically be restricted to the musical sounds produced in narrowed bronchi. The word 'crepitation', derived from the latin *'crepitare'*, to crack or rattle, is an unambiguous term which can be appropriately used to describe all non-musical crackling sounds. The adoption of the terms 'rhonchus' and 'crepitation', as defined below, allows the term 'râle' to be discarded and for the sake of clarity this policy has been followed in the description of added sounds originating in the bronchi and lungs.

Added sounds heard on auscultation of the chest are therefore of three types: (1) rhonchi, (2) crepitations and (3) pleural sounds.

1. RHONCHI. These are musical sounds of high, medium or low pitch produced by the passage of air through narrowed bronchi, particularly where the degree of narrowing is not uniform throughout the bronchial tree. Rhonchi caused by mucosal oedema or spasm of the bronchial musculature are usually superimposed upon the expiratory phase of the respiratory murmur, which is always prolonged when rhonchi are present. Rhonchi heard during inspiration are more often due to secretion in the bronchi and may disappear, or at least become less numerous, after coughing. In many patients with bronchitis and asthma rhonchi may be present during both inspiration and expiration. The pitch of a rhonchus is related to the size of the bronchus in which the sound is produced, low-pitched rhonchi originating in larger bronchi and high-pitched rhonchi in smaller bronchi.

2. CREPITATIONS. These are non-musical sounds with a 'crackling' quality. In most cases crepitations are produced by secretions dislodged by the flow of air into or out of bronchi, alveoli or pulmonary cavities. Sounds of this type often increase in number temporarily after a short cough, but may become less numerous or even disappear completely for a time, after a prolonged bout of coughing. They are usually superimposed on the inspiratory phase, particularly its second half, and are seldom heard during expiration.

Occasionally, crepitations seem to be unrelated to the presence of secretions, as, for example, when they occur in diseases which cause thickening of the alveolar walls such as allergic and fibrosing alveolitis. In these conditions numerous crepitations may be heard throughout inspiration, which persist unchanged after coughing and are often accompanied by high-pitched rhonchi at the end of inspiration.

Three descriptive terms are applied to crepitations, namely fine, medium and coarse. *Fine crepitations* may be audible in the early stages of pneumonic consolidation and in acute miliary tuberculosis. *Medium crepitations* are typically present in pulmonary oedema, and appear to be produced by transudate in the alveoli and smaller air passages. *Coarse crepitations* are heard in conditions such as resolving pneumonia (in which a resolving exudate is being discharged into the bronchi), bronchiectasis, lung abscess, advanced pulmonary tuberculosis and allergic or fibrosing alveolitis. When arising in large cavities, crepitations often have a very coarse, 'metallic' quality.

Another distinct type of crepitation may be heard over a pneumothorax when fluid is present in the pleural space. These sounds, which have a 'tinkling' quality, seem to be related to the level of intrapleural pressure and their presence usually indicates that the air in the pneumothorax is under tension. Tinkling crepitations are often audible only during coughing, which creates the sounds by agitating the fluid in the pleural space.

3. PLEURAL SOUNDS. A *pleural rub* is a 'leathery' or 'creaking' sound produced by movement of the visceral pleura over the parietal pleura, when both surfaces are roughened by fibrinous exudate. It is usually heard at two separate stages in the respiratory cycle, towards the end of inspiration and just after the beginning of expiration. A pleural rub may be inaudible during normal breathing but can be easily heard when the patient is asked to breathe deeply. A rub may also become more distinct when a 'bell' type of chest piece is applied with firm pressure to the chest wall.

It is sometimes difficult to distinguish between a low-pitched rhonchus, coarse crepitations and a pleural rub. If there is any doubt as to the nature of the sound, auscultation should be repeated after a forceful cough, when rhonchi or crepitations will usually alter in character or disappear, while a pleural rub will remain unchanged.

A *'pneumothorax click'* is a rhythmical sound, synchronous with cardiac systole, which may be heard with or without the aid of a stethoscope when a shallow left pneumothorax is present between the layers of the mediastinal pleura below the pulmonary hilum. The mechanism by which the click is produced is not fully understood and may not be the same in every case. The most likely explanation is that with each cardiac systole there is a momentary, sharp impact between the two layers of the pleura, which produces a sound similar to that heard when fingers are snapped. The pneumothorax space may then amplify the click by acting as a sounding box.

**Technique of auscultation.** A stethoscope must have a satisfactory acoustic performance and the examination must be carried out carefully and systematically. The design of stethoscope recommended for routine clinical use is described on p. 127. With this instrument the examiner has the choice of a bell or diaphragm. As most of the sounds reaching the chest wall from the bronchi and lungs are in the low-frequency range, the bell should normally be used in preference to the diaphragm. Another reason for selecting the bell for respiratory auscultation is that stretching of the skin under the diaphragm during deep breathing is apt to produce a scraping sound which may be difficult to distinguish from that of a pleural rub.

Auscultation should be carried out with the patient relaxed, breathing deeply and fairly rapidly, but maintaining as far as possible the normal time relationship between inspiration and expiration. He should be asked to keep his mouth open, and, in particular, to avoid pursing his lips during expiration.

The following information can be obtained from auscultation:

(a) The type and intensity of the breath sounds.
(b) The type and number of any added sounds and their position in the respiratory cycle.
(c) The quality and intensity of the conducted voice sounds.

To ensure that small localised lesions are not overlooked, auscultation must be performed with the chest piece of the stethoscope placed in a large number of positions on the chest wall. It is important to compare the findings in equivalent positions on the two sides, anteriorly from just below the clavicle down to the sixth rib, laterally from the axilla down to the eighth rib, and posteriorly from above the level of the spine of the scapula down to the eleventh rib. Alternate auscultation on the two sides is particularly essential for gauging the intensity of breath sounds and voice sounds. Auscultation within 2·5 cm of the midline, either anteriorly or posteriorly, may give misleading information in regard to the type of breath sounds and voice sounds, particularly in the upper half of the chest, where the stethoscope may pick up sounds transmitted directly from the trachea and main bronchi to the chest wall. Bronchial breath sounds heard in these situations should therefore be disregarded.

Auscultation should be carried out in two stages. In the first stage, attention should be directed to breath sounds and added sounds, and in the second stage to the voice sounds. A systematic method of listening to the *breath sounds* and *added sounds* is essential. With the patient breathing regularly and fairly deeply, the observer should concentrate separately on the inspiratory and expiratory phases, noting their quality and intensity, and also on the type, number and position of any added sounds. He should also note if there is any gap between the end of the inspiratory murmur and the beginning of the expiratory phase. Finally, it may be necessary to repeat auscultation in certain situations during and after coughing.

The quality and intensity of the *voice sounds* should be noted and compared in the same positions as the breath sounds. 'One, one, one' is preferable to 'ninety-nine' as it produces a more continuous sound of slightly longer duration and of lower and more uniform pitch; these qualities facilitate the recognition of changes in the character of sounds transmitted to the chest wall. Where there is an increase in the intensity of the voice sounds or an alteration in their quality (e.g. aegophony) it will be necessary to test for whispering pectoriloquy.

The technique of auscultation may have to be modified to meet the needs of individual cases. Examples of this are:

1. When abnormal breath sounds are heard, the extent of the lesion should be carefully mapped out by moving the chest piece of the stethoscope with each breath from the normal towards the abnormal zone and noting, or marking with a skin pencil, the level at which the breath sounds change.

2. A patient with severe pleural pain should not be asked to take frequent deep breaths when an attempt is being made to elicit bronchial breath sounds or crepitations. It is preferable in such patients to test the voice sounds first. If an area is found in which the voice sounds are increased or aegophony is present, the patient should be asked to take one or two deep breaths and bronchial breath sounds will usually be elicited in the same area. Similarly, auscultation during a single breath after a short cough is often a more useful way of eliciting crepitations than auscultation during a series of deep, pain-producing breaths.

3. Auscultation after coughing is often a useful procedure in other circumstances. It may help to show whether an added sound is a low-pitched rhonchus, a series of coarse crepitations or a pleural rub (p. 188). When the breath sounds are diminished or absent over a lobe or segment thought to be involved in pneumonia, this may be due to bronchial obstruction by secretions, and bronchial breath sounds often become audible when these secretions are dislodged by coughing. When pulmonary cavitation is suspected, inspiration after a forceful cough may produce a low-pitched 'suction' sound as air re-enters the cavity.

4. Auscultation during forced expiration with the mouth open is a valuable method of detecting rhonchi which are inaudible during normal expiration. This procedure should always be practised in suspected cases of chronic bronchitis or bronchial asthma, in which rhonchi elicited in this way may at times be the only clinical abnormality.

### THE INTERPRETATION OF AUSCULTATORY FINDINGS

1. *High-pitched bronchial breath sounds* are heard over areas of pneumonic consolidation, over a collapsed lung or lobe when the peripheral bronchi are obstructed by secretions, and over a lung compressed by a large pleural effusion or a tension pneumothorax. In all these conditions the *voice*

*sounds* have the quality of aegophony and are usually increased in intensity. Whispering pectoriloquy is always present.

2. *Low-pitched bronchial breath sounds* are heard over localised areas of pulmonary fibrosis, e.g. in chronic pulmonary tuberculosis, chronic suppurative pneumonia or bronchiectasis. In all these conditions the *voice sounds* are increased in intensity and whispering pectoriloquy is often present.

3. *'Amphoric' bronchial breath sounds* are heard over large, superficial pulmonary cavities and occasionally over a pneumothorax. In these conditions *the voice sounds* are usually increased (less often with a pneumothorax) and whispering pectoriloquy is always present.

4. Breath sounds are *diminished* or *absent* over a pleural effusion, thickened pleura, a pneumothorax or a collapsed lung, lobe or segment where the major bronchus supplying it is obstructed. The breath sounds are symmetrically diminished over both lungs in emphysema, this abnormality usually being accompanied by prolongation of the expiratory phase. In these conditions the *voice sounds* are decreased in intensity in proportion to the diminution of breath sounds.

5. *Rhonchi* are heard diffusely over both lungs in bronchial asthma and in most cases of acute and chronic bronchitis. In asthma the rhonchi are typically medium- or high-pitched, expiratory and continuous. In bronchitis they are typically low- or medium-pitched, both inspiratory and expiratory, and not continuous. A localised rhonchus may be heard over a partially obstructed large bronchus. If the obstruction is caused by a fixed lesion, such as a tumour or foreign body, the rhonchus is usually louder during inspiration and is not altered by coughing. If caused by secretions, the obstruction is immediately relieved by coughing, which causes the rhonchus to disappear.

6. *Crepitations* are heard whenever there is an abnormal amount of liquid of any type, e.g. mucus, pus, serous transudate or blood, in the bronchi or lungs, or in pulmonary cavities in communication with the bronchial tree. With localised pulmonary lesions, such as pneumonia, lung abscess, bronchiectasis or tuberculosis, the crepitations are confined to the lobes or segments involved. In diffuse abnormalities such as pulmonary oedema and chronic bronchitis, they may be audible over the whole of both lungs but because of the effect of gravity are usually more numerous over the lung bases. Persistent coarse crepitations are heard over fibrosing alveolitis and tinkling crepitations over a pneumothorax.

7. A *pleural rub* is heard over areas of 'dry' pleurisy. It disappears as soon as the visceral and parietal pleura are separated by fluid, but often remains audible above an effusion. If dry pleurisy involves the pleura adjacent to the pericardium, a 'pleuro-pericardial rub' may also be heard. This is a rather misleading term since the pericardial element in the sound is not due to pericarditis. It is caused merely by roughened pleural surfaces adjacent to the pericardium being moved across one another by cardiac pulsation. A

## TABLE 3

### Summary of Typical Physical Signs in the More Common Respiratory Diseases

| Pathological Process | Movement of Chest Wall | Mediastinal Displacement | Percussion Note | Breath Sounds | Vocal Resonance | Accompaniments |
|---|---|---|---|---|---|---|
| Consolidation: as in lobar pneumonia | Reduced on side affected | None | Dull | High-pitched bronchial | Increased (with aegophony) Whispering pectoriloquy | Fine crepitations early Coarse crepitations later |
| Collapse due to obstruction of major bronchus | Reduced on side affected | Towards lesion | Dull | Diminished or absent | Reduced or absent | None |
| Collapse due to peripheral bronchial obstruction | Reduced on side affected | Towards lesion | Dull | High-pitched bronchial | Increased (with aegophony) Whispering pectoriloquy | None early—coarse crepitations later |
| Localised fibrosis and/or bronchiectasis | Slightly reduced on side affected | Towards lesion | Impaired | Low-pitched bronchial | Increased | Coarse crepitations |
| Cavitation (typical signs only when cavity is large and linked with bronchus) | Slightly reduced on side affected | None, or towards lesion | Impaired | 'Amphoric' bronchial | Increased Whispering pectoriloquy | Coarse crepitations |
| Pleural effusion Empyema | Reduced or absent (depending on size) on side affected | Towards opposite side | Stony dull | Diminished or absent (occasionally high-pitched bronchial) | Reduced or absent (occasionally increased with aegophony) | Pleural rub in some cases (above effusion) |
| Pneumothorax | Reduced or absent (depending on size) on side affected | Towards opposite side | Normal or hyper-resonant | Diminished or absent (occasionally faint high-pitched bronchial) | Reduced or absent | Tinkling crepitations when fluid present |
| Bronchitis: Acute Chronic | Normal or symmetrically diminished | None | Normal | Vesicular with prolonged expiration | Normal | Rhonchi, usually with some coarse crepitations |
| Bronchial asthma | Symmetrically diminished | None | Normal | Vesicular with prolonged expiration | Normal or diminished | Rhonchi, mainly expiratory and high-pitched |
| Diffuse lobular pneumonia | Symmetrically diminished | None | May be impaired | Usually harsh vesicular with prolonged expiration | Normal | Rhonchi and coarse crepitations |
| Diffuse pulmonary emphysema | Symmetrically diminished | None | Normal or hyper-resonant | Diminished vesicular with prolonged expiration | Normal or reduced | Rhonchi and coarse crepitations from associated bronchitis |
| Interstitial lung disease | Symmetrically diminished | None | Normal | Harsh vesicular with prolonged expiration | Usually increased | Crackling crepitations uninfluenced by coughing |

pleuro-pericardial rub may, however, be impossible to distinguish from a pericardial rub. When a typical pleural rub is audible laterally this suggests that the central rub is pleuro-pericardial, but as pleurisy and pericarditis may coexist such a conclusion is open to fallacy.

## Other Physical Signs

*Forced expiratory time* (FET) is measured by placing the chest piece of a stethoscope over the trachea and timing the duration of forced expiration following a full inspiration. This is normally less than four seconds. A prolonged FET is indicative of diffuse airways obstruction, and is a feature of chronic bronchitis, emphysema and bronchial asthma.

The *'coin test'* may occasionally be of value in confirming the presence of a pneumothorax when the air pressure in the pleural space is above atmospheric level. It is carried out by placing a coin on·the posterior chest wall and tapping it with a second coin while another observer listens with a stethoscope in front. When the test is positive, a ringing sound is heard; when negative, a dull thud.

*Hippocratic succussion* is the name given to the splashing sound which is produced by shaking the chest of a patient with both air and fluid in the pleural space. Care should be taken not to confuse gastric with pleural splashing.

# THE METHODS IN PRACTICE

## Interpretation of Physical Sings

The physical signs found in the more common respiratory diseases are shown in Table 3 (opposite). It must be emphasised, however, that these signs are not necessarily present in every case. An area of consolidation or collapse may, for example, be too small to give rise to the classical pattern of physical signs. Furthermore, the picture may be confused by the coincidence of two groups of signs, as when consolidation or collapse is accompanied by pleural effusion. Difficulties are also apt to arise when the differential diagnosis rests on the observer's estimate of the position of the mediastinum. In patients with pulmonary collapse or pleural effusion mediastinal displacement of a sufficient degree to be recognised clinically is an inconstant feature and, even when present, may be difficult to detect with certainty since the trachea and cardiac apex beat are not always readily palpable.

# FURTHER INVESTIGATIONS

From the history and clinical examination it is possible in many cases to make a reliable and reasonably complete diagnosis. This applies, for example, to conditions such as bronchial asthma, chronic bronchitis and emphysema, and to some cases of pneumonia and pulmonary infarction. In many conditions, however, information required to expand and clarify the diagnosis must be obtained by other methods. By means of radiology the precise anatomical position of a lesion can be determined, and from this and other features its pathology may be deduced. Bacteriological and cytological examination of sputum and pleural fluid may provide even more reliable data, by means of which a clinical diagnosis can be elaborated into an aetiological diagnosis, for example by the identification of the organism responsible for an acute pneumonia or by the finding of carcinoma cells in a pleural effusion. In a few cases a diagnosis cannot be completed without more formidable investigations, such as bronchoscopy, bronchography, pleural biopsy and even thoracotomy.

In a rather different category are those cases in which clinical examination fails to reveal any abnormality whatever and the diagnosis depends entirely on specialised investigations, particularly radiology. The two most important diseases in this group are pulmonary tuberculosis and bronchial carcinoma, neither of which may give rise to any clinical abnormality in the early stages. It is important to appreciate this point and to advise radiological examination of the chest whenever one of these conditions is suspected from the history, even if no abnormal physical signs can be detected.

Even when a precise diagnosis has been made, it is often desirable to measure the effects the disease is having on respiratory function. Investigations of this type are useful for the assessment of fitness for work and suitability for certain forms of treatment, such as thoracotomy in bronchial carcinoma or corticosteroids in bronchial asthma.

A full account of all the special methods of investigation cannot be given here, nor is it possible to indicate in any detail the information they can be expected to provide. The summary which follows is therefore intended to serve only as a rough guide to the value of each investigation and the indications for its use.

### Radiological Examination

1. *Radiographs* (postero-anterior and lateral) should be obtained whenever pulmonary or pleural disease is suspected. This examination may disclose a lesion or lesions undetected by physical examination. It will also show where a lesion is situated, and in many cases indicate its pathology.

2. *Fluoroscopy* provides information about the movement of the diaphragm and the position of the oesophagus. It is of particular importance in patients with bronchial carcinoma. Unilateral diaphragmatic paralysis or a localised displacement of the barium-filled oesophagus would, by demonstrating mediastinal invasion, contraindicate an attempt at surgical treatment.

3. *Tomography* is a special radiographic technique by means of which an opacity or part of an opacity lying in one particular plane can be visualised

clearly, even when there are superimposed opacities in different planes. This technique is of value in the detection of pulmonary cavities and in demonstrating local variations in density (e.g. calcification) within a pulmonary lesion. It can thus be helpful in distinguishing between a tumour and a tuberculous focus.

4. *Pulmonary angiography* can be used to detect vascular abnormalities in the lungs. A series of chest radiographs is taken in rapid succession after the injection of contrast medium into the main pulmonary artery through a cardiac catheter.

5. *Radiographic examination of the nasal sinuses* is an important part of the investigation of chronic infection of the upper respiratory tract.

**Examination of the Sputum.** This examination, or that of laryngeal swabs if no sputum is available, is an important diagnostic measure in all suspected bronchopulmonary infections, particularly pneumonia and tuberculosis. In all such cases a direct film, appropriately stained, should be examined microscopically and suitable culture media inoculated. Sputum may be examined for malignant cells if bronchial carcinoma is suspected, but the results are not uniformly reliable.

**Intradermal Tests.** *The tuberculin test* is chiefly of value in excluding present or past tuberculosis infection. A positive test is of diagnostic significance only in children. *The Kveim test* confirms a diagnosis of sarcoidosis. *Skin sensitivity tests* may indicate the aetiology of allergic rhinitis, asthma and pulmonary eosinophilia and assist in the management of these conditions.

**Examination of the Blood.** *The total and differential white cell counts* may give guidance as to the nature of a radiographic abnormality, e.g. whether it is an area of pneumonic consolidation or an eosinophilic infiltrate. *Blood culture* and *examination of serum for viral and other antibodies* may be of value in determining the aetiology of a pneumonic illness.

**Bronchoscopy.** With a rigid bronchoscope the bronchi can be inspected as far as the segmental orifices. A flexible (fibreoptic) bronchoscope may be of value in the detection of more peripheral lesions. Bronchoscopy is an essential investigation whenever bronchial carcinoma is suspected, and often the diagnosis can be confirmed histologically by biopsy. It is also a valuable method of investigating other causes of bronchial obstruction, e.g. inhaled foreign body, tuberculous lymph nodes.

**Bronchography.** In this examination radiographs are taken after the whole bronchial tree has been outlined by an opaque medium. The main indication is in the diagnosis of bronchiectasis and the precise determination of its degree and distribution.

**Pleural Aspiration and Biopsy.** Cytological and bacteriological examination of pleural fluid often provides information which reveals the cause of the effusion. Pleural biopsy taken from the site of aspiration is of particular value in the diagnosis of tuberculous and malignant effusions.

**Thoracoscopy.** The examination of the pleural surfaces with a telescope after air has been introduced into the pleural space, may show pleural abnormalities from which tissue can be removed for histological examination. This technique need, however, only be used when examination of pleural fluid and pleural biopsy by the ordinary method are unhelpful.

**Lymph Node Biopsy.** Removal of a supraclavicular or, less frequently, an axillary lymph node may provide histological proof of the diagnosis in bronchial carcinoma, sarcoidosis, reticulosis and, occasionally, pulmonary tuberculosis. A lymph node can also be removed from the vicinity of the trachea and main bronchi by the technique of *mediastinoscopy*.

**Lung biopsy.** If the nature of a diffuse pulmonary abnormality cannot be determined by other methods, a histological diagnosis can be made by needle or drill biopsy of lung. A similar technique can be used for the diagnosis of localised peripheral pulmonary lesions. Thoracotomy is occasionally required for the diagnosis of pulmonary or mediastinal lesions if the results of all other investigations are negative or inconclusive.

**Tests of Respiratory Function.** Disturbances of ventilation, distribution, diffusion and respiratory work can be measured, but many of these tests require complex facilities, which are not generally available. For practical purposes, respiratory function can be adequately investigated by the following procedures:

1. The measurement of *oxygen tension* ($PaO_2$), *carbon dioxide tension* ($PaCO_2$) and pH in a sample of arterial blood obtained from the brachial or femoral artery. The estimation of $PaCO_2$ by the rebreathing method[1] does not require arterial puncture, and can be performed at the bedside in 10 minutes without special training or expensive equipment. $PaCO_2$ is normally 36-44 mm Hg, and is always increased when there is inadequate alveolar ventilation.

2. The estimation of *forced expiratory volume* ($FEV_1$) and *forced vital capacity* (FVC). This requires either a recording spirometer, or a standard spirometer incorporating an electronic timing device. The $FEV_1$ is the largest volume which can be expired, from full inspiration, in one second, and provides information about ventilatory capacity. In health the $FEV_1$ may be 3·5 litres or more, and amounts to at least 80 per cent of the FVC. In diseases such as bronchial asthma and emphysema, which produce narrowing of the air passages during expiration, both $FEV_1$ and FVC are reduced but the reduction in $FEV_1$ is proportionately greater, i.e. the $FEV_1$/FVC ratio is reduced, perhaps to 40 per cent or less. In diseases such as diffuse fibrosis and ankylosing spondylitis, which render the lungs or chest wall more rigid, the $FEV_1$ and FVC are reduced proportionately and the normal $FEV_1$/FVC

[1] Campbell, E. J. M. & Howell, J. B. L. (1959), *A Symposium on pH and Blood Gas Measurement*, ed. Woolmer, R. F. London: Churchill.

ration of 80 per cent is preserved. These simple measurements are thus of value in distinguishing between one type of respiratory disorder and another, as well as in providing an index of its severity. Serial measurements can also be used to assess improvement or deterioration.

The *peak expiratory flow rate* (PEFR), which correlates closely with the $FEV_1$, can also be used for the assessment of airways obstruction. The apparatus required for this measurement (a peak flow meter) is portable and easy to operate, and is eminently suitable for use in general practice. The normal range of PEFR in healthy adults is 500–650 litres per minute.

**Pulmonary radio-isotope scanning.** Perfusion scanning of the lungs following the intravenous injection of isotope-labelled macro-aggregated albumen can be used to detect and delineate unperfused areas of lung. This technique is of considerable value in the diagnosis of pulmonary embolism, particularly if combined with ventilation scanning following the inhalation of an isotope-labelled gas.

CHAPTER 7

# The Alimentary and Genito-Urinary Systems

'Every pain has its distinct and pregnant signification if we will but carefully search for it.'

JOHN HILTON, *Rest and Pain*, 1863

The diagnosis in many diseases of the viscera is more often dependent upon careful analysis of the history and is less often supported by physical signs than is the case elsewhere. Pain is particularly prominent among the symptoms which are encountered both in the alimentary and genito-urinary systems, and thorough interrogation on the lines indicated on page 29 is essential before complicated investigations are initiated. Nothing is more frustrating for a radiologist than to be asked to conduct a 'complete barium series' without being given any indication of the lesion suspected. The request is still more futile if the cause of the symptoms turns out to be something which might well have been recognised if an adequate history had been taken. It is also possible that unnecessary investigation may lead to the discovery of a symptomless abnormality such as a hiatus hernia to which the patient's complaint may be incorrectly attributed. The history is therefore so important that considerable space is devoted to symptoms and in particular to an amplification of the analysis of pain. However, the physical examination must not be neglected for after a careful history has been recorded, inspection, palpation, percussion and auscultation may each provide essential information.

## THE HISTORY

### Cardinal Symptoms of Alimentary Disease

The principal complaints can conveniently be studied in four main groups; firstly, those due to depression or exaggeration of normal sensations; secondly, those due to disturbance of motility; thirdly, those due to disturbance of function; and fourthly, pain. It must be borne in mind that organic disease may be present without any such symptoms, and its presence may be suspected only after the development of some secondary feature such as anaemia or jaundice. Equally it must be remembered that, in the absence of an organic cause, the mental state of a patient may lead to symptoms through the influence of autonomic nervous control of the gut.

#### Depression or Exaggeration of Normal Sensations

Conscious sensations do not normally arise from most of the viscera. There is, however, greater awareness of those parts which are in more immediate communication with the exterior—the mouth, pharynx and oesophagus, the urethra, bladder and rectum. In addition to the frequent sensations arising in these areas, there are a number of other common occurrences attributable to the alimentary tract which do not necessarily indicate any abnormality. Among these are appetite, hunger, belching, acid regurgitation, heartburn, epigastric fullness after a big meal, borborygmi and flatus. However, depression or exaggeration of these normal phenomena may be of pathological significance. Examples are the loss of appetite (anorexia) which may accompany the development of a gastric carcinoma; abnormal hunger in some patients with peptic ulcer; excessive belching due to aerophagy, a habit which often develops in an effort to relieve abdominal pain or discomfort; acid regurgitation and recurrent heartburn when recumbent or when bending, due to an incompetent cardia as a result of a sliding hiatus hernia; loud borborygmi caused by violent peristalsis induced chemically by the products of the rare carcinoid syndrome; inability to pass flatus when intestinal obstruction is present; a frequent desire to defaecate caused by a growth or by faecal impaction in the rectum.

## Disturbance of Motility

**Waterbrash.** This refers to the sudden filling of the mouth with a tasteless clear liquid, often preceded by transient high epigastric pain. It is due to the regurgitation of saliva which has accumulated in the oesophagus.

**Dysphagia.** Difficulty in swallowing is the main symptom caused by disease of the oesophagus. It is such an important symptom of organic disease that an explanation for it must be found in every case. Less often there is pain.

UPPER DYSPHAGIA. When food is felt to stick behind the cricoid cartilage it is sometimes an effect of a lesion at the lower end of the oesophagus. More often it is due to stricture or a growth at the upper end of the oesophagus or to a neurological or neuromuscular disorder. It may occur in combination with iron deficiency anaemia and atrophic glossitis. Upper dysphagia, regurgitation, gurgling noises and sometimes a swelling low in the neck are characteristic of pharyngoesophageal pouch.

LOWER DYSPHAGIA. When food is felt to stick behind the xiphisternum, a lesion at the lower end of the oesophagus is indicated such as tumour, cardiospasm, or peptic oesophagitis. Meat and other solid foods and especially potato tend to stick first. The chewing habit of the patient largely determines the degree of obstruction necessary to produce symptoms. Regurgitation of food may occur, and though patients often call this vomiting, there is no nausea and the taste is seldom unpleasant. Inhalation of regurgitated food may cause pneumonia.

The site of dysphagia between these upper and lower limits is usually a good indication of the level of the lesion.

GLOBUS HYSTERICUS. This is a psychogenic symptom in which there is a feeling of a lump in the throat which needs to be swallowed. It is present between meals and there is no difficulty in swallowing food.

**Vomiting.** Simple reasoning might lead to the conclusion that vomiting is likely to be due to disease of the stomach. In fact this is very far from the case; it is a symptom of a wide variety of local and systemic disorders, many of which are unassociated with alimentary disease. Instances among the functional and organic disorders of the nervous system, for example, are vomiting due to excitement, disgust or fear, motion sickness, vestibular disorders, migraine, meningitis and intracranial tumour. It also occurs in association with severe pain as in renal colic or some cases of myocardial infarction. Among systemic conditions are febrile illnesses, whooping-cough, chronic renal failure, pregnancy and endocrine disorders such as hyperparathyroidism, severe diabetic ketoacidosis, or a thyrotoxic or Addisonian crisis. Certain drugs are also prone to cause vomiting, some due to a central action such as digoxin, aspirin or morphine, others as a result of gastric irritation such as aminophylline or potassium chloride. In the alimentary system, vomiting may indicate pyloric obstruction but is also associated with such varied conditions as acute gastritis, acute appendicitis, intestinal obstruction and hepatitis. Children are prone to vomit for relatively trivial reasons such as a mild fever. Vomiting is preceded in most cases by nausea, but in some instances of intracranial tumour there may be no warning and vomiting may be projectile. In most cases the cause of vomiting can be discovered by a full clinical history and examination.

Enquiry should be made about the patient's observations as to the quantity, smell, taste, colour and other appearances of the vomitus, the frequency of vomiting and the time of day at which it occurs. These characteristics are discussed on page 451.

**Defaecation.** It is important to find out the frequency of defaecation and whether the bowel actions are occurring at any special times of day or night. Many people do not inspect their stools and therefore only positive observations can be accepted. These should include information about bulk, consistency, colour and other appearances such as recognisable food, blood, pus or slime (p. 452). An opportunity to corroborate patients' observations should be made if any abnormality is suspected and the alleged presence of worms should be confirmed by inspection. It must be borne in mind that individual bowel habit varies normally from once in three days or so to two or three times a day and that bowel action is readily influenced by emotional disturbances.

CONSTIPATION. A recent alteration of bowel habit without change in the mode of living is very suggestive of an organic abnormality in the distal colon, such as carcinoma or diverticular disease. Habitual constipation on the other hand is a common disorder and the diagnosis is supported by the palpation of formed faeces on digital examination of the rectum.

DIARRHOEA. This refers to the frequent passage of loose stools. In geriatric patients diarrhoea is often 'spurious', due to severe constipation resulting in impacted faeces, yet readily recognised if a rectal examination is performed. It should be borne in mind that diarrhoea is sometimes self-inflicted through clandestine purgation and rarely imposed by others emulating the Borgias.

## Disturbances of Function

These include disorders of secretion, digestion, absorption or excretion, some examples of which are mentioned below.

**Disorders of Secretion.** Lack of salivation results in a dry mouth and difficulty in swallowing certain foods. Common causes are nervousness, fever, or treatment with anticholinergic or ganglion-blocking drugs. Rarely the symptom is due to disease affecting the salivary glands such as Sjögren's syndrome.

Lack of the intrinsic factor in gastric secretion leads to pernicious anaemia, occasionally accompanied by vague abdominal discomfort and recurrent bouts of diarrhoea. Extreme over-secretion of gastric acid is found in association with a rare hormonally active adenoma of the pancreas (Zollinger-Ellison syndrome) and it may lead to peptic ulceration of the duodenum and jejunum, and to diarrhoea.

**Disorders of Digestion.** It is probably no exaggeration to state that the term 'indigestion' is invariably misused by patients. Almost any symptom arising from the alimentary tract and other complaints besides may be referred to as indigestion. It is seldom that disorders of the alimentary system lead to a failure to digest food except when there is lack of secretion of pancreatic juice. This may lead to loss of weight and steatorrhoea; undigested fat, starch granules and meat fibres may be seen in a specimen of faeces examined under the microscope.

**Failure of Absorption.** Absorption occurs mainly in the small intestine, disorders of which may lead to steatorrhoea and a wide variety of symptoms which depend upon some of the factors mentioned below. These include anaemia due to iron, folic acid or vitamin $B_{12}$ malabsorption, various other vitamin deficiencies, muscle wasting, weight loss or hypoproteinaemic oedema resulting from the inadequate absorption of amino acids. In addition lack of mineral salts may be manifest clinically as tiredness due to lack of sodium or as tetany and osteomalacia due to a failure of absorption of calcium. Specific absorption defects are also being recognised, such as the recessively inherited glucose-galactose malabsorption, the excessive absorption of iron and copper leading to haemochromatosis and hepatolenticular degeneration respectively, and the failure of absorption of amino acids leading to Hartnup disease, a genetically determined disorder of the nervous system.

**Disorders of Excretion.** This applies particularly to diseases affecting the liver and bile ducts; the retention of bile pigment causes jaundice while the failure of excretion of bile salts, or of some associated factor, results in itching of the skin. Bile pigment (p. 434) is commonly found in the urine when jaundice is due to obstruction of the biliary tract or to hepatocellular disease. Urobilinogen (p. 435) is present in excess in the urine of patients with haemolytic jaundice or in the early or recovery stages of hepatocellular disease.

**Loss of Essential Substances.** Examples include water and electrolyte depletion in cholera, potassium loss from adenomatous polyps and protein losing enteropathy.

### Pain

Pain is a very frequent symptom in disorders of the alimentary system. The common causes are spasm or stretching of smooth muscle, inflammatory or neoplastic lesions, and the effect of a high hydrogen ion concentration in the gastric juice on the nerve endings in the base of a peptic ulcer. Pain may also be caused by ischaemia or congestion as the result of mesenteric vascular lesions. It must be borne in mind that pain of visceral or parietal origin may be identical with respect to site, radiation, character, and severity. A distinction can usually be made by taking other features into account. It is essential that a diagnosis is made if possible on the data provided by the history of pain and by examination. Questions should be framed in such a way as to analyse the complaint of pain in the manner described on page 29.

Radiological examination, exploratory operation or other investigations should always be regarded as confirmatory rather than as primary diagnostic procedures. For example gall-stones may cause abdominal pain, but they are present in 10 to 20 per cent of the adult population and do not usually cause symptoms. Unless clinical methods have led to a diagnosis of pain due to gall-stones, the radiological demonstration of calculi might lead to inappropriate cholecystectomy with its attendant risks, and to neglect of the real cause of the symptoms.

The prime guide to the source of a pain is usually its main site. From the clinical aspect it is therefore logical to consider visceral and other pains on a segmental basis, starting with those in the anterior midline which is the usual reference from unpaired structures, and thereafter dealing with the lateralised pains from paired organs and other causes. The following notes are given as a guide to the analysis of abdominal pain and as an indication of the questions which may have to be posed. The regions of the abdomen, to which reference is made in the text, are described and illustrated on page 210.

### Retrosternal Pain

Pain in this site may arise from the heart (p. 105), pericardium (p. 107), aorta (p. 107), mediastinum (p. 160), sternum, oesophagus and occasionally from a hiatus hernia.

**Oesophageal Pain.** Site—midline retrosternal at the level of the lesion. Radiation—through to midline of back at the level of the lesion. In the presence of oesophagitis, pain may be caused by swallowing; hot fluids are particularly apt to be mentioned.

## UPPER ABDOMINAL PAIN

**Pain of Hiatus Hernia.** Site—epigastric or retrosternal. Radiation— through to the middle of the back, to the jaws and down the arms. Pain is usually due to peptic oesophagitis from acid regurgitation through an incompetent cardia when a sliding hernia is present. Pain of moderate severity may occur on bending or lying down. Conversely it is relieved by standing, stretching or sitting and is eased rapidly, though perhaps temporarily, by alkalies. Heartburn on bending or lying down is common, and there may also be dysphagia and regurgitation. It must be mentioned that a hiatus hernia is often present without any symptoms. Pain may occur in the absence of peptic oesophagitis and it may also be caused by distension of, or strangulation of a para-oesophageal hernia.

**Gastric Pain.** Site—epigastric. Radiation—usually none, but it may pass through to the midline of the back or below the left scapula.

**Duodenal Pain.** Site—epigastric. Radiation—usually none but it may be felt in the midline of the back or below the right scapula.

**Pain of Peptic Ulcer.** This is the only common cause of pain arising from the stomach or duodenum. Steady gnawing pain of slight to moderate intensity tends to recur at predictable times and is eased in 5 to 15 minutes by food, by alkalies or by vomiting. The patient points with one finger to the site of pain in the epigastrium. If the pain sometimes also wakens the patient at night, the source is nearly always a duodenal ulcer. Penetration of a posterior ulcer may lead to accentuation or extension of the pain, especially to the back, and the factors which previously gave relief may become less effective.

**Pain of Perforated Peptic Ulcer.** Intense pain of sudden onset rapidly extends all over the abdomen, and may radiate to the shoulder-tips. The patient, pale and perspiring, tends to lie still; this contrasts with the restlessness of other very severe pains such as that of biliary origin. The clinical picture is modified when leakage is confined locally and does not spread throughout the peritoneal cavity. Some other conditions described below may closely simulate the pain of perforated ulcer. These are gall-stone attacks, acute pancreatitis, severe diabetic ketoacidosis, tabetic crisis and lead colic.

**Biliary Pain.** Site—epigastric, or right upper abdominal. Radiation— through to the back below the right scapula; sometimes felt in the centre of the back, the right shoulder-tip or behind the lower part of the sternum. The pain is commonly severe, causing restlessness, pallor, sweating and often vomiting. The onset is sudden and pain increases to maximum intensity usually in 5 to 15 minutes, though sometimes it is maximal at onset like a perforated peptic ulcer. Subsequently the pain usually remains intense for about 10 to 60 minutes, though it may persist for many hours unless relief is obtained from powerful analgesics. It is rare for pain to come in waves as in intestinal colic, though a few patients experience minor fluctuations in severity (Fig. 3, p. 35).

**Pancreatic Pain.** Site—epigastric. Radiation—may radiate through to the midthoracic region of the back centrally or to the left side. Acute pancreatitis causes severe pain which is apt to be mistaken for that due to gall-stones or to perforation of a peptic ulcer. The incidence is greater in alcoholic subjects and in those with disease of the biliary tract. The diagnosis should be suspected in every upper abdominal emergency, particularly if the patient is more ill than would be expected in the early stages of the alternative conditions.

Chronic pancreatic pain due to tumour is usually felt in the back and may be so much affected by posture that patients may prefer standing to sitting, and sitting to lying. At night they may be unable to sleep unless they sit upright or lean forwards.

**Hepatic Pain.** A considerable variety of gross disorders of the liver may be present without pain, for the parenchyma is insensitive. Conditions which cause a sudden enlargement of the liver such as infective hepatitis or acute congestive cardiac failure often cause pain which is attributed to sudden stretching of the capsule. If a lesion involves the capsule and leads to perihepatitis, there may be pain on breathing accompanied by audible friction which may prompt the unwary to make a diagnosis of pleurisy.

**Pain and Diabetes.** Patients who develop severe ketoacidosis may complain of severe abdominal pain which has variously been ascribed to abdominal cramp associated with salt and water depletion, or to acute enlargement of the liver. In such cases the clinical picture and the findings of large quantities of glucose and ketones in the urine should leave the diagnosis in no reasonable doubt. The smell of acetone in the breath is a very sensitive guide to those who can appreciate it. This diagnosis will not be overlooked if the urine is routinely examined.

**Pain due to Gastric Crisis.** This is now a very rare cause of abdominal pain; it occurs in about 10 per cent of patients with tabes dorsalis. Epigastric pain of sudden onset and usually of excruciating intensity persists for hours or days and is unrelieved by the vomiting which attends it. Some of the other clinical features of the condition will be present such as lightning pains, ataxia, pupillary changes and absent tendon reflexes in the lower limbs.

### CENTRAL ABDOMINAL PAIN

**Small Intestinal Pain.** Site—central abdominal (at umbilicus). Pains of moderate to severe intensity recur for several seconds about three times a minute, with complete freedom between each pain. The patient tends to double up. Though commonly due to inflammatory or obstructive lesions, the rare condition of acute porphyria should be borne in mind; this may be accompanied by port wine coloured urine, polyneuritis and mental changes. It is often precipitated by the administration of barbiturates.

Pain may also be caused by ischaemia of the small intestine. Occlusion of the superior mesenteric artery may cause infarction of the gut, giving rise to sudden severe pain in the central abdomen, often radiating through to the back, accompanied by acute circulatory failure. Chronic ischaemia of the midgut may cause 'intestinal angina' and/or malabsorption. The pain comes on after eating and is usually constant for up to an hour or so, although rarely it is colicky.

**Pain of Lead Colic.** Site—widespread, mid or lower abdominal. The term 'colic' is a misnomer in the sense that the pain is often continuous, and unlike the pain of intestinal colic it is unrelieved by antispasmodic drugs such as atropine.

**Appendicular Pain.** Site—central abdominal initially. Usually persistent pain of mild to moderate severity later accompanied by vomiting without relief. Obstruction of the appendix may cause pain identical with small intestinal colic. When the peritoneum over the appendix becomes inflamed, the site of pain changes, commonly to the right iliac fossa at McBurney's point, situated one-third of the distance along a line from the anterior superior iliac spine to the umbilicus. Sometimes pain may be felt only in the right iliac fossa. Pain may also occur elsewhere if the appendix lies in an unusual position; for example, it may dangle into the pelvis and cause hypogastric pain, often accompanied by diarrhoea and dysuria. Sometimes the leg may be flexed at the hip joint or extension of the right hip joint may be resisted owing to spasm of the psoas muscle. Similarly, if the inflamed appendix is in contact with the obturator internus, resistance will be felt and pain will be produced by attempts to rotate the thigh when it is flexed at the hip. The appendix may lie behind the ascending colon and give rise to pain which may erroneously be thought to be renal in origin.

**Colonic Pain: Proximal Hemicolon.** Site—central abdominal. In practice, painful lesions of the proximal half of the colon are very rare unless the pathological process has extended to surrounding structures.

### LOWER ABDOMINAL PAIN

**Colonic Pain: Distal Hemicolon.** Site—hypogastric. Most painful colonic lesions are in the distal hemicolon, and the pain is felt in the hypogastrium or left iliac fossa. The pain is of moderate intensity, but can be severe; it is intermittent with longer intervals than in small intestinal colic, the pains lasting a minute or so with periods of freedom for a minute or a few minutes. Sometimes pain is felt in the right iliac fossa due apparently to distension of the caecum.

**Pain in the Urinary Bladder.** Site—suprapubic. Pain is associated with a desire to urinate and therefore seldom causes any diagnostic difficulty. Inflammation of the bladder trigone, or a calculus at the lower end of a ureter may each cause pain referred to the tip of the penis. A calculus in the bladder is apt to irritate the sensitive trigone while the patient is ambulant, and therefore gives rise to greater frequency and dysuria by day than by night.

**Uterine Pain.** Pain is felt low in the abdomen and may radiate through to the lumbosacral area of the back, for example in labour pains or dysmenorrhoea.

### PAIN IN THE PERINEAL AREA

**Rectal Pain.** Site—correctly localised to rectum. Pain is not commonly caused by organic lesions which more frequently result in tenesmus—an abnormally frequent desire to defaecate and a sensation that evacuation is incomplete. The most common pain felt in the rectum is proctalgia fugax. The term refers to brief severe spasms of pain which have no organic cause and which are probably due to cramp in the sacrococcygeal muscles.

**Anal Pain.** Accurately localised and most commonly due to a fissure.

**Prostatic Pain.** Site—perineal. Diseases of the prostate are very common, yet pain is rare. Hesitancy in starting to void urine followed by a poor stream and frequency of urination is usually due to senile hyperplasia. Pain may be due to prostatitis and is made worse by local pressure such as that exerted during digital examination of the rectum or during defaecation.

**Urethral Pain.** Site—urethral. A burning pain is correctly localised and is felt during urination.

### LATERALISED PAIN

**Splenic Pain.** Pain does not arise from the spleen unless perisplenitis is present. If the spleen is not palpable, then it is only by careful consideration of the problem as a whole that the erroneous diagnosis of left-sided pleurisy may be avoided. Mistaking for pleurisy the rub over a splenic infarct in a patient with infective endocarditis, for example, might cause a delay in treatment which could have serious consequences.

**Renal Pain.** Site—in the back between the twelfth rib and the iliac crest. Diseases which affect the capsule or the pelvis of the kidney are often painful, while those that are confined to the parenchyma cause pain only by acute stretching of the capsule.

A persistent low-grade pain or discomfort is sometimes associated with a stone in the renal pelvis, hydronephrosis, tumour or polycystic disease. A more severe pain of sudden onset, accompanied by chill or rigor, is characteristic of acute pyelonephritis. The similar, but usually much more intense and continuous pain of 'renal colic' is caused by acute distension of the renal pelvis and kidney due to calculous or other obstruction of the ureter. Periodic increase in the high pressure in the renal tract due to peristaltic activity in the pelvis and ureter may account for the superimposition of an even more excruciating pain in about half of the cases. Radiation may occur anteriorly to the hypochondrium or down to the groin and into the genitalia.

**Pain in the Testis and Epididymis.** Site—testicular. Radiation to the groin and lower abdomen where the pain may be so intense that its testicular origin may be obscured. Pain due to injury is brief, but that due to torsion is prolonged and is felt initially in the iliac fossa. The pain of acute inflammation and torsion is ultimately accompanied by local swelling and tenderness.

**Ovarian Pain.** Pain is felt in the iliac fossa on the affected side in such conditions as endometriosis or malignant tumours.

### Abdominal Pain Originating in Other Structures

Pain in the front of the abdomen at various levels may also be caused by collapse of a vertebra or other disease of the spine. Unilateral disease of a vertebra, prolapsed intervertebral disc or tumour affecting the nerve may give rise to pain on one side of the abdomen. Associated features such as aggravation by certain movements are usually present to indicate the source of the pain; there may be tenderness over the affected bone and segmental sensory and motor changes. In other instances herpes zoster, epidemic myalgia or abdominal aneurysm may create diagnostic difficulties by causing abdominal pain.

## Cardinal Symptoms of Disease of the Genito-Urinary System

### Pain

Notes on pain involving kidney, bladder, prostate, urethra, testicle and epididymis, ovary and uterus will be found on pages 205 and 206.

### Disturbances of Urination

As part of the routine history enquiry should be made for symptoms related to urination. The more common disturbances are dysuria (pain on passing urine), frequency, polyuria, nocturia, oliguria, abnormal colour of the urine, cloudy or offensive urine, a poor stream or sudden cessation of the flow.

**Dysuria and frequency** are almost diagnostic of cystitis, but may be due to prostatitis, tumour of the bladder or stone at the lower end of the ureter.

**Pneumaturia** is diagnostic of vesico-colic fistula.

**Polyuria.** An osmotic diuresis is caused by glucose in diabetes mellitus, by urea in chronic renal failure and by sodium from the use of thiazide diuretics. Polyuria may also be due to lack of, or failure to respond to antidiuretic hormone and to the effect of parathormone on the renal tubules in hyperparathyroidism. It may occur as a result of psychogenic polydipsia.

**Nocturia.** The necessity to pass urine during the sleeping hours may be a life-long habit. As a newly developing symptom it may be due to insomnia or to a number of organic causes such as polyuria. Other reasons for nocturia may be less obvious. Thus obstruction to the urinary outflow by an enlarging prostate may leave some residual urine after voiding so that the bladder refills too quickly. In such cases straining for some time may be necessary to start the flow, and then the stream may be poor. Nocturia in the elderly is also a common symptom of cardiac failure; the diuresis results from the excretion of oedema fluid due to the improved renal circulation which occurs with rest in bed. Necessity to pass urine in somewhat increased quantities at regular intervals throughout the day and night is a frequent feature of chronic renal failure, and the urine will be found to have a low specific gravity which may be fixed around 1·010 (isosthenuria).

**Oliguria.** This means the passage of too little urine to maintain the constancy of the 'milieu interieur'. The minimum quantity of urine which is necessary to achieve this objective varies with the diet, the amount of exercise taken, the metabolic rate and the efficiency of renal function. Thus almost 200 ml might be sufficient for a normal man at rest on a protein-free diet, whereas 2000 ml might be insufficient for maintaining a normal 'milieu' when chronic renal failure is present.

**Poor stream.** This indicates a stricture and it is a common complaint in the elderly male due to hyperplasia of the prostate gland.

**Stress incontinence.** Many females, especially those who have borne children, suffer from urinary incontinence due to the stress of laughing, coughing, sneezing or lifting a heavy weight. It is due to the development of a cystocele, a weakness in the anterior wall of the vagina, often accompanied by some prolapse of the uterus.

**Neurological Disturbances of Bladder Function.** The symptoms which result from diseases interrupting the nervous control of the bladder depend upon whether the sensory or motor pathways are affected.

*Sensory Disturbance.* Dilation of the bladder with dribbling incontinence results from inability to feel that the bladder is distended; it occurs characteristically in tabes dorsalis and sometimes in diabetic neuropathy.

*Impairment of Voluntary Control.* Urgency or precipitancy is the term applied to the main symptom; the desire to pass urine must be obeyed at once or incontinence will occur, yet the patient cannot urinate at will. Multiple sclerosis is the most common neurological cause of urgency in Britain.

*Combined Damage of Sensation and Voluntary Control.* This occurs with spinal cord lesions. The bladder fills to a certain pressure and then empties reflexly; by experience and training the patient may be able to control the emptying by raising the intravesical pressure at suitable intervals by manual compression of the lower abdomen. Unfortunately in some cases the bladder is overactive and contracted so that urinary incontinence is more or less continuous.

In addition the bladder may become overdistended in the early days of acute cerebrovascular accidents and rarely in poliomyelitis and extensive polyneuritis.

### Disturbances of Sexual Function

The menstrual history should include a note of age at the menarche or the menopause and details of the menstrual cycle. These are the frequency, regularity and duration of the menses, and whether blood loss is small, normal or excessive. The date of the last menstrual period should be noted. The occurrence and the nature of any vaginal discharge must be ascertained, while a complaint of intermenstrual bleeding should lead without delay to examination by a gynaecologist. Dyspareunia (pain during sexual intercourse) or failure to achieve an orgasm often occurs in the female and is frequently due to or may lead to psychological difficulties. Failure of erection (impotence) or premature ejaculation are equivalent symptoms in the male. The longer these symptoms persist, the more difficult they are to eradicate. These subjects may be avoided by the patient (and the doctor) because of embarrassment but if there is any indication of a difficulty the patient should be encouraged to speak about it. The opportunity can be provided, once rapport has been established, by asking if sexual intercourse is satisfactory. Thereafter any problem can be discussed frankly as already indicated on pages 8 and 21.

## THE PHYSICAL EXAMINATION

### Mouth and Throat

The examination of the mouth and throat is described on page 77. It is of particular relevance to the alimentary system to know whether the teeth provide an adequate chewing surface or, if the patient is edentulous, whether dentures are used for eating.

### Oesophagus

There is no bedside method of examination. However, when there is a complaint of dysphagia it can be helpful to watch the act of swallowing solids and liquids. The reproduction of the symptom may confirm the organic nature and the site of the lesion, and if swallowing is immediately followed by a distressing bout of coughing, a fistula between the trachea and the oesophagus may be diagnosed with some confidence.

### Abdomen

For purposes of description the abdomen is conveniently divided into nine regions by the intersection of imaginary planes, two horizontal and two sagittal. The upper horizontal plane (transpyloric) lies at a level midway between the suprasternal notch and the symphysis pubis. The lower plane passes through the upper borders of the iliac crests. The sagittal planes are indicated on the surface by lines drawn vertically through points midway between the pubis and the anterior superior iliac spines (Fig. 38).

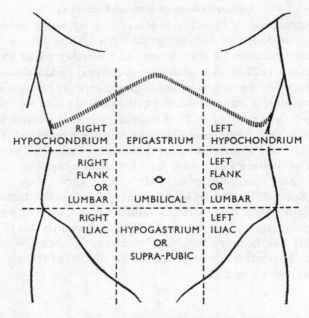

FIG. 38    Regions of the Abdomen.

Whenever possible patients should be examined in a good light and in warm surroundings, warmth being particularly important as it facilitates muscle relaxation. The patient should lie comfortably supine with the head resting on one or two pillows in order to relax the muscles of the abdominal wall. An extra pillow or two may be necessary to prop up a patient with a severe kyphosis. Clothes must be removed so that there is complete exposure from the xiphisternum to the pubis. The chest and the legs should be suitably covered. For the examination of patients in bed, all the bed-clothing except for the sheet should be pulled down as far as the knees. The sheet can then be folded back to the pubis and the nightdress drawn up to the chest. The examination then follows the routine sequence of inspection, palpation, percussion and auscultation.

## Inspection

**Skin Lesions.** Any abnormality of the skin should be noted and the reasons for scars ascertained if these have not already been divulged. In elderly patients senile warts, ranging from pink to brown or black, and haemangiomas (Campbell de Morgan spots) are so common that they could be considered as normal changes as age advances. If striae are present an appropriate reason for them should be determined (p. 94).

**Veins.** Collateral veins (p. 143) may be visible if the inferior vena cava is obstructed; these are usually tortuous dilatations of the superficial epigastric veins in which the blood flows upwards instead of down towards the groins. In the presence of hepatic cirrhosis dilated collateral veins may radiate from the umbilicus (caput Medusae) as a result of blood flowing from the portal vein through collateral vessels along the falciform ligament.

**Hair.** Secondary sexual hair appears at puberty; its absence or complete disappearance after this time should lead to a search for signs of hypopituitarism, cirrhosis of the liver or hypogonadism. Adrenal virilism in the female leads to a male distribution of pubic hair.

**Movements and Contour.** In males particularly, quiet respiration is predominantly diaphragmatic, so that the abdominal wall moves out during inspiration. In the presence of acute peritonitis respiratory movements of the abdomen usually cease.

Pulsation in the epigastrium is usually transmitted from the abdominal aorta (p. 124). Much less frequently is it caused by the right ventricle, the liver or an abdominal aneurysm. Careful inspection and palpation for the type, timing and direction of the thrust will easily distinguish between these possibilities.

The shape and symmetry of the abdomen should be observed. A scaphoid abdomen is due to starvation, wasting diseases or dehydration. Protuberance may be due to obesity, gaseous distension, ascites, pregnancy or other swellings. In obesity the umbilicus is sunken, whereas in other conditions it is flat or even projecting. Visible enlargement of the bladder, uterus or ovary shows a characteristic shape as these structures rise out of the pelvis, the swelling being predominantly central in contrast to the bulging of the flanks in ascites. Distension of the stomach due to pyloric obstruction causes bulging of the upper part of the abdomen; tangential inspection is the best means of seeing the slow waves of gastric peristalsis passing from the rib margin on the left, across the midline, and subsiding beneath the right upper rectus. Activity may be stimulated by a drink, by massage or by flicking the skin over the area. Confirmation may be obtained by placing the observer's hands over the lower ribs, and giving the patient a quick shake from side to side, when a sound like that due to shaking a hot-water bottle which contains water and air is heard and is known as the succussion splash. The sound may also be evoked by quick dipping movements of the hand over the upper abdomen. Similar sounds may be evoked from a normal stomach for an hour or two after food or drink. Small intestinal peristalsis may normally be seen through a thin abdominal wall, and it may become unduly prominent in the presence of intestinal obstruction. It is recognised as writhing movements in the centre of the abdomen. Visible bulges may also be due to gross enlargement of the liver, spleen or kidneys, or to large tumours.

### Palpation

The examiner's hands must be warm. When they are cold, then by far the quickest method of warming them is by immersion in hot water. If there are no facilities for warming, the hands should be rubbed together vigorously and the temperature of the skin of the patient's abdominal wall should be brought into equilibrium with that of the examining hand by light palpation all over. It may help to prepare the patient and to reduce the shock of a cold examining hand if it is first placed upon the patient's forearm. An assessment of obesity can be made by grasping a double thickness of skin and subcutaneous tissue between the fingers and thumb.

**Light Palpation.** Muscle tone should be tested by light dipping movements over symmetrical areas commencing at the point most remote from the site of any pain. The patient's face should be watched for any grimace indicative of local tenderness. Resistance due to increased muscle tone commonly accompanies organic lesions, particularly when pain is present, and it may be restricted to one side or to any quadrant of the abdomen according to the

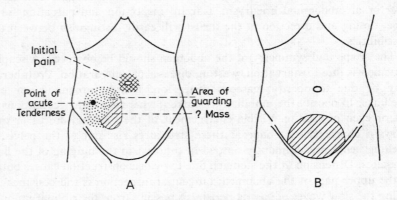

FIG. 39   THE USE OF DIAGRAMS IN CASE RECORDING.
A. Pain, tenderness, guarding and mass in patient with acute appendicitis and appendix abscess.   B. Tumour arising from the pelvis. This could be a bladder, uterine or ovarian swelling.

organ affected or the area over which the peritoneum is involved. Another sign of some value in this context is *rebound pain*, indicating inflammation of some part of the peritoneum. Rebound pain is elicited in the affected region by the sudden release of pressure of the hand which has been applied firmly over an area of the abdomen which may even be remote from the pain.

Generalised rigidity of the abdominal muscles is commonly due to the inability of a nervous patient to relax. This cause can usually be suspected by the circumstances, and confirmed by variability in the resistance and transient relaxation during the earliest phase of expiration. The tendency can be reduced by ensuring that the patient is warm and comfortable and that the examiner's hand is not cold, and by gaining the patient's confidence by very light palpation at first. Generalised rigidity due to acute peritonitis is persistent and is accompanied by tenderness; the abdomen does not move with respiration and bowel sounds cease.

**Deep Palpation.** The abdomen should now be palpated more deeply. The predominant use of the finger-tips is apt to induce muscular resistance and lead to inefficient results. Using the flat of the hand, the gut can be displaced and abnormal masses may be felt. The liver edge and the lower pole of the right kidney are often palpable in normal persons.

Enlargement of the bladder, ovary or uterus, often already suspected from inspection, may be confirmed as a dome-shaped swelling rising above the pubis. It should be possible to identify the normal colon in the left iliac fossa; the caecum and sometimes the transverse colon may also be palpable particularly if they contain faeces. The massaging effect of feeling for these structures often causes them to contract and to become more readily palpable. The aorta is often palpable and it may be slightly tender. If any mass is present, then its characteristics should be identified so that all the points mentioned on page 48 have been observed. It must be borne in mind that a

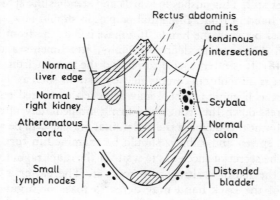

FIG. 40  PALPATION OF THE ABDOMEN
Some 'normal' findings which are often misinterpreted.

hard craggy lump, indistinguishable at first from a malignant tumour, may be due to faeces in a constipated patient in which case the lump disappears or changes its position after the next bowel action. Faeces are commonly palpable in the sigmoid colon; in severe constipation, irrespective of whether it is due to bad habit or to organic obstruction, faecal masses may be palpable throughout the colon or in any part of it.

Caudal movement on inspiration means that the structure or mass is not part of the abdominal wall. It does not necessarily mean that it is intraperitoneal, for both the kidneys and the pancreas move with respiration, although not so freely as the liver or the spleen. An upper abdominal mass which does not move with respiration either arises from or has become attached to the parietes (the walls of a cavity or organ). Masses which are superficially situated in the abdominal wall continue to be palpable when the muscles are contracted by raising the head off the pillow or by blowing against resistance.

Tightening the muscles in this way is an important method of identifying the intersections of the recti abdominis. An intersection frequently misleads the unwary beginner into believing that a tumour has been felt. Parietal masses situated deep to the muscles of the abdominal wall and also swellings in the abdominal cavity, are less easily felt when the muscles are contracted.

**Bimanual Palpation.** A bimanual technique should always be used for palpating the liver, kidneys, spleen and intra-abdominal masses. Examination couches are generally made at a convenient height. When the patient is in bed it may be necessary in the interests of comfort and efficiency to sit or kneel beside the bed, especially while examining the nearside of the abdomen. One hand should be placed posteriorly in the gap between the twelfth rib and the iliac crest, with the finger-tips lateral to the erector spinae. There is usually space enough for one to three fingers which should be pressed firmly over this area and kept still. This pushes forwards and steadies the structures to be felt by the other hand in front. Bimanual palpation should now easily appreciate any solid mass between the hands. If a mass is felt, the front hand should be moved in all directions to define its limits, attachments and other characteristics (p. 48). It is often useful to remind the patient from time to time to relax. If there is difficulty in complying, suggestions such as 'lie heavily on the bed' or 'relax as if going to sleep' may achieve the desired result; if not, it is helpful to press down the front hand firmly immediately after the height of inspiration, for at this moment the abdominal muscles will be relaxed.

The liver, spleen and kidneys should be examined in turn by a bimanual technique. The secret of success is to wait for the diaphragm to push down the organ onto the hands waiting to receive it. Thereafter a quick forward movement of the back hand may detect a mass or organ, which might not otherwise be felt, by bumping it against the hand in front.

**Palpation of the Liver.** A satisfactory position of the hands can usually be achieved if the examiner sits on the edge of the bed or kneels beside it. The front hand should be placed flat with the fingers pointing upwards and placed so that the sensing fingers (index and middle) are lateral to the rectus muscle (Fig. 41). The hand should be firmly pressed inwards and upwards and it should be kept steady while the patient takes a deep breath through the mouth. At the height of inspiration the inward pressure on the front hand is released while the upward pressure is maintained. At this movement the tips of the fingers should slip over the edge of a palpable liver. It should be noted whether the edge is sharp and flexible as is normal, or whether it is rounded, firm, irregular or tender. The surface of a palpable liver should then be felt for irregularities using the finger-tips and keeping them steady in a new position each time the patient takes a deep breath. Irregularities may be felt as the liver slides under the finger-tips with each respiration. Two common errors should be avoided. One is to feel for the liver with the hand placed horizontally. In this position the palm of the hand is pressing backwards the

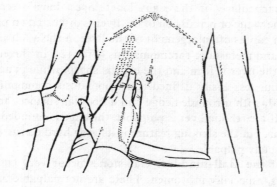

FIG. 41   Palpation of the Liver.

edge which it is desired to feel. This is particularly the case in those people in whom the right lobe of the liver lies almost vertically. The second error is to start feeling too high up with the front hand; a palpable liver cannot always be appreciated between the two hands unless it is much harder than normal. This is because the posterior surface of the liver, unless it is enlarged, does not usually reach down as far as the back hand. It should also be noted that forward rotation of the liver will bring down the anterior margin though the edge may be difficult to feel; the level of the lower border must then be judged by the much less reliable feeling of a sense of resistance. The fact that the liver is palpable for a distance of three or four fingerbreadths below the costal margin does not necessarily mean that it is abnormal. The significance of the finding must be judged by the characteristics mentioned above and by the slope of the edge. A normal liver is often palable, especially in adult women

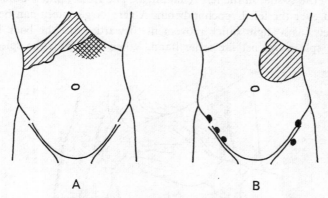

A        B

FIG. 42   THE USE OF DIAGRAMS IN CASE RECORDING.

A. Abdominal mass and enlarged liver in patient with gastric carcinoma and hepatic metastases.
B. Splenomegaly and lymphadenopathy in a patient with Hodgkin's disease.

and children particularly if the right lobe slopes down steeply from the epigastrium. The value of percussion of the liver is discussed on page 219 .

The common causes of enlargement of the liver in the adult in Britain are cardiac failure and metastatic carcinomatosis (Fig. 42). In chronic congestive cardiac failure the liver is firm and the edge is sharp, while in acute failure it is also tender but less easily defined. Carcinomatosis commonly causes the liver to feel hard, with a rounded edge and a nodular surface, and there may be tenderness. If a cirrhotic liver is palpable, the edge is rounded and perhaps slightly irregular, but the striking feature is its very hard consistency, and the spleen is also usually palpable.

**Palpation of the Gall-bladder.** Gall-stones occur very commonly with advancing years, especially in women. These are not palpable unless a single very large stone is present. Stones, however, are often associated with attacks of acute cholecystitis, with tenderness below the right costal margin midway between the xiphisternum and the flank. If the examiner's hand is placed over this situation and the patient is asked to take a deep breath, inspiration may be sharply arrested due to a sudden accentuation of pain (sometimes described as Murphy's sign).

Enlargement of the gall bladder in the absence of jaundice is due to obstruction of the cystic duct leading to mucocele or empyema. Obstruction of the common bile duct leads to jaundice; if the gall-bladder is also enlarged, the obstruction will be due to causes other than gall-stones since in most cases of cholelithiasis the wall of the gall-bladder is thickened and toughened by changes due to chronic cholecystitis and it cannot stretch (Courvoisier's law). Carcinoma of the head of the pancreas is the most common cause of palpable enlargement of the gall-bladder in the presence of obstructive jaundice.

**Palpation of the Spleen.** This should be done bimanually with one hand supporting the tissues in the left renal angle. The front hand should be firmly placed flat over the left hypochondrium. A very large spleen can be detected immediately, as a slight quick movement forwards with the back hand will bump the spleen against the other hand. When the tip of the spleen is just

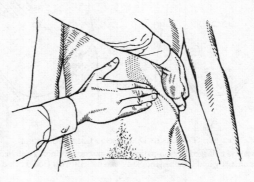

Fig. 43    Palpation of the Spleen.

beneath, at, or just below the costal margin, the front hand should be placed an inch or two below the ribs and then pressed upwards towards the left axilla, so that the fingers either touch the spleen or come to lie beneath the costal margin (Fig. 43). When the patient takes a deep breath through the open mouth, an enlarged spleen will bump against the tips of the index and middle fingers. At the height of inspiration, the pressure on the hand should be released so that the finger-tips slip over the pole of the spleen, confirming its presence and feeling its surface and consistency. It is almost invariable that an enlarged spleen retains its shape. Therefore if a lump is felt below the left costal margin which does not feel smooth and rounded, it should be regarded as something other than the lower pole of the spleen. On rare occasions it is easier to feel the tip of the spleen with the patient lying on the right side and with the left hip and knee flexed at a right angle.

When the spleen is large enough to be felt in the loin it is often stated that it may be mistaken for a large kidney. This difficulty does not arise if the mass is examined properly. The features which are particularly characteristic of a spleen are that the fingers can usually be pushed deep to the anterior edge and under the lower pole, and the postero-lateral edge can generally be appreciated in the loin. It will not be possible to insert the fingers between the firm, flat mass and the costal margin. In addition, a very large spleen tends to point towards the right iliac fossa and may cross the midline and one or two notches may be felt on the anterior edge. An enlarged kidney rarely crosses the midline; it fills the loin diffusely, and unless a lump projects from it, the fingers cannot be inserted deep to the mass at any point.

**Palpation of the Kidneys.** A bimanual technique similar, except for two differences, to that described for the liver and the spleen should be employed. Firstly the front hand should be laid lightly over the abdomen in a position suitable for deep palpation just lateral to the spine (Fig. 44). Secondly the patient should be asked to take a deep breath, and immediately after the end

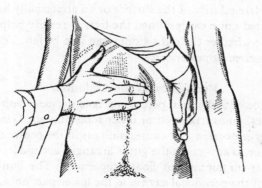

FIG. 44   Palpation of the Kidney from the Opposite Side.

of inspiration the front hand should be pressed firmly back against the hand behind. If pressure is applied before a breath is taken the kidney may be prevented from descending as it is not pushed down by the diaphragm with the same force as the liver and spleen. When a kidney is felt between the two hands, its presence should be confirmed by a brisk flexion movement of the fingers of the hand in the renal angle; this will bump the kidney forward on to the front hand. An alternative position of the hands is shown in Figure 45. A normal kidney has a very firm consistency and the surface is smooth. The lower half of the normal right kidney is often palpable, especially in slim women. The normal left kidney is less often palpable, especially if the other one cannot also be felt. By tilting the upper borders of the palpating hands towards one another it is sometimes possible to squeeze the right kidney down below the hand. Then by pressing the lower borders of the hands towards one another and releasing the pressure of the upper fingers, but without otherwise moving the hands, the kidney may slide back above both hands. In making

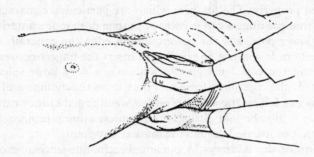

FIG. 45    Palpation of the Kidney from the Same Side.

this manœuvre an excellent idea of the normal size and consistency of the kidney can be obtained. Owing to the varying thickness of the parietes, enlargement of a kidney, unless it is gross, is difficult to judge without a good deal of practice. Irregularity of the surface or an abnormally hard consistency may be appreciated quite easily. When the liver is readily palpable, it may be difficult to decide whether the right kidney can also be felt. Tenderness of the kidney is usually greatest posteriorly.

### Percussion of the Abdomen

The main value of abdominal percussion is to decide whether distension is due to gas, ascites, an ovarian cyst or other solid tumour. Gaseous distension is resonant. A large *ovarian cyst* causes dullness in the centre of the abdomen and resonance due to any gas in the gut is arranged around it. In the presence of *ascites* the gas-containing gut floats uppermost. The liquid flows to the dependent part of the peritoneal cavity, to the lower part on standing, to both flanks on lying supine and to one side when reclining. This shifting dullness should be sought in confirmation of ascites. It is usually simplest to detect it by examining the patient supine and then when rolled on to each side in turn. The presence of small quantities of free fluid in the peritoneal cavity cannot be determined with certainty, for slight changes in percussion note may be due to gravitational shift of normal bowel. Two abnormal conditions in particular should be borne in mind as they are apt to simulate slight ascites; firstly the pot belly and dilated small intestine in patients with steatorrhoea, and secondly pneumoperitoneum. A moderate accumulation of ascites should already have been suspected from inspection and palpation. If the abdominal muscles are well relaxed, a characteristic wobbly sensation similar to that of handling a partly filled rubber water-bottle, may also have been noted. An additional useful sign is dipping over the liver or spleen if either of these organs is palpable. The examiner's hand is laid over the abdomen, and quick dipping movements are made so that the palms of the fingers dart in towards the organ. The sudden displacement of liquid gives a tapping sensation on the surface of the liver or spleen comparable to the patellar tap (p. 360). Conversely, by this manœuvre it may also be possible to detect and to map the outlines of enlarged organs or of tumours which cannot be felt in the ordinary way because the abdomen is so distended. Very large accumulations of ascites or large liquid-containing cysts may give a palpable thrill. In order to detect this, one of the examiner's hands is placed flat on the patient's flank. The other flank is then flicked or tapped, and a shock wave is transmitted to the palpating hand. A third person, or the active participation of the patient, is required, for a hand should also be placed in the midline of the abdomen to prevent any ripple from passing through the fat of the anterior abdominal wall. In a thin patient this is not necessary.

Resonance to percussion is valuable evidence that a swelling contains or is overlain by gas.

Percussion is a poor second-best method of seeking for enlargement of the *spleen,* but its employment may be necessary when adequate relaxation of the abdominal muscles cannot be achieved or if it is doubtful whether the tip can be felt. Normally the spleen lies against the posterolateral wall of the abdominal cavity beneath the ninth, tenth and eleventh ribs. As it enlarges, it remains closely applied to this wall, growing forwards, downwards and eventually medially, the tip emerging somewhere beneath the left costal margin. The patient should therefore be asked to take in a deep breath and hold it while the area just above the costal margin is percussed from front to back. The position of the underlying spleen may be detected by impairment of the percussion note.

Percussion of the borders of the *liver* is likely to lead to gross under-estimation of its size. Although the upper border may be raised by a greatly enlarged liver, the change from resonance to dullness is dependent upon the level of the diaphragm and the state of the lung and pleura. The apparent level of the lower border of the liver varies with the amount of gas in the colon. Even when light percussion is employed it will be observed that a palpable lower border may be 3 or 4 cm below the edge detected by percussion. Thus a combination of pulmonary emphysema and gaseous distension of the colon may make it almost impossible to detect the liver by percussion. However, when palpation is uninformative owing to rigidity of the abdominal muscles, percussion may be some value in determining the position of the lower border of the liver. During this procedure also, the patient should take a deep breath and hold it. Absence of liver dullness may be of contributary diagnostic value when gas has leaked from a perforated peptic ulcer.

## Auscultation of the Abdomen

Movement of the bowel contents by peristaltic activity of the gut creates characteristic gurgling sounds which may be heard from time to time by the unaided ear. Through the stethoscope they can be heard every 5 to 10 seconds, though the interval varies greatly in relationship to meals. Bowel sounds disappear in paralytic ileus (obstruction) which is usually secondary to peritonitis. They increase in frequency and intensity in the presence of diarrhoea due to disorders of the small intestine, and when there is much blood in the bowel from a bleeding peptic ulcer; the noise may be so loud in the rare carcinoid syndrome as to cause social embarrassment. When mechanical obstruction is present, not only are the sounds increased in frequency and intensity, but gaseous distension of the gut adds a tinkling quality to the sounds. Attention should be paid to the pitch of the sounds which, like rhonchi in the bronchial tree, vary in accordance with the size of the tube involved.

Systolic murmurs due to strictures of mesenteric or renal arteries may be audible but owing to the distracting effects of the bowel sounds, a conscious effort must be made if bruits of vascular origin are to be heard. A venous hum is occasionally present in the liver area due to turbulence in a well-developed collateral circulation from portal hypertension. Friction sounds resembling those of pleurisy may rarely be heard over an area of perisplenitis or perihepatitis.

## Examination of the Groins

After examining the abdomen it is convenient at this point to palpate the groins for the femoral pulses and for abnormal lymph nodes. The normal variation in size and consistency of the latter can be appreciated only by making this a routine practice. At the same time, hernias may be observed but their presence cannot be excluded unless the groins are examined while the patient is standing.

**The Examination of Hernias.** The principles described on page 48 for the examination of swellings apply to hernias but emphasis has to be placed on certain anatomical features. Hernias occur at the site of operation scars and at points of anatomical weakness. All hernias bulge more when the pressure within them is raised. Hernias of the abdominal wall are therefore more prominent in the erect position, and an impulse can be felt in the hernia when the patient coughs. It must be remembered, however, that both of these features also apply to a saphenous varix. After the identification of a hernia, an attempt should be made to replace the contents by the application of gentle sustained pressure. An obstructed hernia cannot be reduced and a strangulated hernia is tense and tender and shows no impulse on coughing.

An *indirect inguinal hernia* bulges through the internal inguinal ring and may extend down the inguinal canal into the scrotum or labium major. It therefore lies above the pubic tubercle, whereas a *femoral hernia* lies in the femoral canal below and lateral to the tubercle. These hernias usually contain small intestine which is neither resonant to percussion nor transilluminant.

A *direct inguinal hernia* bulges forward above the inguinal ligament and does not extend to the scrotum. It protrudes through the fascia transversalis medial to the inferior epigastric artery and lateral to the rectus sheath. Following reduction, pressure over the mid-inguinal point will obliterate the cough impulse in an indirect inguinal hernia but not in a direct hernia.

An *umbilical hernia* bulges through the fascia around the navel. It is very common in babies and usually disappears spontaneously. It is also frequently encountered in women who have borne many children. Divarication of the recti is also common in multiparous women and becomes evident immediately the supine patient attempts to sit; the intra-abdominal pressure rises and the region of the linea alba bulges between the recti abdominis.

An *epigastric hernia* is common and is visible as a small swelling not usually more than 1 cm. in diameter. It is due to a piece of extraperitoneal fat bulging through a defect in the linea alba. By gentle massage with the finger-tip it is often possible to reduce such a hernia and then the small defect in the tendon can be felt.

*Incisional hernias* may form at the site of any operation on the abdomen, especially if the wound has been complicated by sepsis.

*External hernias at other sites* are comparatively rare.

## Examination of the Male Genitalia

In the male, examination of the genitalia conveniently follows palpation of the groins. The penis and scrotum are inspected and the testes, epididymes and vasa deferentia palpated. Minor degrees of hypospadias (p. 410) occur once in every 300 boys. Other conditions which should be borne in mind are syphilis and gonorrhoea, and enlargement of the groin lymph nodes should lead to careful search for a chancre or a urethral discharge in cases in which these conditions might not otherwise have been suspected. Both testes are atrophic in hypogonadism and one may atrophy after orchitis due to mumps. An empty scrotum on one or both sides should lead to a search for incompletely descended testes in the inguinal canal or for ectopic testes in sites such as the groin or above the pubis outside the line of normal descent of the testicle.

Examination of a scrotal swelling should follow the principles laid down on page 48. The first objective must be to confirm that the swelling is of the scrotum and its contents rather than an inguinal hernia. Since the scrotum contains paired structures, the two sides should be compared; its accessibility enables the exact site of origin of a swelling or other change to be accurately determined by careful palpation. Finally an indication of the pathology will be provided by the consistency of the swelling and by the presence or absence of signs of inflammation.

Swellings within the scrotum commonly contain a clear liquid, a fact which can be confirmed by transillumination (page 52). A hydrocele, a spermatocele and a cyst of the epididymis are differentiated by their relationships to the testis as illustrated in Figure 46. The possibility that a hydrocele may obscure

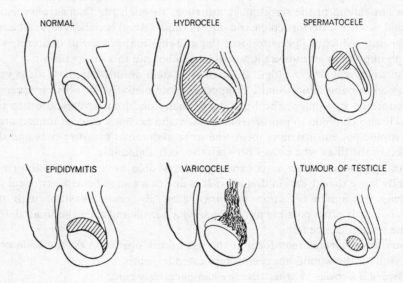

FIG. 46    Swellings of the Scrotum.

a testicular tumour must not be overlooked and in each case the testis must be palpated with care. Infections other than syphilis and mumps affect primarily the epididymis and tuberculosis produces a characteristic nodular change within the epididymis accompanied by thickening of the cord. Shortening of the cord is a characteristic of torsion of the testis, so that the lesion comes to resemble a strangulated hernia. The differention is made by the pain which is felt in the iliac fossa and is constant from the outset in torsion of the testis.

Examination of the genital organs in the female is described on page 226. It is not a routine procedure.

### Examination of the Rectum
Because digital examination of the rectum is slightly disagreeable to the

patient and a little extra trouble for the doctor it is often omitted from the routine physical examination. There is no doubt that many have suffered from the consequences of the neglect of this simple procedure. The student should seize every opportunity to make a rectal examination in order to become familiar with the feel of the normal structures. Male students must ask a nurse or a female colleague to be in attendance when the patient is female. Digital examination of the rectum should be included in all cases of doubt and in particular in the following circumstances:

1. *Alimentary problems*
    Suspected appendicitis; pelvic abscess; peritonitis.
    All cases of abdominal pain in which the cause is obscure.
    Diarrhoea or constipation; mucus or blood in the stools.
    Anal irritation or pain; tenesmus or rectal pain.
    Bimanual examination of a lower abdominal mass.
    In the search for tumours or transperitoneal metastases either
        diagnostically or in making a decision about treatment.

2. *Genito-urinary problems*
    Dysuria; haematuria; haematospermia; epididymo-orchitis.
    In lieu of gynaecological examination in virgins.

3. *Miscellaneous problems*
    In the search for a cause of backache, root pains in the legs or diffuse
        bone pains.
    In all cases of pyrexia of unknown origin.

**Digital Examination.** The patient should be informed that it is necessary to examine the back passage. If the examiner is right-handed, the patient should lie in the left lateral position with a maximal degree of flexion of the spine and legs consistent with comfort. The buttocks should be at the edge of the couch or bed. The examiner's right forefinger, preferably protected by a fingerstall or a suitable glove, should be smeared with a lubricant. In a good light the perianal skin should be examined for intertrigo or for evidence of scratching, thrombosed external piles or fistulae. Fistula-in-ano should lead to a search for pulmonary tuberculosis or for disease of the small or large gut. The possibility of a chancre or of gonorrhoea must also be borne in mind.

The patient should be informed that the finger within the rectum will cause a sensation similar to that of opening the bowels. After asking the patient to relax, the forefinger tip is placed on the anal margin and with steady pressure on the sphincter is moved to point upwards and slightly forwards. The finger is then inserted gently through the anal canal into the rectum (Fig. 47a and b). Resistance at the anus is commonly due to spasm induced by nervousness, and

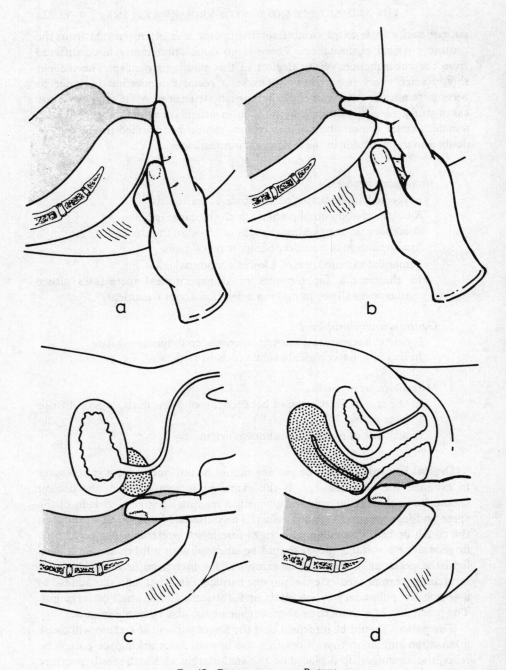

FIG. 47   EXAMINATION OF THE RECTUM

The finger is inserted as shown in (a) and (b).   The hand is then rotated and the most prominent features
are the prostate in the male (c) and the cervix in the female (d).

this can sometimes be overcome by asking the patient to strain down in an attempt to defaecate. If spasm is associated with local pain, the presence of an anal fissure should be suspected; a local anaesthetic suppository may be required before a satisfactory examination can be made. Rarely, tightness is due to a fibrous stricture or a growth or to Hirschsprung's disease in the infant (p. 400). Beyond the anal canal, the direction of the rectum is upwards and backwards along the curve of the coccyx and the sacrum. The exploring finger should then feel round the whole extent of the rectum. The normal rectum should be empty and the wall should be smooth and soft. In cases of habitual constipation the rectum is full of firm faeces, though in elderly patients, especially after barium radiographic studies of the alimentary tract, faecal impaction in the rectum may cause spurious diarrhoea and faecal incontinence. An obstructing carcinoma of the upper rectum will produce a ballooning of the empty cavity below. Posteriorly the coccyx and sacrum can be felt through the rectal wall, while anteriorly from below upwards, the membranous urethra, the prostate and often the base of the bladder may be felt in the male, while the firm round cervix uteri can be felt projecting backwards in the female (Fig. 47c & d). The normal prostate is smooth and has a fairly firm consistency with the contours of miniature buttocks represented by the lateral lobes and a median groove between them. When the prostate is palpated the patient should be informed that he will probably feel the desire to pass urine. Prostatic hyperplasia in the adult, which may be responsible for obstruction of the urinary outflow, commonly causes a palpable enlargement. The prostate is abnormally small in hypogonadism due to castration, treatment by oestrogens, hypopituitarism, Klinefelter's syndrome or other causes. Tenderness, accompanied by other local and systemic symptoms and by a change in the consistency of the gland, may be due to prostatitis or an abscess. A hard, irregular gland, which may be fixed to the mucosa or the surrounding structures, and usually without a detectable median groove, is characteristic of carcinoma. It must be remembered that piles which are not thrombosed and normal seminal vesicles cannot be felt.

Any deviation from normal should be noted, and lumps in particular should be examined by the systematic method described on page 48. For this purpose it is sometimes helpful to palpate bimanually with the other hand laid flat over the abdomen. A faecal mass is commonly palpable and this should be movable and may be indented. If several masses are present, the examination should be repeated after the patient has defaecated. Metastases or a tumour in a loop of colon lying in the lower part of the peritoneal cavity may otherwise be mistaken for faeces. The finger after withdrawal should be examined for blood, and the colour of the faeces should be noted. A sample of faeces from the finger-stall can be tested chemically for occult blood (p. 453).

**Proctoscopy.** Visual examination of the rectum and anal canal is an extension of the digital method. It is essential for the diagnosis of inflammatory lesions and of piles. Through the proctoscope it is also possible to inspect any palpable lesions, to remove polypi and to take specimens for biopsy. The patient should be asked to kneel with the feet over the edge of a firm couch, then bend forward with the shoulders down and head turned to one side on a pillow. The examination is facilitated if the thighs are placed perpendicular to the couch and the knees and feet are separated, while the lumbar spine is extended. The forefinger and thumb of one hand separate the buttocks, while with the other, a warmed and well-lubricated proctoscope is gently inserted in the same directions as described for digital examination. Similar instructions should be followed for sigmoidoscopy, but owing to the technical difficulty of passing the instrument round the rectosigmoid junction in many cases, the sigmoidoscope should be reserved for those trained in its regular use. The surface of the normal rectum can be closely compared to the appearance of the buccal musoca—clean, shiny, smooth, reddish pink with clearly visible submucosal veins here and there.

For the detection of piles the patient should lie in the lateral position and be asked to strain down as the proctoscope is gradually withdrawn. Under these conditions the piles will be distended with blood and their extent can be fully appreciated. The lateral position is suitable also for sigmoidoscopic or proctoscopic examination of the feeble, elderly and infirm.

### Gynaecological Examination

The peculiarly intimate nature of a gynaecological examination not only makes it difficult to combine with routine abdominal examination, but also renders it more likely to raise medico-legal problems than any other form of medical examination. The patient's consent must, of course, always be obtained, and a suitable third person should be present during examination.

For the comfort of the patient and for ease of interpretation of the examination, it is important that the bowel and bladder should be empty. The patient should lie comfortably on her back with her head on pillows so as to relax the abdominal muscles. The hips and knees should be flexed, the thighs abducted, and illumination arranged so that a good light falls upon the vulva. The examiner is advised to wear rubber gloves which should be smeared with a suitable lubricant. The labia minora should be separated by the forefinger and thumb of one hand, bringing into view the clitoris anteriorly, then the urethra, the vagina and finally the anus posteriorly. Any discharge from the urethra or vagina should be swabbed; one specimen should be sent for culture and another smeared on to a glass slide for microscopical examination. Direct microscopy of a smear is particularly useful in the confirmation of infection due to *Trichomonas vaginalis*; a stained smear may give conclusive evidence of gonorrhoea or thrush infection.

The lateral walls of the vulva on either side of the vagina should be palpated for abnormalities of Bartholin's glands. In parous women two fingers should then be turned palmar surface down and spread, to test for laxity of the superficial muscles, and to allow inspection of the vaginal walls for prolapse when the patient is asked to strain down. The index finger of the other hand and in most cases the middle finger too should then be inserted into the vagina. The cervix uteri is readily felt, being circular, with a small central os in the nulliparous patient. The normal cervix points downwards and slightly backwards. In parous women, the cervix is usually larger and the os a good deal bigger and often palpable as a transverse slit.

Bimanual palpation is now made. With the middle finger at the os and the forefinger in the anterior fornix, the other hand is placed flat on the abdomen and worked down towards the pubis. The position and other characteristics of the uterus can then be identified between the hands. Each fornix should now be palpated in turn with particular regard to tenderness and swellings of the Fallopian tubes and ovaries. The bladder lies immediately anteriorly. In the posterior fornix, abnormalities may be appreciated in the pouch of Douglas, and faecal masses may be identified by the fact that they become indented.

Digital examination should be supplemented by inspection of the vagina and uterine cervix through a vaginal speculum. At this stage it is now routine practice to take a smear from the cervix using an Ayres spatula. Cytological examination of such smears is an important screening procedure in the early detection of cancer of the cervix.

Vaginal examination of virgins should if possible be avoided, and minors should not be examined without the consent of a parent or guardian. In these circumstances adequate information can often be obtained by digital examination of the rectum.

## EXAMINATION OF URINE, VOMIT AND FAECES

Testing of the urine is an essential part of every clinical examination. Vomit should be inspected and the stools also if there is any indication to do so. The little extra effort involved is often productive of much useful evidence. The details of this important part of the examination are described in Chapter 12.

## FURTHER INVESTIGATIONS

In many cases it will be possible to make a satisfactory diagnosis by clinical examination alone. In others further investigations will be required either to confirm the clinical opinion, or to establish a diagnosis when this has not been possible otherwise. The following notes are given as a rough guide to the main procedures available and to the indications for their use.

### Alimentary System

**Alimentary Tract.** Radiological examination by the use of barium sulphate emulsion or sometimes other contrast media is of particular value.

The oesophagus, stomach and duodenum can be outlined by a barium meal, thus demonstrating such lesions as oesophageal stricture, cardiospasm, hiatus hernia, peptic ulceration and carcinoma. Errors of interpretation can however occur, particularly at the cardia. By following the barium through the alimentary tract, changes may be demonstrated in the pattern of the small intestine which may indicate such processes as regional enteritis or the malabsorption syndrome. The looping of the small intestine is so complex, however, that gross lesions may be overlooked. Barium enema is a reasonably reliable method of demonstrating tumours, diverticula and chronic inflammatory conditions, but lesions of the rectum and in the region of the rectosigmoid junction are difficult to delineate. Sigmoidoscopy should therefore precede barium enema, and indeed may obviate the necessity for it. With this exception endoscopy, i.e. oesophagoscopy and gastroscopy, is usually delayed until a lesion has first been located or sought by radiological examination. In the case of dysphagia, oesophagoscopy may be required even if the barium swallow is negative, unless a neurological or neuromuscular cause is beyond reasonable doubt. In iron-deficiency anaemia associated with occult blood in the stools, examination may be necessary both by barium meal and barium enema. Normally the enema should be carried out first as the barium is usually evacuated promptly and examination by barium meal can, if the diagnosis is still in doubt, be conducted without further delay. In acute abdominal conditions radiographs of the abdomen taken in the erect and lying positions, may be most helpful by showing such features as gas under the diaphragm following perforation of the gut or gaseous distension and fluid levels in the bowel proximal to an obstruction.

Biopsy specimens may be taken through the oesophagoscope, proctoscope or sigmoidoscope. Pieces of mucous membrane may also be obtained blindly from the stomach and the small intestine by being sucked into a capsule at the end of a flexible tube. Exfoliative cytology is occasionally helpful in suspected neoplasm of the stomach; deposits of the centrifuged gastric juice are examined for malignant cells by a pathologist experienced in this technique.

Chemical examination of the stools for occult blood by a simple tablet test (p. 453) is often positive in the presence of ulcerative, inflammatory or neoplastic lesions of the alimentary tract. A persistently positive test may therefore be a valuable guide to the necessity for a complete investigation of the alimentary tract, and if necessary may lead to laparotomy in patients with unexplained iron-deficiency anaemia or obscure abdominal symptoms.

The main tests of function are those for gastric secretion and intestinal absorption. The pentagastrin secretion test is of great importance for the demonstration of achlorhydria and of considerable value in the management of patients with a duodenal ulcer. Intestinal absorption may be assessed in many ways, but the principles involved are simple and are enumerated below. The absorption, metabolism and excretion of any individual substance is so complex, however, that several tests are usually employed in conjunction.

1. The stools may be examined microscopically (p. 453 ) and biochemically for evidence of failure to digest or absorb food, especially fat and protein.

2. Blood may be tested for the appropriate rise in concentration of a substance given by mouth, e.g. glucose.

3. Urine may be collected for the estimation of substances which, after absorption, are largely excreted by the kidneys, e.g. xylose. Folic acid and vitamin $B_{12}$ absorption tests may help to differentiate between disease of the jejunum and ileum, as hydroxocobalamin is absorbed solely in the ileum. The validity of these tests on the urine is dependent upon normal renal function.

**Liver.** The main emphasis in most cases is on confirmatory biochemical tests of the synthetic and the excretory functions of the liver, as the most common problem is to distinguish between hepato-cellular and obstructive jaundice. Assessment of synthetic activity includes estimations of serum proteins, various precipitation and flocculation tests on the serum which depend upon differential protein changes, the prothrombin concentration in the blood and its response to the parenteral administration of vitamin $K_1$. The excretory functions include the estimation of serum bilirubin, alkaline phosphatase and cholesterol, and the bromsulphthalein test. In addition, when the liver cells are damaged, the concentration of substances normally contained within them, such as glutamic pyruvic transaminase (G.P.T.), may rise in the serum.

Percutaneous biopsy of the liver may provide valuable histological information, though the procedure should not be undertaken lightly as it involves a small but definite risk to life from haemorrhage as a result of the bleeding tendency which may be present with diffuse hepatic disease. When obstructive jaundice is present the dangers are increased by the risk of the more lethal biliary peritonitis in which the symptoms are slow in onset and difficult to recognise.

Radiological investigations may be of value in cirrhosis of the liver by the demonstration of filling defects in the oesophagus due to varices, or by the more elaborate procedure of portal venography, during which the portal venous pressure may be measured. Portal venography may also demonstrate space occupying lesions such as tumours or abscesses in the liver though selective hepatic arteriography is better for this purpose. Space occupying lesions may also be detected by a radioisotope scan or by means of ultrasound.

**Biliary tract.** Radiological examination is of great value in confirming the clinical diagnosis of gall-stones. It must be borne in mind, however, that calculi are often present without symptoms. They may be seen on a routine radiograph, but many gall-stones are radiotranslucent and a contrast technique of cholecystography or cholangiography is necessary. The fact that the dye used for cholangiography is also excreted by the kidneys accounts for the confusion which may arise from simultaneous opacification of the right renal pelvis, particularly when hepatic function is poor. If the serum bilirubin is above 2·5 mg per 100 ml neither the gall-bladder nor the ducts are likely to be visualised.

**Pancreas.** Tests of exocrine secretion may be made by collecting pancreatic juice through a tube passed through the mouth or nose into the duodenum. Extensive disease of the pancreas may also damage its endocrine function, with the development of overt or latent diabetes. Hence a glucose tolerance test is particularly useful in distinguishing between malabsorption due to pancreatic disease in which there is a diabetic type of curve and that due to diffuse disease of the small intestine in which there may be an abnormally small and sustained rise in the blood sugar.

Acute pancreatitis is accompanied by a transient but often marked increase of the serum amylase, but it should be noted that this may also rise during other abdominal crises, especially when there is a perforated duodenal ulcer. Radiological examination may show displacement of the stomach and duodenum by swelling of the pancreas and absence of gas in the middle of the transverse colon.

## Urinary System

**Kidney.** One kidney is sufficient to maintain normal renal function. When there is clinical evidence of renal failure, disease of both kidneys must be present, though this may in some cases be temporary. A simple estimate of renal failure may be made by measuring the rise in the blood levels of the nitrogenous waste products, especially urea while the bicarbonate falls in proportion to the rise in acid metabolites.

The glomerular filtration rate may be assessed by measuring the renal clearance of endogenous creatinine. Tubular function can be judged approximately by determining the power of the kidneys to acidify and to form concentrated or dilute urine (pp. 427 and 428). Histological examination of the glomeruli and tubules in specimens obtained by percutaneous biopsy can be made by the ordinary light or the electron microscope. The main indication for biopsy is in the differentiation of the causes of the nephrotic syndrome.

Total plasma flow can be estimated by the clearance of para amino-hippuric acid. The demonstration of a renal artery stenosis leading to a reduction in blood flow to one kidney may be of importance in a patient with arterial hypertension. The presence of such a lesion may be indicated by an audible vascular bruit. Radiologically an intravenous pyelogram (I.V.P.) usually shows a greater concentration of dye on the affected side, while the radioactivity over the kidney after an intravenous dose of radiohippuran is less. The renal arteries and their branches may be outlined by aortography. The function of each kidney can be assessed separately by collecting urine through ureteric catheters.

**Urinary Tract.** The urethra, bladder and ureteric orifices can be seen endoscopically. On radiological examination, shadows of both kidneys can usually be seen on a plain film of the abdomen; calcification in the parenchyma and radio-opaque calculi will also be visible. An outline of the renal pelvis, ureters and bladder can be obtained by I.V.P. or retrograde pyelography. Such investigations are indicated in a great variety of congenital, infective and neoplastic conditions and when the presence of calculi is suspected.

### Genital System

Comparatively few investigations of the genital system are available or are indeed necessary, as for most purposes the structures concerned are reasonably accessible to clinical examination. In either sex appropriate specimens may be required to confirm the diagnosis of venereal infection or to identify the cause of discharges.

The investigations of sterility may require seminal analysis or testicular biopsy in the male, and insufflation of air or injection of radio-opaque oil into the genital tract in the female. Pregnancy can be confirmed by immunological and other tests whereby the presence of chorionic gonadotrophin in the patient's urine is demonstrated. The diagnosis can be made in this way at a much earlier stage than is possible by clinical means but it must be borne in mind that positive results are also obtained when a hydatidiform mole or a chorionepithelioma is present.

Microscopical examination of the lining of the uterus after dilatation of the cervix and curettage (D. & C.) is a routine procedure in the investigation of abnormal vaginal bleeding, and biopsy of the cervix or the cytological examination of cervical smears is invaluable in the early detection of carcinoma (p. 227). The laparoscope can be used to inspect the pelvic organs and is particularly useful in the elucidation of the cause of lower abdominal pain.

## THE METHODS IN PRACTICE—AN EXAMPLE

### The Examination of the Acute Abdomen

The 'acute abdomen' is a term which is applied to disorders of sudden onset, sometimes of dramatic severity and often requiring prompt surgical treatment. The most common examples are acute appendicitis, perforation of a duodenal ulcer and acute intestinal obstruction. The principles of examination are identical with those already described. Perhaps the main justification for a special section is to point out some differences in emphasis. These are determined by the acute and rapidly changing situation and by the necessity for an immediate decision about appropriate action. The life of the patient may be at stake.

**The History.** The history is of paramount importance. Pain is nearly always a symptom of the acute abdomen and careful analysis of its features (p. 29) will commonly lead to the diagnosis. Severe pain may require alleviation but such action must not be taken until a diagnosis has been made, unless it has been decided to operate, because the suppression of pain may mask the deterioration of serious disease. Enquiries about previous abdominal symptoms such as pain, nausea, vomiting and disorders of defaecation, urination or menstruation, are also particularly relevant.

**The Physical Examination.** General as well as abdominal examination is essential, for an abdominal emergency may be mimicked by disease of almost any other system, for example, basal pneumonia, herpes zoster, diabetic keto-acidosis, tabes dorsalis, glaucoma or myocardial infarction.

The patient's behaviour, position in bed or facial appearance may be of diagnostic value. Thus the severe pain of biliary or renal calculus usually causes restlessness while that of perforation of a peptic ulcer induces the patient to lie still. The child with intestinal colic draws up his legs and screams with each wave of pain. Flexion of the right hip due to spasm of the ilio-psoas muscle occurs in some cases of acute appendicitis. Jaundice, in its early stages, may readily pass unnoticed, especially in artificial light, unless the sclera is carefully inspected.

Abdominal examination should follow the usual sequence. Inspection is of particular importance as a means of recognising local or general distension, the impaired movement of the abdominal wall in acute peritonitis, the visible peristalsis of intestinal obstruction or bruising indicative of recent trauma. The scar of a previous abdominal operation should stimulate enquiry about the reason for its presence if this is not already known.

Palpation provides the most important information. It should be light at first and should start at a point furthest removed from the site of pain. Rigidity, guarding and tenderness are common clues to the source of trouble. Rebound pain indicates the presence of peritonitis. In the case of obstruction of the pelvic colon, rebound pain confined to the right iliac fossa may be the only indication of imminent rupture of an overdistended caecum.

Percussion is of limited value, but resonance over distended gut or disappearance of liver dullness after perforation of an ulcer may be useful signs. Auscultation is of special value. In acute peritonitis the abdomen is silent, while intestinal obstruction gives rise to abnormally loud, resonant and frequent peristaltic sounds. Examination of the acute abdomen must always include a search for hernias and a digital examination of the rectum. A vaginal examination may also be necessary. The need for testing of the urine for bile or for porphyrins should be borne in mind, and microscopy may lead to the detection of a urinary cause for the symptoms. Pyrexia and leucocytosis strongly suggest an inflammatory lesion. Finally radiological investigations, especially films taken with the patient upright and supine if intestinal obstruction is suspected, and, in other situations, emergency barium studies, an intravenous pyelogram or a cholangiogram.

On completion of the examination it will frequently be possible to make a firm diagnosis. Failing this, it should be possible to decide whether the essential disorder is due to infection, perforation, obstruction or vascular occlusion. Thereafter laparotomy may be indicated but in many cases it will be necessary to keep the patient under careful observation and repeat the examination at appropriate intervals. By this means any alteration, either deterioration or improvement, can be assessed and a decision then taken either to operate as in acute appendicitis, or to initiate further investigation as in subacute intestinal obstruction, or to continue to keep the patient under observation because the pathological process appears to be resolving as in many cases of acute cholecystitis on treatment with antibiotics.

# CHAPTER 8
# The Nervous System

'Discard in the first instance all attempts to identify or to name, and try
instead to read the malady, tracing the symptoms to the seat of their
cause, and discerning the nature of the morbid process by their character
and course.'

GOWERS, 1892

After a period of study of modern neurophysiological concepts, students often
approach clinical neurology with an exaggerated idea of its difficulties. This is
confirmed and compounded if their initial explorations are confused and
misdirected by the use of polysyllabic and eponymous signs and the division of
neurological disorders into rigidly labelled compartments.

The study of neurology is founded on those principles of clinical medicine,
which are outlined in Chapter 1 of this book. No other clinical discipline
offers so exemplary an illustration of the logical and scientific foundations on
which medicine is based. Deviations from normal neural function are
observed. The nerve pathways and tracts whose interruption would cause
such functional disturbances are inferred. Where possible the precise anatomical sites of lesions are then determined. In the light of the distribution of
lesions, the history of the patient's illness and collateral evidence of disease in
other systems, the causal pathological process is deduced. This diagnostic
process defines a logical sequence which should always be followed. Though
increasing facility will enable the steps to be made more rapidly, there are no
short cuts; no signs are pathognomonic of disease processes.

The nervous system is organised functionally in a hierarchical fashion.
Hughlings Jackson introduced the concept of different roles subserved by
different levels of the nervous system. Peripheral effectors and receptors are
supplied by nerves whose function is restricted, which originate from the
spinal cord and dorsal root ganglia and which are arranged in a segmental
fashion. Connections within a spinal cord segment between afferent and
efferent nerve fibres enable reflex motor responses to occur as a result of
certain sensory stimuli. Activities within the spinal cord are modified by
influences deriving from 'higher' levels such as the basal ganglia or cerebellum which function as co-ordinating centres. The highest level of activity is
represented in the cerebral cortex which is concerned with the elaboration of
ideas, with the complex patterns of learned movements and with the
integration and interpretation of sensory information. This organisational
pattern is of fundamental clinical importance. Dissolution of neural activity
at different levels produces different patterns of disability as is illustrated in
the section on the motor system (p. 277).

Neurological lesions may produce deviations from normal function in three ways: (1) they may give rise to positive phenomena, i.e. there may be overaction of part of the nervous system, as for instance in Jacksonian epilepsy where convulsive movements of a limb result from an irritative lesion affecting the motor cortex; (2) abnormal function may occur because of a 'release' of lower levels of nervous activity from restraints or inhibitions which in normal circumstances are imposed by the functions of higher levels. A common example of this is the increased tone seen in limbs after damage to the pyramidal pathway; (3) 'negative' features result from the loss of normal neural functions as, for example, the muscle paralysis and impaired sensation which follow damage to a peripheral nerve. Sometimes damage to nerve pathways will concurrently cause patterns of positive, release and negative phenomena which are distinctive, as, for example, the tremor, rigidity and hypokinesis of the Parkinsonian syndrome.

The significance of some signs may cause difficulty during the neurological examination. The results of examination often depend on the patient's cooperation and subjective responses to stimuli as well as on the examiner's interpretation based on his experience of normality. It should be recognised at the outset that with the most careful and meticulous examination some signs are less reliable and more difficult of interpretation than others. There are 'soft' and 'hard' neurological signs, using these terms to denote reliability by analogy with currencies. An extensor plantar response denotes a lesion of the corticospinal pathways. This is the paradigm of a 'hard' neurological sign. The assessment of deep pain sensation by pinching the patient's calf depends on the patient's reaction and personality and, unless deviation from the normal response is marked, little reliance can be placed on this sign in isolation. Such difficulties are obviated to some extent since it is rarely necessary to base one's pathophysiological interpretation on single signs. Several abnormalities elicited during the examination will add weight to each other. A lesion in the posterior lobe of the cerebellum is more certainly diagnosed if intention tremor in the limbs on one side of the body is accompanied by a jerking type of nystagmus on looking to the same side. It is important, however, that this process of assessing signs in combination in order to localise lesions should not lead to a false importance being given to indeterminate observations. It is even more dangerous to attribute significance to findings in order to complete a pattern which is 'typical' of a disease. It sometimes occurs that an immediate prejudice is formed in favour of a diagnosis and thereafter signs are elucidated which support this diagnosis. When a young patient presents with paralysis of the legs (paraparesis), it may be immediately assumed that the diagnosis is disseminated sclerosis. Examination of the optic discs in such a case reveals pallor of the temporal halves of the discs relative to their nasal halves which is a normal phenomenon. If, however, this normal variation is recorded as 'bitemporal pallor', putatively a sign of disseminated sclerosis, then a spurious significance is given to a normal finding and the diagnosis of disseminated sclerosis is made on flimsy grounds and a potentially remediable lesion such as a spinal cord tumour may be missed. This type of thinking is tautological. Signs are invented to fit the intuitions of the observer who then adduces such counterfeits as confirmation of the diagnosis to which he is already committed. This is the antithesis of good medical practice.

The clinician must appraise each of his observations in the light of his knowledge of normal variations and then decide whether a given finding is abnormal. There is little point in saying that a patient's optic discs look pale; the observer must make up his mind whether the discs are abnormally pale or not. The statement that tendon reflexes are brisk says little more than that they are present and enables no useful inferences to be drawn. A decision that tendon reflexes are pathologically brisk implies a lesion of the pyramidal pathways. It is legitimate sometimes to say that one does not know whether a finding is beyond normal limits but in such instances the indeterminate findings should not be given undue weight when evaluating the sites of lesions. Throughout the neurological examination, the need for the constant exercise of judgment regarding the significance of signs, must always be exercised.

## THE HISTORY

Taking a history from a patient with neurological disease follows closely those principles outlined in Chapter 1. Each symptom must be carefully analysed; in the case of headache, the nature of the pain, its distribution, time relationships and precipitants should be delineated (p. 29). Blackouts or fits should be assessed as described on p. 37. A complaint of double vision is an important feature which becomes much more informative if the direction of displacement of the two images, direction of gaze in which they are maximally separated and the variation, if any, of the diplopia are analysed (p. 254). Many patients complain of dizziness. Some of these will suffer from a hallucination of movement which can legitimately be called vertigo. But the word 'dizziness' is also used for very varying conditions by patients. Epilepsy, syncope, hypoglycaemia or anxiety may be described as dizzy turns. Thus to record that a patient suffers from dizziness without considerable elaboration is of little diagnostic value.

The object of taking a neurological history should be to plot in the mind's eye the course of the patient's illness in terms of its severity and its time relationships and the process of interpretation by the clinician should be applied while doing so in terms of the possible physiological and anatomical implications of previous or present symptoms. Thus the process of taking a history is an active one, in the course of which hypotheses are formulated (p. 16), not merely the passive record of the narrative of an illness.

Clinical examination will often enable lesions of the central nervous system to be localised with precision, but the nature of the pathology of the lesion can be intelligently surmised only in the light of the development of the illness. In general, lesions which suddenly affect the nervous system, cause maximal disability within a few hours and after a static period of days or weeks then show a tendency to improve, are due to vascular disturbances. Lesions of insidious onset and slow but inexorable progression are often due to degenerative disorders or to tumours of the central nervous system. A remittent history wherein episodes of disability are followed by periods of marked improvement and well being with later recurrence of symptoms elsewhere in the nervous system suggests a diagnosis of disseminated sclerosis.

**Direct Questioning** After evaluation and recording of the patient's history specific questions should routinely be asked about headache, fits, visual difficulties, weakness, tingling or numbness of the limbs and disturbances of micturition or defaecation.

## THE PHYSICAL EXAMINATION

The technique and the order of the physical examination is highly variable. An individual clinician's method is as characteristic of him as his golf swing. Many neurologists begin at the head and work down to the feet. In this way the examination of the central nervous system can be interspersed with that of other systems. Though the order in which the examination is carried out may be varied, the findings should be recorded in a systematic and conventional way (p. 467).

### General Observations

Whilst a patient is giving the history, observation should be made of those features which are outlined in Chapter 4. Signs of disease of other systems may be relevant to a patient's neurological disorder. During the course of listening to the history, observation of the patient's face will often suggest the nature of neurological disabilities or may lead to relevant direct questioning of the patient and augmentation or expansion of the history. There may be cranial nerve palsies such as ptosis, squint or facial weakness. The cheeks may show the typical pigmented papules of adenoma sebaceum and hence point to tuberose sclerosis as the cause of epilepsy in a child. Poverty of facial expression observed during the diagnostic interview may be due to depression or to the hypokinesis of Parkinsonism. Facial grimacing may point to a diagnosis of chorea. A facial weakness which develops during the course of the patient's history may be a strong diagnostic pointer to myasthenia gravis. The pouting lips and transverse smile of myopathic weakness may indicate the presence of one of the primary diseases of muscle.

During this period of observation an estimate will be made of the patient's intellectual and speech function as well as of mood and personality. The detailed examination of specific nerve functions should be preceded by assessment of the patient's intellectual function, speech and gait.

## INTELLECTUAL FUNCTION

Usually the coherence and circumstantial detail volunteered by the patient during his history will indicate whether intellectual function is within normal limits and in many cases a formal clinical assessment is unnecessary. However, when the patient's narrative or conduct or evidence from his relatives suggests that there may be intellectual deterioration, an assessment should be made as described in the examination of the mental state (p. 22). Attention should therefore be paid to the patient's orientation, memory, attention and concentration, fund of general information and powers of abstraction. The examiner's approach must be flexible and tailored to the patient's previous level of intellectual function and educational background, as a patient whose professional achievements were high may still be functioning competently even when there has been some deterioration in his capability. A mathematician, although demented, may still possess a facility for calculation which is greater than the examiner's. In contrast, a man whose inherent intellectual gifts were poor should not be expected to perform as well during testing as his more talented fellow.

## SPEECH

In the assessment of speech it is first necessary to determine whether the patient suffers from a defect of language or of speech production. Impairment of language functions is manifest by inappropriate usage of words or a disturbance of the appreciation of the symbolic value of words. This may occur as part of a generalised intellectual disturbance; incoherence of thought processes is mirrored in incoherence of speech (p. 22). Such a defect should be perceived when taking the history and the associated widespread intellectual defect would become more apparent during the testing of general intellectual function. Specific difficulty with language function is called dysphasia. It may be that words are used appropriately but that speech production is impaired either because of a defect in articulation (dysarthria) or because of alteration in the quality or reduction of volume of speech (dysphonia). A total inability to fulfil these functions is denoted by the prefix 'a' — hence aphasia, anarthria and aphonia respectively.

### Dysphasia

This specific language difficulty results from a lesion affecting the speech area in the dominant hemisphere (Fig. 48). The examination of speech function should therefore be preceded by an assessment of the likely side of the dominant hemisphere. When a patient is right handed, the decision is usually easy. In the vast majority of right-handed people language function is

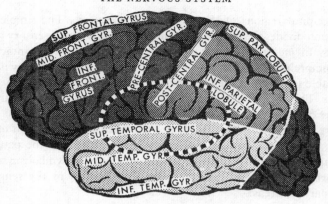

Fig. 48  THE CEREBRUM. The dotted line indicates the approximate extent of the 'Speech Area' in the dominant hemisphere.

represented in the left hemisphere. Occasional exceptions to the rule occur in those people who claim to be right handed because they have been trained in early childhood preferentially to use the right hand though their natural inclinations are left handed. This will usually become apparent on questioning the patient. However, the situation is more complicated in those who preferentially use the left hand, in at least half of whom language functions are served by the left hemisphere. The remaining half comprise genetically determined left handers and the right hemisphere is concerned with language. Patients are asked which hand they use for writing, though this perhaps is one of the more misleading indices of hand preference since many left-handed people, particularly those of middle age, were forced to write with the right hand at school. One needs to know which hand the patient uses for cutting bread; which hand would be used to catch a ball; and which foot would normally be used for kicking a ball. Since hand preference, in most instances, is congruous with the side of the dominant eye, one should ask the patient which eye he would use for sighting a rifle. One may present him with a rolled up newspaper telling to look through it as if it were a telescope. The patient will almost always place the simulated telescope to the dominant eye. This eye dominance test is invalidated if there be a marked discrepancy of visual acuity in the two eyes. In many clinical circumstances, these problems of dominance are largely irrelevant. If the patient has a dysphasic defect accompanied by a right hemiplegia, it is clear that the left hemisphere is affected and that it is dominant for speech. Sometimes, however, it may be a matter of importance to determine which is the hemisphere concerned with speech if surgical removal of part of a hemisphere is contemplated.

Those areas which are principally concerned with speech function are shown in Figure 48 and include the inferior frontal, superior temporal, and parieto-occipital regions of the dominant hemisphere. The simplest clinical classification divides dysphasia into motor (expressive) and sensory (receptive) categories. In *motor dysphasia* internal speech is preserved intact and the patient comprehends language satisfactorily. He knows what he wishes to say but is unable to say it, in the absence of any affection of the peripheral speech apparatus. This type of disturbance arises from discrete lesions in the inferior part of the frontal lobe.

*Sensory dysphasia.* This is the term used when comprehension of speech is impaired. This is always accompanied by derangement of the patient's own use of language since the learned conventions of verbal symbolism and syntax are disturbed. Sensory dysphasia arises from lesions in the temporal and temporo-parietal areas.

*Global Dysphasia.* Very commonly in clinical circumstances there is a combination of both motor and sensory dysphasic difficulties which is referred to as global or central dysphasia.

**Examination of language function.** This should include careful attention to the patient's speech when he gives his history and to his responses to questions during the course of examination. Inappropriate usage of words, the use of nonsense words or the formulation of sentences in which the word order is unconventional betray an underlying defect of language function. It should be remembered during the appraisal of dysphasia that very well known or automatic speech is often surprisingly well preserved in the presence of severe dysphasia. Patients may be able to count fairly well, may be able to say 'yes' and 'no' quickly and confidently and they may be able to swear with fluency.

Comprehension of spoken speech would be tested by asking patients to carry out commands. The level of difficulty of these commands can gradually be raised. One may start by asking the patient to close his eyes or raise an arm and go on to make the command more difficult by asking the patient consecutively to touch his nose with his left thumb and thereafter to bow his head. Patients are commonly thought to suffer from a purely motor dysphasia when in fact they have a mixed or global dysphasia. The responses to these simple commands will often reveal that in addition to impaired production of speech there is impaired comprehension thereof.

During the assessment of language function the ability to speak and to comprehend the spoken language is supplemented by tests of the patient's ability to read. Impaired ability to read (*dyslexia*) often results from a lesion in the dominant parietal lobe. This may be associated with an inability to write (*dysgraphia*) which may result from lesions of the frontal or parietal lobes.

## Dysarthria

Speech may be normal in its use of language but may still be difficult to comprehend because of defective articulation (dysarthria). The impaired intelligibility produced by dysarthria is largely due to the imprecise enunciation of consonants. In the English language vowel sounds, though important, vary markedly in duration and character in different dialects. Speech may remain intelligible despite quite marked alterations in vowel sounds but becomes very difficult to understand if consonants are imperfectly formed. The production of clearly defined consonants requires precise, co-ordinated movements of the lips, tongue and palate. Before seeking the origin of dysarthria in terms of neural dysfunction the mechanical integrity of all these structures should be established. Ill-fitting false teeth commonly cause slurring of consonants; a cleft palate will give rise to a nasal speech quality similar to that produced by a palatal palsy.

It is sometimes possible to define which of the executive speech organs is primarily affected. A rapidly vibrating tongue is required to produce the rolled 'R' and weakness of tongue movements cause a lisp due to imperfect pronunciation of 'Rs'. The enunciation of 'Ps', 'Bs' and 'Ms' demands finely co-ordinated movements of the lips.

Dysarthric difficulties vary in severity from complete inability to articulate (*anarthria*) to very minor slurring of consonants. In the latter case attention to the patient's spontaneous speech may leave the examiner in doubt as to whether dysarthria is present. The patient should then be asked to repeat such well known 'tongue-twisters' as 'Royal Irish Constabulary', 'The Leith police dismisseth us', 'Red leather, yellow leather', to emphasise his problem. Slurring of speech, even when of minor degree, is easily recognised by lay, as well as professional, observers. The patient himself is often unaware of his dysarthria even when his speech is badly affected.

Having established the presence of dysarthria the clinician must then determine the site of the neural lesions which may underlie it. This requires the same sort of analysis of motor function as outlined on page 287. Dysarthria may occasionally arise from intrinsic weakness of the articulating muscles due to myopathy; it may occur as a result of lesions at the myoneural junction in myasthenia gravis where characteristically the dysarthria becomes more marked as the patient continues to speak. Diffuse lesions of the lower brain stem leading to bulbar palsy and bilateral upper motor neurone lesions causing supranuclear bulbar palsy give rise to dysarthria. In Parkinsonism, impairment of voluntary movements may affect speech as it does other motor functions. Cerebellar defects too may cause a distinctive type of dysarthria in which the slurring of consonants is accompanied by a staccato, interrupted cadence of speech referred to as 'scanning' dysarthria.

## Dysphonia

Normal speech not only involves the articulation of learned language but also requires a method of sound production or phonation. Phonation depends on an adequate flow of air passing from the lungs through the glottis, causing vibration of the vocal cords. Impairment of phonation (dysphonia) may result from disordered function of the vocal cords or from respiratory dysfunction leading to inadequate expiratory air flow. Lesions of both vocal cords and respiratory musculature may be combined. Dysphonia is characterised by an alteration in quality (often a hoarseness) of the voice or by a loss of voice volume or both features may be evident.

Dysphonia is the result of neurological disease in only a minority of cases; other more common causes are described on page 162. Dysphonia may rarely result from primary diseases of muscle or may be due to myasthenia gravis when it tends to be variable. More often it results from damage to neural structures, such as bilateral lesions of the vagus nerve in bulbar palsy or bilateral upper motor neurone lesions above the level of origin of the vagus nerves causing supranuclear bulbar palsy. Dysphonia may be a manifestation of impaired movements in Parkinsonism wherein speech tends to be low in volume and monotonous.

### Miscellaneous Disorders

Though most speech disorders will fit into the broad categories outlined above, the examination should also include a detailed analysis of the rhythm and cadence of speech.

**Stammering or stuttering.** This comprises an abrupt halt to the flow of speech together with repetitive utterance of sounds or syllables or of the initial consonants of words. This disorder usually arises in childhood and is more common in boys. It is not associated with organic neurological disease but can be mimicked occasionally by patients with expressive dysphasia and sometimes the delayed initiation of speech seen in Parkinsonism may superficially resemble a stammer.

**Undue slowness of speech** (bradylalia). This occurs in some patients with depression, Parkinsonism or myxoedema. It should be emphasised that the rate of verbal utterance varies greatly from individual to individual and only profound slowness of speech should be regarded as pathological.

**Rapid verbal delivery of speech.** This is a manifestation of temperament rather than of any organic disease. It may be particularly noticeable in some patients with hypomania.

**Echolalia.** Echolalia is a term used to describe the automatic repetition by the patient of the examiner's utterances. This imitative repetition is a normal stage of development of language in childhood. When it occurs in adults, it is usually a manifestation of widespread cortical disease.

**Palilalia.** This rare disorder of speech differs from echolalia in that the patient here repeats the terminal part of his own utterances. Either the last sentence, the last phrase, or even the last word may be reiterated again and again, often at an increasing rate. It is best exemplified, rather flippantly, in 'My father was a gramophone maker but it hasn't affected me, affected me, affected me'. The disorders of neural function which produce this speech phenomenon are ill understood. It tends to occur in widespread cerebrovascular disease but also occurs in patients suffering from post-encephalitic Parkinsonism.

## Summary

Spontaneous speech should be listened to attentively and if necessary language or articulatory function should be tested. The appraisal of speech defects should first determine the type of disturbance, whether it be due to dysphasia, dysarthria or dysphonia or to one of the miscellaneous disorders discussed above. It should also be emphasised that these categories are not exclusive. Some patients may exhibit several types of speech disturbance concurrently. Patients with general paresis of the insane may suffer from generalised intellectual deterioration as well as some degree of dysphasia and may also be dysarthric. Patients with Parkinsonism are frequently dysphonic, often dysarthric and they may show the features of bradylalia or palilalia.

Having assessed the type of speech disturbance, the clinician should then determine the level in the central nervous system at which a lesion might cause such a disorder.

## GAIT

Inspection of a patient's gait is an integral part of the neurological examination and should never be omitted if the patient is fit enough to walk. It is appropriately considered during the general examination of the nervous system rather than under a specific heading such as the motor system, since normal walking depends also on intact proprioception and normally functioning higher centres such as the cerebellum and the extrapyramidal system. A careful examination of gait will often lead to an accurate deduction of the nature of a patient's neurological deficit.

A patient with a hemiparesis will often exhibit a characteristic gait. The affected arm will usually be held flexed at the elbow and adducted across the chest while the leg on the same side is stiff and swings forward in a circular fashion rather than being lifted from the ground. Paraparetic patients, i.e. patients with upper motor neurone lesions of both legs, show a slow, stiff movement of each leg in turn with the feet remaining in contact with the ground.

Foot drop due to a lower motor neurone lesion will often be detected as readily by the ear as by the eye, for patients so affected tend to lift the foot high to clear the toes from the ground and as it is returned, there is often a loud slapping noise. Unilateral foot drop may be due to compression of the common peroneal nerve or to a prolapsed intervertebral disc. Bilateral foot drop may be due to a generalised polyneuropathy. A high-stepping gait affecting both legs is seen in patients who have lost postural sensation in the feet due to diseases such as tabes dorsalis. Instability of a knee joint, or wasting and weakness of the muscles around the knee joint leading to hypotonia, may cause the patient to fling the leg forward in a flail-like manner as he walks. Such lesions may be seen in patients suffering from the after-effects of poliomyelitis. A waddling gait (p. 324) results from a weakness of the gluteal muscles in primary diseases of muscles (myopathies); it is occasionally also seen in lesions of anterior horn cells.

A patient who walks unsteadily on a wide base or in a drunken, reeling manner may have a disease of the cerebellar hemispheres. Lesions confined to one posterior lobe of the cerebellum cause the patient to stagger or drift towards the affected side when he tries to walk in a straight line, or may become apparent if the patient is observed as he turns. Lesions at the lower end of the vermis are uncommon and cause a jerky rocking of the trunk from side to side, akin to a man walking along a tightrope. Various combinations of gait disturbances may occur, a common example being unsteadiness due to a cerebellar lesion combined with spastic stiffness of the legs in disseminated sclerosis.

A patient suffering from Parkinsonism will usually exhibit a slow shuffling gait, each step being smaller than normal. One of the earlier signs of this disease is an absence of arm swinging on walking. Some patients with Parkinsonism tend to take increasingly rapid, small steps forward in an attempt to maintain an upright posture. This type of gait is called festinant. Some patients with encephalitis lethargica or post-encephalitic Parkinsonism show odd interruptions of their forward progression; they may halt, spin round on their axis and then continue forward.

Bizarre gaits may be due to hysteria (p. 28) and walking may be disturbed by diseases of the locomotor system (p. 322).

After general inspection of the patient and assessment of intellectual function, speech and gait, the clinician should proceed to examine the cranial nerves. The junior student may find the understanding of this section is facilitated by reading first about the examination of the motor system, the sensory functions and the reflexes.

## THE EXAMINATION OF THE CRANIAL NERVES

Cranial nerves should be examined individually and systematically in consecutive order. Some carry special afferent fibres like the distance receptors of the optic, olfactory and auditory nerves. Others are concerned with exteroceptive sensation (pain, temperature and touch) and proprioceptive sensation (muscle and joint sense and deep pressure). Some cranial nerves contain efferent fibres to voluntary muscles and resemble spinal nerves in this regard. Others also contain visceral efferent fibres which, being part of the autonomic system, innervate smooth muscle and regulate glandular secretion. In order to test cranial nerves effectively a knowledge of their functions and their anatomy as well as their connections with higher levels of the central nervous system is essential. These features will be outlined for each cranial nerve, the tests of function described and then an interpretation given of the findings.

## The Olfactory (First Cranial) Nerve

The olfactory nerve subserves the sense of smell. Its receptors are situated high in the nasal cavity whence thin filaments pass centrally, through the cribriform plate, where they are extremely vulnerable to injury, to the olfactory bulbs. Second order neurones arise here, run through the olfactory tract and divide into the medial and lateral olfactory striae. Some of the medial group cross to the opposite side; the remainder pass to the medial surface of the cerebral hemisphere. The lateral striae pass to the temporal lobe. The sense of smell is essential for the appreciation of flavours and hence a patient whose sense of smell is impaired may complain of a loss of taste.

### TESTING THE SENSE OF SMELL

Loss of sense of smell is much more commonly due to nasal disease than to neurological causes and hence before examining the sense of smell the patient should be questioned about nasal disorders such as hay fever, sinusitis and catarrh and his nasal passageways should be inspected.

The sense of smell should be tested separately in each nostril, the other being occluded by finger pressure. The patient, with his eyes closed, is asked to sniff test substances through each nostril in turn and to name the odours. Irritating, pungent substances should be avoided since these stimulate the trigeminal nerve rather than the olfactory nerve. Ammonia, vinegar and menthol are, therefore, inappropriate. Easily recognised substances such as coffee, cocoa, oil of almonds or vanilla are suitable. If bottles of these are not available, toothpaste or soap from the patient's bedside locker will serve equally well in most circumstances.

### INTERPRETATION

*Loss of the sense of smell (anosmia)*, if due to a neurological lesion, is most commonly the result of trauma. Head injuries, even of minor degree, accelerate the brain differentially from the skull. The thin olfactory filaments are thus subjected to shearing strain and are readily torn. Less common causes of anosmia are lesions within the anterior cranial fossa. Tumours in this area may arise from the frontal lobe or in the olfactory groove itself and usually involve both the olfactory and optic nerves. Tumours arising near to the pituitary gland may cause bilateral anosmia at an early stage. Chronic basal meningitis of tuberculous, syphilitic or neoplastic origin may also involve the olfactory pathways.

*Increased olfactory acuity* is rarely due to organic disease though it is occasionally a feature of the premonitory phase of migraine. Perversion of smell (parosmia) is nearly always of psychological origin though it occasionally occurs from the ingestion of certain drugs such as phenytoin.

*Olfactory hallucinations*, usually of an unpleasant nature, are characteristic of fits arising in the uncinate gyrus of the temporal lobe and then are often accompanied by smacking gustatory movements of the lips.

Disturbances of function of the first cranial nerve are uncommon, but the sense of smell should be meticulously examined whenever a patient's history suggests a lesion in the anterior cranial fossa.

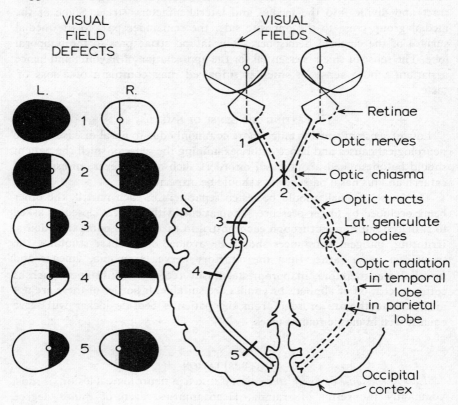

FIG. 49  Visual Field Defects.

1. Total loss of vision in one eye due to a lesion of the optic nerve. 2. Bitemporal hemianopia due to compression of the optic chiasma. The upper quadrants are usually first affected. 3. Right homonymous hemianopia from a lesion of the optic tracts. 4. Upper right quadrantic hemianopia from a lesion of the lower fibres of the optic radiation in the temporal lobe. Less commonly a lower quadrantic hemianopia occurs from a lesion of the upper fibres of the optic radiation in the anterior part of the parietal lobe. 5. Right homonymous hemianopia with sparing of the macula from a lesion of the optic radiation in the posterior part of the parietal lobe.

## The Optic (Second Cranial) Nerve

The basic anatomy of the visual pathways is shown in Figure 49. The examination can begin by *inspecting the optic nerve-head and fundus by ophthalmoscopy* as described in Chapter 11.

Alteration in the colour of the disc may be very important. There is a wide normal colour variation and there will be a small group of patients in whom the colour changes will not be extreme enough to enable diagnoses to be made with certainty. Pathological pallor when present indicates *optic atrophy* (Plate VII). Pallor is due to gliosis in the optic nerve head together with an associated loss of some small blood vessels. There is confusion in the terminology which is applied to optic atrophy. Primary optic atrophy is a term generally used to describe a pathologically pale disc with well defined margins. Secondary optic atrophy usually refers to a pathologically pale disc with irregular or blurred margins. Some people, however, subdivide this latter group into 'secondary' and 'consecutive' categories. Consecutive optic atrophy is then the label given to pale discs of irregular outline associated with disease of the retina or choroid; secondary optic atrophy is applied to these changes when they are the sequel to a period of raised intracranial pressure. Unfortunately these two terms are used in directly contrary ways by other authorities, one man's 'secondary' is another's 'consecutive' and vice versa. It is best to describe the disc's appearance and then deduce from the history or other features the likely nature of any antecedent condition. There is usually some loss of visual acuity associated with optic atrophy. This is not necessarily of severe degree. When there is marked loss in visual acuity due to optic atrophy, this is reflected in an impaired direct pupillary response to light on the affected side (p. 254).

A heightened pink colouration of the disc (often referred to as hyperaemia) makes the disc less easily distinguished from the surrounding retina and hence is attended by difficulty in defining the edges of the disc. Hyperaemia of the disc is a sign of swelling of the optic nerve head and will usually be attended by obliteration of the optic cup, congestion of the veins and, if the changes be of recent, acute occurrence, by haemorrhages radiating out from the disc. Swelling of the optic nerve head may be a manifestation of raised intracranial pressure when it is called *papilloedema* Plate VII; it may arise from an intrinsic lesion of the optic nerve when it is known as *papillitis*. The ophthalmoscopic appearances of these two conditions are indistinguishable. They are differentiated by associated changes in visual acuity and in the visual fields. Papilloedema of recent onset usually produces little or no change in visual acuity, but the visual field of the affected eye will reveal enlargement of the blind spot. With more profound and prolonged papilloedema there is often concentric constriction of the whole visual field. On the other hand papillitis due to intrinsic lesions of the optic nerve, such as a retrobulbar neuritis, is attended by severe diminution in visual acuity; if visual fields are delineated, a central scotoma can be demonstrated.

## EXAMINATION OF VISUAL ACUITY

Visual acuity should be measured for both near and distant vision. The latter should be estimated by the ability of the patient, with each eye in turn to read standard Snellen types at a distance of six metres. The results are recorded as 6/6, 6/18, etc., the latter meaning that at 6 m, the patient can just read what he should be able to read at 18 m. Near vision is tested by using standard reading charts such as the Jaeger card. Each of the patient's eyes is covered in turn. He is allowed to wear spectacles should he need them. He should be asked, with each eye, to read the smallest print he can manage. The result is recorded by noting the chart number of the passage read.

### EXAMINATION OF VISUAL FIELDS

During examination of the second cranial nerve it is customary to assess visual function throughout the visual pathways from the retina to the

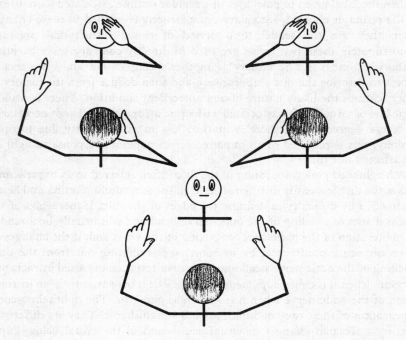

FIG. 50   Testing the Visual Fields.

occipital cortex. The defects in the visual fields resulting from lesions of the visual pathways is shown in Fig. 49. At the bedside it is possible to obtain a rough assessment of the visual fields by the technique of *confrontation* (Fig. 50). This is based on a direct comparison of the patient's visual field with the examiner's, presumed normal, field. The patient sits upright and directly faces the examiner whose eyes should be approximately two feet away from the patient. The patient is then instructed to close or cover one eye and to look directly into the opposite eye of the examiner. Thereby the patient's left visual field will correspond exactly to the examiner's right visual field. The examiner, throughout the test, monitors the fixation of the patient's gaze since if he looks away from the examiner's eye the test is invalidated. The clinician then proceeds to test the outer limits by bringing a target into the field of vision from the periphery at several points on the circumference. The direction of approach should be distributed over upper and lower quadrants and nasal and temporal aspects of the visual fields. The test object should be moved on a plane mid-way between the patient and the examiner. A finger is a satis-factory target but a more accurate assessment may be made by using a pin with a large head (e.g. a hat pin). This has the advantage of enabling an estimate to be made of the extent of the visual fields to different coloured objects. The clinician should supply himself with pins with white, red and green heads. The visual fields for coloured objects are concentric with, but smaller than, those for white objects. When using a pin the distraction caused by movement of the examiner's hand is minimised if the pin is stuck into the end of a pencil. After mapping out the peripheral extent of the fields, the hat pin can be used to plot gaps in the central areas of the fields (scotomata).

If the patient is unable to cooperate by fixing his eye on the examiner's, other techniques may be used roughly to map out hemianopic or quadrantic field defects. The patient may be asked to look at the examiner's nose with both eyes open. The examiner then stretches out both arms and moves his fingers asking the patient to point to the hand which he sees moving. When the patient, as the result of disturbed consciousness or because of a dysphasic defect is unable to cooperate at all, it is possible to demonstrate gross defects in his visual fields by rapidly moving one hand towards the patient's face from the side. This menacing stimulus will usually evoke reflex blinking when it is perceived from a normal visual field but the patient will not blink when he is menaced from a hemianopic side.

A patient suffering from a lesion in a parietal lobe may see the test object perfectly well when presented in isolation in each visual half field but will consistently fail to perceive an object in one half of his visual field when stimuli are presented simultaneously and bilaterally. This is called an inattention hemianopia.

In most cases confrontation will map out visual defects with sufficient precision for clinical purposes but when minor defects are present or when the shape of the visual defect is important in localisation the visual fields should be mapped out more accurately by using a tangent (Bjerrum) screen and a perimeter.

## The Oculomotor, Trochlear and Abducens (Third, Fourth and Sixth Cranial) Nerves

During the close inspection of the eyes and their movements which examination of the third, fourth and sixth cranial nerves requires there should be concurrent observation of local abnormalities of the eye (pp. 72–75). The examination of the functions of these three nerves requires a fairly detailed knowledge of the anatomy and physiology of the nerves and the muscles they supply. There are interconnections between the nuclei of the three nerves and pathways to them from higher centres of control. As with every other motor activity the clinical examination is designed to establish the sites of lesions. Some basic considerations are an essential preliminary to an understanding of the techniques employed in the examination and the interpretation of signs.

**Ocular Muscles** The principal voluntary muscle of the upper eyelid is the levator palpebrae superioris. Fibres of the orbicularis oculi and involuntary (tarsal) muscles are also found in the network of muscle fibres in the eyelids.

The involuntary muscle fibres in the iris subserve two functions. Concentric fibres form the sphincter pupillae which constricts the pupil; radial fibres within the iris dilate the pupil. The ciliary muscle, when contracted, causes an increase in convexity of the lens.

Six external ocular muscles supply and move the eye ball. Whenever movement of the eye occurs there is participation to a greater or lesser extent of all the external ocular muscles but individual muscles are particularly responsible for individual movements of the eyes and a knowledge of these is important in testing eye movements. It can be seen from Figure 51 that the lateral rectus is almost solely responsible for turning the eye outwards (abduction) and the medial rectus for adduction of the eye ball. When the eye lies in the mid position the movement of the eye in the vertical plane is a function of four muscles. The inferior oblique and superior rectus are responsible for upward movement, the superior oblique and inferior rectus for

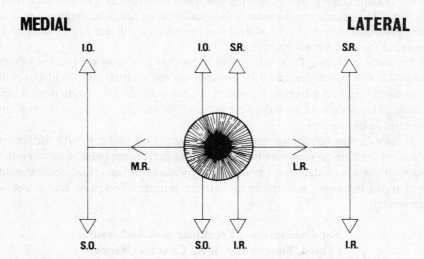

FIG. 51   TESTING OF OCULAR MOVEMENTS

Medial and lateral rectus (M.R. and L.R.) move the eyes medially and laterally respectively. With the eyes in the mid position inferior oblique (I.O.) and superior rectus (S.R.) elevate the eye and superior oblique (S.O.) and inferior rectus (I.R.) depress the eye. When the eye is turned medially inferior oblique moves the eye upwards and superior oblique moves it downwards. When the eye is turned laterally superior rectus elevates the eye and inferior rectus depresses it.

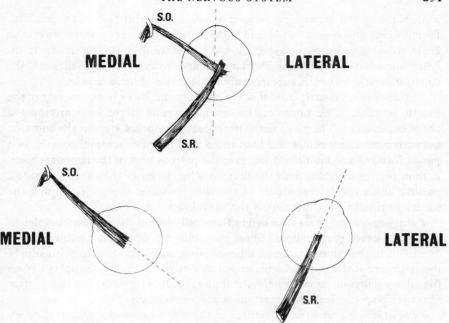

FIG. 52   To show the actions of the superior oblique (S.O.) and superior rectus (S.R.) muscles. The dotted line represents the optical axis. It will be seen that when the eye is turned medially, superior oblique is a depressor of the eye. When the eye is turned laterally superior rectus elevates the eye. The actions of inferior oblique and inferior rectus are similar.

downward movement. Upward and downward movements of the eyes in the mid position do not separate the actions of these muscles. The actions of the four muscles are easily elucidated if Figure 52 is studied. Here it can be seen from the planes of action of the oblique muscles that when the eye is adducted the superior oblique is a pure depressor of the eye and the inferior oblique is almost solely responsible for elevation of the eye. When the eye is turned outwards, or abducted, the superior rectus bears the main responsibility for upward movement and the inferior rectus for downward movement.

**Nerve Supply.** The *oculomotor* or *third cranial nerve* originates in a series of nuclei in the mid-brain whence fibres run anteriorly in close relationship to the red nucleus, the substantia nigra and the pyramidal pathways in the cerebral peduncle. After leaving the mid-brain the third nerve enters the cavernous sinus on its lateral wall, there lying lateral to the internal carotid artery. It then enters the orbit through the superior orbital fissure and separates into branches which supply the levator palpebrae superioris, the superior, medial and inferior recti and the inferior oblique muscles.

The *trochlear* or *fourth cranial nerve* arises from its nucleus anterior to the aqueduct of Sylvius in the mid-brain just below the third nerve nuclei. The fourth nerve passes posteriorly and is the only cranial nerve which leaves the brain stem on its posterior aspect. It too passes through the cavernous sinus, lying immediately below the third nerve and enters the orbit through the superior orbital fissure. It supplies only the superior oblique muscle.

The *abducent* or *sixth cranial nerve* arises in the lower pons anterior to the fourth ventricle. The fibres of the seventh cranial nerve loop around the abducent nucleus. The sixth nerve fibres leave the brain stem at the junction between pons and medulla and then run a very long intracranial course. As it passes forward and laterally it lies over the petrous part of the temporal bone. It then pierces the dura near the dorsum sellae to enter the cavernous sinus, passing along the lateral aspect of the sinus to enter the orbit through the superior orbital fissure and supply the lateral rectus muscle.

*Parasympathetic fibres* take origin from cells within the nuclear complex of the third nerve. Preganglionic fibres pass with the fibres of the third nerve. Most run to the ciliary ganglion whence postganglionic fibres arise to supply the sphincter of the pupil. A smaller number of parasympathetic fibres bypass the ciliary ganglion to end in episcleral ganglia. It is thought that these latter fibres are responsible for the reaction of accommodation.

*Sympathetic fibres* arise in centres in the hypothalamus and run through the mid-brain, pons, medulla and cervical cord and emerge through the ventral roots of the first two or three segments of the thoracic spinal cord. These fibres then ascend through the sympathetic chain to the superior cervical ganglion. From here postganglionic fibres arise and ascend in the carotid plexus and enter the orbit with the ophthalmic artery to terminate on the radial (dilator) muscle of the iris. Sympathetic fibres also supply the tarsal muscles and the orbital muscle (Müller's muscle) which latter tends to hold the eye forward in the orbit.

*Internuclear connections* Connecting the nuclei of the three ocular nerves to each other and to other nuclear masses, particularly the vestibular nuclei, is the medial longitudinal bundle which co-ordinates the activity of the motor nerves to the eye. A schematic diagram of this system is shown in Figure 53. Near to the sixth nerve nucleus in the pons is a centre, the parabducens nucleus, which co-ordinates conjugate lateral movements of the eyes. Fibres from this centre run to the sixth nerve nucleus on the same side. Other fibres cross the mid line and run in the medial longitudinal bundle to that part of the contralateral third nerve nucleus which supplies the medial rectus. Thus a mechanism is provided for retaining the optical axes parallel when the eyes are turned conjugately to the side. A lesion of the medial longitudinal bundle anywhere along its course between the pons and mid-brain will obviously cause a weakness of adduction on attempted lateral conjugate gaze and this is the characteristic clinical phenomenon of internuclear ophthalmoplegia. Such lesions may be unilateral or bilateral. If the medial longitudinal bundle is damaged in the mid-brain, impaired convergence will

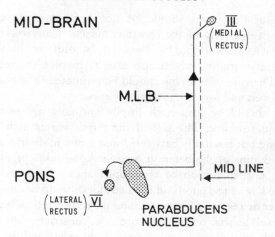

**FIG. 53** Co-ordination of Lateral Gaze. Fibres from the parabducens nucleus run to the immediately adjacent sixth nerve nucleus. Other fibres run in the medial longitudinal bundle (M.L.B.) to that part of the third nerve nucleus on the opposite side which activates the medial rectus. Thus the lateral movements of the abducting eye and medial movements of the adducting eye can be synchronised.

accompany the defect of lateral conjugate gaze. When a lesion lies in the lower part of this tract, in the pons, fibres to the adjacent sixth nerve may also be interrupted so there will be defective abduction as well as restricted adduction on lateral deviation. The weakness of abduction may be reflected by nystagmus in the abducting eye. This type of nystagmus confined to, or more marked in the abducting eye on attempted lateral gaze, is known as ataxic nystagmus and denotes a pontine lesion.

*Supranuclear Connections.* There lies in the cortex of the frontal lobe at the posterior end of the second frontal convolution an area which when stimulated causes conjugate deviation of the eyes away from the stimulated side. Fibres from this area probably run through the anterior part of the internal capsule, through the basal ganglia to terminate in the pontine centres co-ordinating lateral gaze. Damage to these frontal centres, paralysing or weakening their function leads to an inability to turn the eyes away from the side of the lesion.

There are also centres in the occipital cortex concerned with conjugate eye movements but these are much less well defined than are those in the frontal area and their clinical role is not clear.

### EXAMINATION

*Inspection.* The examination should be prefaced by a detailed inspection of the eyes. The size of the palpebral fissures and any asymmetry between the two should be noted. Minor degrees of asymmetry often are seen in normal people. Drooping of one or other eyelid should be observed and any variation in the degree of the ptosis should be noted; it may be accompanied by compensatory overactivity of the frontalis muscle. Conversely any widening of the palpebral fissures should be observed. Involuntary movements of the eyelid, particularly spasms which also usually involve the orbicularis oculi, may be seen. The rate of blinking should be estimated. The patient should be asked fully to open and forcibly to close his eyes.

The pupils should be inspected. Pupils normally are round, regular in outline and equal in size. The size of the pupils varies with the amount of ambient lighting but is usually between 3 and 5 mm in diameter. Pupils which are less than 3 mm in diameter in average conditions of illumination are called meiotic and dilatation of the pupils above 5 mm is referred to as mydriasis. The size of the pupils on the two sides should be compared.

**Pupillary reflexes.** If a light is shone on to the retina, the pupil on the same side, as well as that on the opposite side, constricts. The reaction of the pupil on the side stimulated is called *direct light reflex* and the constriction of the other pupil is the *consensual light reflex*. The speed and extent of constriction should be assessed in each eye separately, shielding the other from the light while doing so in order to test both direct and consensual reflexes. The light should approach from the side in order to avoid an accommodation response. The *reaction of accomodation* refers to the constriction of the pupils which accompanies convergence of the eyes when the patient looks at a near object. The patient should be asked to relax his accommodation by gazing into the distance at, say the roof. He is then asked to shift his gaze to fix on the observer's finger, held near the patient's nose. Alternatively the patient may be asked to keep his gaze fixed on the clinician's finger which at first is held several feet away and is then brought nearer and nearer to the patient's face. The significance of abnormal pupillary reflexes is discussed on pages 257 and 258.

**Ocular Movements.** During inspection of the eyes the direction of any deviation of the optical axes of the eyes from parallel should be noted. The patient should be asked to move the eyes upwards, downwards, medially and laterally. He should then be asked also to look upwards and laterally, upwards and medially, downwards and medially, and downwards and laterally. He should first perform these movements on request. He should then be asked to follow with his eyes a target held by the examiner who moves it in the six directions listed. The patient should first make conjugate movements with both his eyes open. In some instances each eye should then separately be tested, the other being covered by the examiner's hand. He should be asked specifically whether he sees double when his eyes are deviated into the positions outlined above. If double vision is present, he should be asked in what direction of gaze the objects seem to be most widely separated. In the position of maximal separation of the images the more peripheral of the two images is the false image and is attributable to the eye whose movement is impaired. By covering the eyes alternately and asking the patient to say when

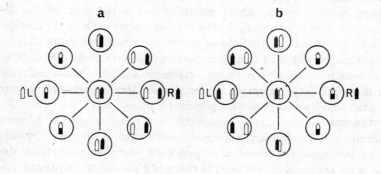

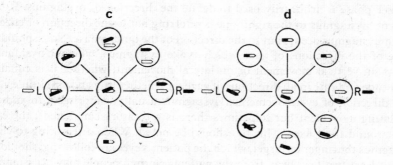

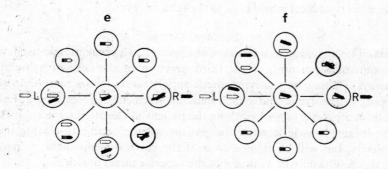

◻ Image seen by left eye.

◼ Image seen by right eye.

⬤ Normal binocular fusion of images.

FIG. 54   DIPLOPIA

The diagram shows the direction of diplopia in paralysis of the individual external ocular muscles of the *right* eye. The muscles involved are: (*a*) lateral rectus; (*b*) medial rectus; (*c*) superior rectus; (*d*) inferior rectus; (*e*) superior oblique; (*f*) inferior oblique.

the outer image disappears it is possible to establish which eye is at fault. The weakened muscle is that which normally moves the affected eye in the direction in which maximal double vision occurs. These principles are illustrated in Figure 54. If diplopia has been present for more than a few months it may be difficult to obtain clear cut answers about the direction of gaze in which maximal separation of images occurs. Occasionally double vision is absent despite obvious ocular paresis; this is particularly common when strabismus (squint) has been present for many years.

**Nystagmus.** Whilst ocular movements are being tested the presence of nystagmus, i.e. involuntary rhythmic oscillations of the eyes, should be observed. Nystagmus is described as 'pendular' when the oscillations about a central point are equal in rate like the swing of a pendulum. Nystagmus is said to be 'jerking' when there are quick and slow phases of unequal duration. The quicker phase is arbitrarily used to define the direction of nystagmus. If one talks of 'nystagmus to the right' one is referring not to the direction of gaze in which nystagmus occurs but to the direction of the quick phase. Note should be made of the directions of gaze which evoke nystagmus, whether nystagmus occurs on vertical movement or on lateral movement, whether it is equal in amplitude and rate in all directions of gaze, or whether rate and amplitude vary with direction of eye movements. Nystagmus usually comprises a to and fro oscillating movement but sometimes there is a rotatory component; the eyes turn around their axes. This too should be noted. When attempting to elicit nystagmus the finger or target, which the patient's eyes are following, should be held at least two feet away from the patient. Normal people may occasionally exhibit jerking movements of the eyes at the extremes of gaze and particularly so when the test object is held close to the subject's eyes.

## INTERPRETATION

**Ptosis.** This may due to a lesion of the levator palpebrae muscle itself, of its neuromuscular junction, of the third nerve or of the cervical sympathetic pathways. Damage to the sympathetic supply rarely causes more than slight drooping of the eyelid and sympathetic involvement can easily be differentiated from a paretic ptosis by asking the patient to elevate the eye voluntarily. If the levator muscle is weak the patient will be unable to elevate the lid completely, but will be able to do so if the cervical sympathetic is involved since this results only in weakness of the superior tarsal muscle.

Ptosis may accompany some myopathies, notably dystrophia myotonica (p. 71). Ptosis is commonly present, often bilateral but unequal and usually variable in myasthenia gravis (Plate VI). If this condition is suspected and there is little spontaneous variation during the period of observation it may be helpful to ask the patient to look at an object held above his head whilst holding the head still. This causes continued elevation of the eyelids and after a period the ptosis will become more marked in patients with myasthenic weakness.

When ptosis is an accompaniment of a third nerve palsy there will usually also be dilatation of the pupils and a pattern of defective ocular movements attributable to a third nerve lesion (p. 258).

Widening of the palpebral fissure or fissures may occur because of lid retraction in thyrotoxicosis. Unilateral widening may indicate a paresis of the orbicularis oculi on that side caused by a seventh nerve lesion.

Spasmodic closure of the lids is often a psychogenic phenomenon but may occasionally occur in Parkinsonism. In the latter condition blinking is infrequent.

**Constriction of the pupils.** This may be due either to paralysis of the sympathetic system or to stimulation of the parasympathetic system. Some drugs such as prostigmin, by inhibiting the action of cholinesterase, cause constriction of the pupil. Constriction of a pupil may be due to a lesion of the cervical sympathetic when it will usually be accompanied by a degree of ptosis and with enophthalmos and impaired sweating on the same side, comprising *Horner's syndrome* (Plate VI).

**Dilatation of the pupils.** This is occasionally a manifestation of an anxiety state and can also result from stimulation of the sympathetic system or paralysis of parasympathetic nerves. Drugs such as atropine and homatropine paralyse cholinergic nerves and therefore give rise to mydriasis whilst amphetamine and similar drugs dilate the pupil by sympathetic stimulation. Enlargement of the pupil may result from blindness due to damage to the optic nerve.

**Abnormal Pupillary Reflexes.** Impairment or absence of the pupillary reaction to light may be due to interruption of afferent or efferent sides of the reflex arc. Since both pupils constrict in response to light shone into one eye afferent lesions can easily be distinguished from damage to efferent pathways. If a pupil constricts when light is shone into the opposite eye, (i.e. the consensual light reflex is preserved), the motor pathway for constriction to that eye is intact and the damage must lie on the sensory side of the reflex arc. Lesions of the optic nerve such as acute retrobulbar neuritis, damage the afferent side of the arc. In such cases there will be no direct light reaction but the consensual light reaction will be observed. This is the *'amblyopic light reaction'*. The afferent side of the reflex arc is impaired also in the *Argyll*

FIG. 55. To show the light reflex pathway in the midbrain and the probable site of the lesion in the Argyll Robertson pupil. The pupillary reflex to accomodation involves a different pathway through the lateral geniculate body and the occipital cortex.

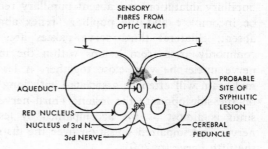

*Robertson pupil* where the affected pupils tend to be small and characteristically the two pupils are unequal and irregular. Here there is loss of the light reaction but preservation of the reaction to accommodation. A lesion in the pretectal area would explain most of the phenomena of the Argyll Robertson pupil (Fig. 55). Isolated loss of reaction to accommodation with preservation of the light reflex is uncommon but may occasionally occur in some cases of brain stem encephalitis. Loss of reaction to both light and accommodation may be due to structural damage to the iris itself, occasioned by trauma or by inflammatory lesions, which prevent the pupil from changing size. The motor pathway serving pupillary reflexes may be damaged by a complete third nerve palsy when both reactions to light and to accommodation will be lost.

A relatively common abnormality of pupillary reflexes, usually seen in adult women, is the *tonic pupillary reaction (Holmes-Adie syndrome)*. In this condition the reaction to light appears absent and the reaction to accommodation is delayed and sustained in a tonic fashion after convergence ceases. In some instances the light reaction is present but is delayed and sustained. This is a benign condition but it needs to be differentiated from the Argyll Robertson pupil. Absence of ankle jerks and other tendon reflexes may accompany these tonic pupillary reactions.

**Disorders of Ocular Movements.** Disordered ocular movements may result from lesions of ocular muscles (myopathies), neuromuscular junctions, ocular nerves and their nuclei, or from interruption of internuclear and supranuclear connections. Analysis of the defects in ocular movements will help to decide whether they fit a pattern of muscular or neural involvement, and if neural, which nerves are implicated. *Myopathies* tend in the early stages to affect all the muscles equally and partially, presenting a generalised restriction of eye movements. Ptosis accompanies this general impairment in the rare condition of ocular myopathy and a similar picture may be manifest in dystrophia myotonica.

*Myasthenia gravis* usually affects ocular muscles variably. Characteristically the ocular paresis associated with myasthenia gravis is associated with ptosis but there are no pupillary abnormalities.

*Lesions of the third cranial nerve,* if complete, cause ptosis, weakness of superior, medial and inferior recti and inferior oblique muscles, as well as pupillary dilatation and absent pupillary reflexes. Third nerve lesions may be incomplete and the pupillary reflex abnormalities and ptosis may be absent. Bilateral third nerve palsies are usually incomplete and most commonly arise from lesions within the mid-brain where the two third nerve nuclei lie very close together. A lesion of one third nerve in the mid-brain will often be associated with long tract signs (usually pyramidal) on the side opposite the lesion. Third nerve damage within the cavernous sinus is almost always accompanied by lesions of the fourth, and sixth nerves and impaired sensation over the distribution of the first division of the fifth nerve (p. 260).

*Lesions of the fourth cranial nerve* are rare in isolation but affection of the superior oblique muscle commonly results from trauma to the orbit causing dislocation of the trochlea through which the tendon of the superior oblique muscle runs. The fourth nerve may be involved, together with the third and sixth nerves in diffuse lesions of the brain stem such as multiple sclerosis and acute vitamin B₁ deficiency (Wernicke's encephalopathy). The fourth nerve is also involved together with the third and sixth nerves in lesions within the cavernous sinus.

*Lesions of the sixth cranial nerve.* Paralysis of the lateral rectus may be due to a lesion affecting the muscle itself, its neuromuscular junction or the sixth nerve, the last being a common accompaniment of raised intracranial pressure whatever the cause. In such instances the sixth nerve palsy constitutes a false localising sign. If the sixth nerve is involved in the brain stem it is usually associated with a seventh nerve palsy on the same side and' crossed pyramidal signs.

*Internuclear Disturbances.* These are discussed on page 252.

*Supranuclear Disturbances.* Irritative lesions of the frontal lobe, such as occur when an epileptic discharge arises there, cause conjugate deviation of the eyes away from the side of the lesion. An infarct in this area may not only cause hemiplegia but in the early stages also function as an irritative lesion. Thus, immediately after a stroke it may be observed that the patient's head and eyes are turned towards the paralysed limbs. Later there is often a paralysis of function and the patient will find difficulty in conjugate deviation of his eyes towards the paralysed side.

*Nystagmus.* A full discussion of the nature and significance of nystagmus can be found in *The Principles and Practice of Medicine*, Macleod, 11th ed. pp. 816–819. Nystagmus may be caused by visual disturbances, by lesions of the labyrinth or of the central vestibular connections or by brain stem or cerebellar lesions. Pendular nystagmus is usually due to a loss of macular vision but is occasionally seen in diffuse brain stem lesions. Jerking nystagmus which is of constant direction regardless of the direction of gaze suggests a labyrinthine lesion or a cerebellar disturbance. Nystagmus which changes direction with the direction of gaze suggests a widespread central involvement of the vestibular nuclei. Jerking nystagmus absent with the eyes in the mid position but which develops only on lateral gaze and whose fast component is in the direction of gaze indicates a lesion of the brain stem or cerebellum. Nystagmus which is confined to one eye suggests a peripheral lesion of the nerve or muscle responsible for movement in the appropriate direction or it may be due to a lesion of the medial longitudinal bundle. Nystagmus which is restricted to the abducting eye on lateral gaze, ataxic nystagmus, is due to a lesion of the medial longitudinal bundle between the pons and mid-brain as in disseminated sclerosis. Nystagmus which is present on vertical gaze may be due to a lesion in the mid-brain at the level of the superior colliculi.

### The Trigeminal (Fifth Cranial) Nerve

The trigeminal nerve carries both motor and sensory fibres. The motor nucleus is situated near the floor of the fourth ventricle in the lateral part of the pons from whence the motor root emerges near to the sensory root and passes below the trigeminal (Gasserian) ganglion to leave the skull through the foramen ovale. After joining the mandibular division of the sensory nerve it supplies the muscles concerned with mastication, the masseters, temporals and pterygoids. The masseters elevate the jaw as, to a lesser extent, does the temporal muscle. The pterygoid muscles depress and protrude the jaw when acting together and when one acts alone it causes the jaw to move laterally away from the side of the contracting muscle.

The sensory part of the trigeminal nerve carries exteroceptive sensation from the face, the anterior part of the head and inside the mouth via:

1. *The ophthalmic division* which supplies the skin of the forehead, the root of the nose and the scalp as far back as a line joining the ears. It also supplies the cornea, conjunctiva and the intraocular structures as well as the mucosae of the frontal, sphenoidal and ethmoidal sinuses and of the upper part of the nasal cavity. It lies on the lateral wall of the cavernous sinus as it passes from the orbit to join the trigeminal ganglion.

2. *The maxillary division* supplies the skin of the nose, cheek and upper lip, the mucosae of the maxillary sinus, posterior part of the nasal septum and the lower part of the nasal cavity. The upper teeth and gums, the hard and soft palate receive sensory fibres from this division.

3. *The mandibular division* supplies the skin of most of the jaw, other than its angle, the mucosae of the cheek, jaw, floor of the mouth and the tongue. It also supplies the lower teeth and gums.

The cells of origin of the sensory part of the nerve lie in the trigeminal ganglion. *Tactile impulses* conveyed in the central processes of these cells pass into the substance of the pons to terminate in the principal sensory nucleus of the fifth nerve. After synapsing here fibres carrying tactile sensation proceed to the thalamus in the ascending tracts of the fifth nerve which lies near the medial lemniscus. *Impulses concerned with pain, temperature and some concerned with tactile sensation* terminate in the nucleus of the descending, or spinal tract which extends downwards from the principal sensory nucleus, through the pons and medulla into the spinal cord where it reaches the third cervical segment. Here nerve fibres from different parts of the face are grouped in the following manner. The area around the mouth is supplied by fibres which synapse with second order neurones lying in the highest part of the descending root. Concentric areas spreading outwards from the mouth are supplied by fibres which synapse at progressively lower levels in the descending tract. The outermost segment of the face is represented by fibres which descend to the lowest part of the tract. These arrangements give rise to the so called 'onion-skin' distribution of facial sensory representation (Fig. 56). The fibres arising from the neurones in the descending tract, cross to the opposite

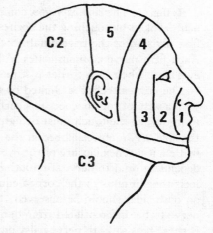

FIG. 56    Pain Fibres to the Head. Areas marked 1 to 5 indicate the central distribution within the spinal tract of the fifth cranial nerve. 1 is represented in the pons, 2 the pontomedullary region, 3 the lower medulla, 4 and 5 the upper cervical cord. The areas labelled C.2 and C.3 derive from the spinal segments directly.

side and pass upwards to the thalamus and thence with those from the body, to the sensory cortex.

## EXAMINATION

*Sensory Functions.* Light touch and pain sensation is tested in the territory of the three sensory divisions using cotton wool and pin prick respectively. Temperature sense can also be tested. The methods of examination conform to those for sensory testing in general (p. 292). The two sides of the forehead, of the cheeks, and of the jaw should be compared.

Sensory deficits occasionally may involve the periphery of the face whilst sparing the central area, or the converse may occur. In addition to testing sensation in the major divisions some comparison should be made between the sensation in the 'snout' area, around the nose and mouth, and sensitivity at the periphery of the cheek.

*Motor Functions.* This starts with inspection of the muscles of mastication. Muscle wasting may be revealed by a flattening of the face above and below the zygoma. In some instances fasciculation may be seen in the masseters and temporal muscles. If there is bilateral weakness of the muscles of mastication the jaw will hang loosely open.

The patient should be asked to open and close his jaw against resistance. As the patient clenches his teeth hard the masseters should be palpated and an estimate made of their bulk and symmetry. When the patient opens his jaw against resistance, if there is unilateral weakness of the pterygoids, the jaw will deviate towards the weakened muscle. If weakness of the pterygoid muscles is suspected patients should be asked to move the jaw laterally against resistance; it may then be found that he can move the jaw towards the affected muscle but cannot deviate it towards the normal side. Facial asymmetry, resulting from a seventh nerve palsy, may give rise to a misapprehension that the jaw is deviated.

**Reflexes.** The *corneal reflex* comprises a brisk contraction of the orbicularis oculi evoked by touching the cornea. The afferent part of the reflex arc is the first division of the trigeminal nerve; the motor limb lies in the facial nerve. Each fifth nerve communicates with both seventh nerves and therefore both eyes close when each cornea is stimulated.

The corneal reflex is elicited by touching the cornea, not the conjunctiva, with a wisp of cotton wool. The cornea is extremely sensitive and is vulnerable to injury, so the touch must be light. The wool should approach the eye from the side, as an object jabbed at the patient from directly in front of his vision will elicit a reflex closure of the eyes which is a response to menace and is not dependent on fifth nerve stimulation. The patient should be asked whether he feels the stimulus to the cornea equally on the two sides and the contraction on both sides should be observed. This will enable lesions of the fifth cranial nerve to be differentiated from damage to the efferent pathway of the reflex. If there be a seventh nerve palsy on the side stimulated there will be no direct response of the orbicularis oculi on that side but the patient will feel the touch on the cornea and there will be a brisk closure of the other eye. The briskness of the direct response on each side should be compared. Impairment of the corneal reflex may be the earliest sign of a lesion affecting the ophthalmic division of the trigeminal nerve and may be observable before cutaneous sensation is demonstrably impaired.

The *jaw jerk* is analogous to the tendon reflexes on the limbs. The afferent and efferent pathways are subserved by the fifth cranial nerve. The effective stimulus is a brisk downward stretch of the masseter muscles which is best evoked by placing the thumb or forefinger over the tip of the patient's mandible and then tapping the examiner's finger downwards with a tendon hammer

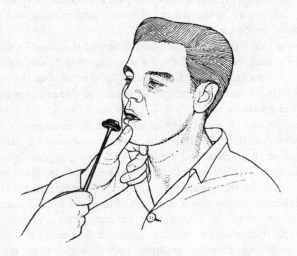

FIG. 57   Eliciting the Jaw Jerk.

(Fig. 57). This manoeuvre should be performed with the patient's jaw hanging open. The reflex response comprises a brisk closure of the jaw.

## INTERPRETATION

**Peripheral Lesions** Trigeminal neuralgia gives rise to no signs. If sensory changes are present, it is likely that there is a structural lesion of the fifth nerve. Multiple sclerosis in young people, or tumours invading the fifth nerve may give rise to episodic trigeminal pain which mimics trigeminal neuralgia. Much commoner than pains caused by neural lesions are those which arise from the structures supplied by the fifth nerve such as dental abscesses or caries, inflammation of the sinuses and abnormalities of the temporomandibular joints.

Herpes zoster (p. 97) often affects the ophthalmic division of the fifth cranial nerve and in elderly people is liable to cause persisting burning pain in the distribution of the nerve. Post herpetic neuralgia is usually accompanied by scars and by slight impairment of sensation over the forehead in the distribution of the affected ophthalmic division.

Peripheral divisions of the fifth cranial nerve may be damaged by trauma, or may be involved in neoplastic processes at the base of the skull. Tumours arising in the post-nasal cavity may erode the base of the skull and cause pain and diminished sensation in one or more divisions of the fifth cranial nerve.

**Central Lesions.** When the fifth cranial nerve is affected more proximally in its course, it is often associated with other cranial nerve signs which indicate the site of the lesion. The first division of the trigeminal nerve may be implicated in lesions within the cavernous sinus, in company with the third, fourth and sixth nerves. Tumours lying in cerebello-pontine angle often impinge on the trigeminal sensory nerve root, giving rise to paraesthesiae and numbness affecting almost all the face on the appropriate side. Lesions here are frequently associated with deafness, cerebellar signs and seventh nerve signs and the combination suggests the site of the affection.

Motor lesions of the trigeminal nerve are much less common. Bilateral involvement of the masticatory muscles may occur as part of a bulbar palsy in motor neurone disease, when wasting and fasciculation may be observed and the jaw jerk may be diminished.

In bilateral lesions of the pyramidal pathways above the level of the pons the jaw jerk is markedly exaggerated. Measured by electrophysiological methods the jaw jerk is always present. It is usually not visible in young people but is commonly seen in people above the age of 50 and the decision as to whether a jaw jerk is merely present or is pathologically exaggerated is sometimes difficult.

## The Facial (Seventh Cranial) Nerve

The facial nerve consists of two parts. The larger motor component supplies all the muscles of facial expression. The smaller part (nervus intermedius) comprises sensory and parasympathetic constituents which carry taste fibres from the anterior two thirds of the tongue and visceral efferent fibres to the lacrimal, submaxillary and sublingual glands. There are a few somatic sensory fibres which carry cutaneous sensation from a small area of the external ear.

The motor nucleus of the facial nerve is found in the pons medial to the descending nucleus of the fifth nerve. Efferent fibres loop round the nucleus of the sixth cranial nerve before leaving the pons on its lateral aspect. It is there joined by the nervus intermedius in the cerebellopontine angle near the sixth and eighth nerves. Motor fibres and the nervus intermedius then enter the facial canal. The afferent fibres of the nervus intermedius have their cells of origin in the geniculate ganglion and terminate in the upper medulla. From the geniculate ganglion secretory fibres pass via the petrosal nerves to the lacrimal glands. The facial nerve then runs through the facial canal, gives off two branches and leaves the skull at the stylomastoid foramen. The first branch is the nerve which supplies the stapedius muscle, which limits the movement of the ear drum and ossicles in response to high tone noise. The more distal branch is the chorda typani (Fig. 58) which joins the lingual nerve (a branch of the mandibular nerve) and carries taste fibres from the anterior two thirds of the tongue as well as parasympathetic fibres to the submandibular and sublingual salivary glands.

After leaving the stylomastoid foramen the facial nerve passes anteriorly through the substance of the parotid gland and is then distributed via a number of branches to all the musculature of the face. Among the more important muscles of facial expression are the frontalis which raises the eyebrows, the orbicularis oculi which causes closure of the eyes and the

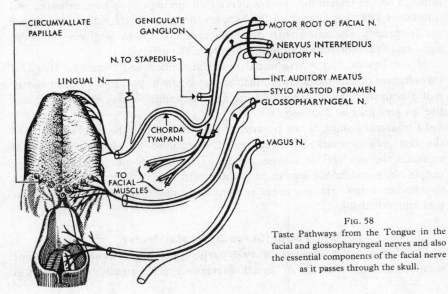

FIG. 58
Taste Pathways from the Tongue in the facial and glossopharyngeal nerves and also the essential components of the facial nerve as it passes through the skull.

corrugator which draws the eyebrows downwards to produce a frowning movement. The nares may be constricted or dilated by muscles supplied by the seventh nerve. The orbicularis oris closes and purses the mouth whose angles are raised by the levator anguli oris. The platysma draws down the lower lip and depresses the chin.

## EXAMINATION

**Motor Functions.** This is the most important part of the assessment of the seventh cranial nerve and should be preceded by careful inspection of the face. Any involuntary movements should be noted. These may take the form of tics or habit spasms which are stereotyped but may comprise very complex movements in certain individuals. In elderly patients spasms may affect one side of the facial musculature.

The play of facial expression whilst the patient gives his history should be observed. Alteration of facial expression with emotion during conversation should particularly be noted since emotional expression may be impaired while voluntary movement is preserved. Signs of facial palsy may be obvious on inspection; there may be a widened palpebral fissure on the affected side; there may be absence of wrinkling on one side of the face causing drooping of the corner of the mouth with a dribbling of saliva and flattening of the nasolabial fold. The two sides of the face should be compared. Bilateral weakness of the facial muscles may be manifest in pouting of the lips and a transverse smile. Movements of the upper part of the face should be compared with activity in the lower face.

Voluntary contractions of facial muscles should be examined. The patient should be asked to frown, raise his eyebrows, wrinkle his forehead and to close his eyes as strongly as possible. The examiner should attempt to open the eyes when the patient is forcibly closing them. The patient should be asked to show his teeth. He should not be asked to smile since in most patients this request evokes an emotional response, i.e. a true smile. He should be required to blow out his cheeks, to purse his mouth and to whistle.

**Sensory Functions.** The exteroceptive sensation supplied by the seventh nerve is unimportant and cannot effectively be tested since the small area of the auditory canal supplied by sensory fibres from the seventh cranial nerve also receives an overlapping supply from the fifth and ninth cranial nerves and the upper cervical nerves. The sensory examination should include testing of taste over the anterior two thirds of the tongue. The primary tastes, sweet, salt, bitter and sour, should be tested using sugar or saccharin, salt, quinine and vinegar respectively. When testing taste the tongue should be protruded, the examiner holding it gently with a swab. The test substances are placed on each side in turn and the patient, whose eyes should be closed, is asked to identify the tastes. He should be instructed not to speak his replies, since when a patient retracts his tongue into his mouth to speak, saliva flows over the tongue carrying taste to both sides, and to the posterior third, of the tongue.

The patient should, therefore, be required to open his eyes and point to the apposite word sweet, salt, sour or bitter, written on a card.

**Secretory Functions.** These are usually not tested formally. If lacrimation is excessive, it will be observed during the taking of the history, while the patient will complain if there is increase or decrease of salivation.

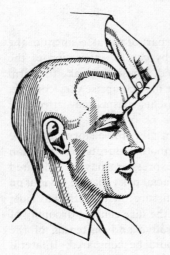

FIG. 59   Eliciting the Glabellar Reflex.

**Reflexes.** The *glabella or nasopalpebral* reflex is elicited by percussion with the finger over the root of the nose, as illustrated in Figure 59. It is important that the tap is light and that the patient is not visually menaced by a direct stab of the fingers from in front. The reflex response to a tap over the glabella is a brisk bilateral closure of the eyes. In most normal people repeated percussion evokes three or four contractions and then the response ceases.

Tapping the upper lip or stroking it with the edge of a wooden tongue depressor normally produces no visible response but may, in pathological conditions (p. 267), give rise to puckering and protrusion of the lips. This response is called the *snout reflex*.

### INTERPRETATION

Impaired facial movements may be due to disturbance of supranuclear motor pathways which influence the activity of the facial nerves, to affections of the seventh cranial nerve itself or to lesions within the facial muscles. The first stage of interpretation involves the assessment and differentiation of lesions at these various levels.

The paucity of spontaneous facial movements and of pliant emotional expressiveness in *Parkinsonism* may at first suggest bilateral weakness of the facial musculature. But the Parkinsonian patient will exhibit no weakness when performing voluntary facial movements on request. A sustained glabellar reflex may help to support the diagnosis of Parkinsonism, but it alone is insufficient evidence on which to base a diagnosis. Some anxious, normal people continue blinking as long as the tapping is repeated and in some patients with Parkinsonism the sustained response is absent.

**Upper Motor Neurone.** *Unilateral lesions* (above the level of the pons) characteristically weaken movements of the lower part of the face more than those of the upper face. This discrepant affection is due to innervation of the upper facial structures from both hemispheres whilst lower facial movements are represented only in the contralateral motor cortex. This pattern of weakness is the rule in upper motor neurone lesions but there are occasional exceptions. A patient who has recently and suddenly sustained a hemiplegia may initially suffer from paresis equally affecting both upper and lower face.

Patients with *bilateral upper motor neurone lesions* may exhibit an obvious snout reflex. Such patients may also show a lability of emotional expression. Their faces sadden and they weep without adequate cause and conversely they brighten and laugh in inappropriate circumstances. In patients with pyramidal lesions a dissociation between emotional and voluntary movements may be observed, for example some patients with a marked lower facial weakness may yet move the paralysed side normally when they smile. The reason for this dissociation is not known but presumably there are alternative pathways subserving emotional movement.

**Lower Motor Neurone.** The facial nerves may be affected anywhere along their pathways from the pons to peripheral branches to give a lower motor neurone palsy. *Bilateral facial weakness* due to neural lesions is much less common than affection of one seventh nerve. Both motor nuclei may be implicated in motor neurone disease causing a bulbar palsy and a few generalised polyneuropathies may extend to involve both seventh nerves. The immunologically precipitated demyelinating polyneuropathy, called the Guillain Barré syndrome, has a particular predilection for the facial nerves.

*Unilateral affection* of a seventh nerve is a common clinical presentation, most frequently arising without known cause in the condition called *Bell's palsy*. It is often possible to localise the site of damage in the nerve with some precision. Interruption of the facial nerve after its emergence from the stylomastoid foramen may be due to trauma or to lesions of the parotid gland. Characteristically these distal lesions involve only some of the muscles of facial expression on the appropriate side. Involvement of the facial nerve proximal to its exit from the facial canal causes a paresis of all the muscles on the corresponding side of the face. Facial asymmetry will be apparent on inspection. Widening of the palpebral fissure and flattening of the facial grooves are quickly recognised. It should be emphasised however, that where a facial palsy has been present for some time the muscles undergo shortening and contracture and in such instances the nasolabial fold and other facial markings may be more deeply etched than on the normal side. Therefore, when ascertaining the presence of facial nerve palsy the diagnosis should not be made on facial appearance alone but should be confirmed by asking the patient to move the facial muscles.

One of the most diagnostically useful accompaniments of a lower motor neurone facial palsy is an exaggeration of a normal reflex; when the patient attempts to close his eye on the affected side there will be restricted movement of the orbicularis oculi but there is a brisk upward movement of the eyeball, often to such an extent that the pupil becomes completely hidden under the eyelid. This phenomenon occurs only in lesions of the seventh nerve and is not a feature of upper motor neurone facial weakness.

The site of lesions within the facial canal can be assessed by the presence of features other than the facial palsy which is common to all of them and which is the only finding in the most distal affections below the chorda typani. Lesions above the chorda typani are accompanied by loss of taste over the anterior two thirds of the tongue and by diminished salivation. Proximal to the nerve to stapedius, hyperacusis in the ear on the same side is added to the other features; such is the picture presented by lesions of the geniculate ganglion. Affection of the geniculate ganglion is rare and in nearly all cases is due to herpes zoster, which is attended by vesicles over the anterior two thirds of the tongue and over the external auditory meatus. Damage to the facial nerve in the most proximal part of the facial canal is uncommon. When it occurs defective lacrimation is added to the manifestations of more distal lesions.

Within the *cerebello-pontine angle* lesions of the motor part of the seventh nerve, together with the sensory and secretory changes due to interruption of the nervus intermedius, are often accompanied by signs of damage to some or all of the eighth, fifth and sixth nerves as well as by cerebellar disturbance. *Pontine lesions* of the seventh nerve affect only its motor component and usually cause a concurrent sixth nerve palsy on the same side together with contralateral pyramidal signs.

**Facial Muscles.** *Myasthenic lesions* tend to affect facial muscles symmetrically and variably with facial weakness and attendant dysarthria becoming more apparent as the patient uses the facial muscles and as the day wears on. *Myopathic weakness* of the face is always bilateral and symmetrical; pouting of the lips, transverse smile, and flattening of the facial creases bilaterally present a characteristic picture. In almost all instances muscles other than the facial muscles will also be affected by the myopathic process.

## The Vestibulocochlear (Eighth Cranial) Nerve

The eighth cranial nerve comprises two components. There are auditory fibres which arise from the cochlea and vestibular fibres which arise from the otolith organs (saccule and utricle) and semicircular canals; the functions of these two elements are distinct so that they need to be considered separately.

**The Cochlear (Auditory) Division.** Sound waves are normally conducted by air to the ear but they may also be transmitted through bone if a vibrating object is in contact with the skull. Central processes from the cochlea within the inner ear enter the skull through the internal auditory meatus near to the facial nerve, pass through the cerebello-pontine angle to enter the brain stem, eventually to synapse in the cochlear nuclei in the lower pons. Second order fibres ascend in the lateral lemnisci of both sides. There are side connections to cell groups such as the superior olive but most fibres pass to the medial geniculate body which constitutes the final sensory relay. From the medial geniculate body the auditory radiations communicate with the anterior transverse temporal gyrus which is the auditory receptive area; each receptive area receives impulses from both ears.

**The Vestibular Division.** The end organs of the vestibular nerves are situated in the semicircular canals and in the utricle and saccule. Fibres are thence carried to the cells of origin in the vestibular ganglia in the internal auditory meatus whose central processes form the vestibular nerve. This passes through the internal auditory meatus in company with the cochlear nerve to enter the upper medulla. The vestibular fibres terminate on the vestibular nuclei whence a new relay of fibres runs to the medial longitudinal bundles of both sides, establishing communications with the third, fourth and sixth nerve nuclei. There is a major connection from the vestibular nuclei to the vermis of the cerebellum. Some fibres pass from the nuclei downwards into the spinal cord to form the vestibulospinal pathway. The vestibular system coordinates the motor reflexes which maintain equilibrium and make the postural adjustments occasioned by movements of the eyes, head and body.

EXAMINATION

**The Cochlear Component.** This should be tested as part of the routine neurological examination. Assessment of the patient's auditory acuity should be preceded by auriscopic examination of the external ear passages and of the drums (p. 76).

Hearing should be tested in each ear in turn by whispering to the patient, with his eyes closed and the other ear occluded by finger pressure on the tragus. Normally a whisper can be heard at a distance of three metres. A wristwatch may also be used and rubbing of the forefinger and thumb together beside the patient's ear provides an alternative stimulus.

If there is some impairment of hearing the next step is to determine whether this results from a lesion within the external auditory meatus or middle ear, i.e. conduction deafness, or whether it is due to a defect of the cochlea or its nerve, i.e. perceptive or nerve deafness. Normally air conduction of sound is more efficient than bone conduction, but when there is conduction deafness, the reverse is the case. A *tuning fork* may be used to make the differentiation, (Rinne's test). A vibrating tuning fork (preferably 256 cycles per second but 128 cycles per second will serve) is held close to the external auditory meatus. Its base is then pressed against the mastoid bone. The patient is asked which of these two stimuli seems to be the louder.

The tuning fork test of hearing should be supplemented by *Weber's lateralising test*; the vibrating tuning fork is applied to the midline of the forehead and the patient is asked whether he hears the sound in the midline or whether it seems to him to come from one or other ear. If hearing is normal the sound appears to arise in the midline. If there is damage to the cochlea or its neural connections the sound will be perceived less well on the affected side and will appear to arise on the healthy side. If there is a lesion in the middle ear or blockage of the meatus, the sound sometimes is referred to the affected ear.

These rules are generally applicable but they are not conclusive for some patients with nerve deafness may have better bone conduction than air conduction. Whenever a patient's hearing is defective he should be subjected to audiometry which measures the degree of hearing loss at different sound frequencies.

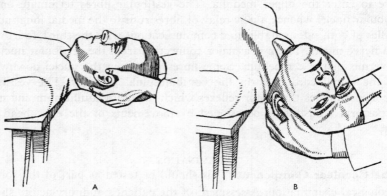

A                                           B

FIG. 60    Testing for Positional Nystagmus.

**Vestibular Function.** This cannot effectively be evaluated at the bedside, but *positional nystagmus* may be sought. The patient is asked to lie on his back, with his shoulders at the end of the bed (Fig. 60). His head, projecting beyond the bed, is supported by the examiner's hands; the head is then fully extended and turned to one side. The patient's eyes should remain open; nystagmus may appear some ten seconds after the head has been positioned and may disappear spontaneously after about a minute. Nystagmus which appears after this manoeuvre and subsides spontaneously indicates a lesion of the otolith organs in the ear which lies inferiorly. Nystagmus which is persistent in this situation usually indicates a lesion affecting the brain stem or cerebellum. After a short interval the test should be repeated with the head extended and rotated to the other side. Nystagmus does not appear as a result of this manipulation in normal people.

### INTERPRETATION

Damage to the cochlear part of the eighth nerve results in diminished hearing and tinnitus. Tinnitus is defined as a subjective awareness of noise, such as a hissing sound, in the absence of an external stimulus. The noise may be high pitched or low pitched and often seems to be originating in the affected ear. Lesions of the vestibular pathways give rise to an abnormal sensation of movement—vertigo. In many instances both components of the eighth nerve are affected together, as in Ménière's syndrome characterised by a combination of tinnitus, deafness and vertigo associated with a progressive dilatation and oedema of the cochlea and the vestibular parts of the labyrinth.

**Deafness.** Conduction deafness most frequently results from blockage of the external meatus by wax or from chronic otitis media. Perceptive deafness most often has its origin in the cochlea in association with advancing years or as a result of damage from measles, from antibiotics such as kanamycin, or from trauma. A blow, blast injury or a noise of high intensity may cause deafness which is particularly marked for high frequency sounds.

**Vertigo.** This may result from a large number of conditions of which the vast majority affect the labyrinth itself or the most peripheral part of the vestibular nerve. In almost all cases these peripheral lesions also involve the cochlea or its nerve; a notable exception to this rule is vestibular neuronitis in which a viral infection causes intense vertigo without deafness or tinnitus.

Vertigo may be due to lesions of the cerebellum and is then usually not associated with auditory loss or with tinnitus. In general, bouts of vertigo, separated by periods of normality, are due to labyrinthine lesions. If paroxysms of vertigo are accompanied by ataxia which persists between the vertiginous episodes the lesion probably lies centrally, in the brain stem or cerebellum. In labyrinthine lesions nystagmus is often prominent only during attacks of vertigo and in general the degree of nystagmus is proportional to the vertiginous disturbance. In central lesions affecting the brain stem or cerebellum there is often persistent nystagmus with relatively slight vertigo.

**Peripheral Lesions.** Assessment of lesions of the cochlear and vestibular divisions of the eighth nerve in its peripheral path requires specialised knowledge and apparatus and includes audiometry, caloric testing and nystagmography.

**Central Lesions.** In the cerebello-pontine angle the commonest lesion is a neuroma of the eighth nerve itself causing tinnitus followed by deafness and occasionally vertigo. Neoplasms of the ninth nerve, meningiomas and tumours arising from the cerebellum may also affect structures in the cerebello-pontine angle where space occupying lesions are often accompanied by cerebellar ataxia, facial palsy, or sensory disturbances of the fifth nerve and, later, raised intracranial pressure.

Perceptive deafness on the same side as the lesion may result from damage to the brain stem by such conditions as infarcts of the pons or plaques of disseminated sclerosis. In most instances intrinsic lesions of the brain stem will be accompanied by other cranial nerve disturbances as well as by long tract signs.

Since auditory impulses are relayed to both temporal lobes unilateral damage to the auditory receptive area usually produces only very transient impairment of hearing.

## The Glossopharyngeal (Ninth Cranial) Nerve

The motor part of this nerve arises in the nucleus ambiguus in the medulla and in company with the tenth and eleventh cranial nerves leaves the skull through the jugular foramen. The ninth nerve supplies the stylopharyngeus muscle which elevates the upper pharynx, in combination with the palato-pharyngeal muscle which is supplied by the tenth nerve.

The glossopharyngeal nerve contains a large sensory component which transmits common sensation from part of the lining of the tympanic cavity and the Eustachian tube. It also carries pain fibres from the pharynx and the tonsillar region and general afferent sensation from the posterior third of the tongue, the soft palate and the uvula. These sensory fibres run back through the medulla to terminate in the nuclei of the fifth nerve. The glossopharyn-geal nerve conveys taste from the posterior third of the tongue and these fibres terminate in the solitary nucleus in the medulla. The ninth nerve also transmits impulses from chemoreceptors and baroreceptors in the carotid body and sinus. It conveys parasympathetic fibres to the parotid gland and partially supplies the submaxillary and sublingual salivary glands.

## EXAMINATION

Many of the functions of the glossopharyngeal nerve are intermingled with those of the tenth cranial nerve. One aspect of the ninth nerve function which can be tested in isolation is taste on the posterior third of the tongue but it is difficult to do so in the manner outlined for the seventh cranial nerve (p. 265) as precise placement of test substances on the back of the tongue is hard to accomplish. Taste in this area is most conveniently, though rarely, tested by applying a weak electric current to the back of the tongue. This normally evokes an acid taste if sensation is intact.

The sensory supply to the posterior third of the tongue and the pharynx can be tested by touching these areas with the point of a long pin or a wooden stick. The procedure is unpleasant and should be performed only when it is important to define ninth nerve function exactly.

Touching the posterior wall of the pharynx evokes its constriction and elevation. This is the 'gag' reflex whose afferent arm is the glossopharyngeal nerve and whose efferent path is the vagus nerve. It may occasionally be absent in normal people. When there is no reflex response to this manoeuvre the patient should be asked if he feels the pharyngeal stimulus, in order to differentiate interruptions of the reflex arc on its afferent side from those affecting the vagal efferent limb. A reflex arc of similar constitution supplies the palatal reflex. When the soft palate is touched it moves upwards. When testing these reflexes the stimulus should be applied to each side in turn.

Motor functions of the glossopharyngeal nerve cannot be tested satis-factorily since paralysis of the stylopharyngeus muscle is not manifest clinically if tenth nerve function is intact.

## INTERPRETATION

Lesions of the ninth nerve are extremely rare in isolation. It may be implicated by lesions at the base of the skull such as fractures or invasive tumours but usually the tenth nerve and some of the other lower cranial nerves will be simultaneously involved. Glossopharyngeal neuralgia is the most important condition solely affecting the ninth nerve. This is felt in the back of the throat and resembles trigeminal neuralgia in its lancinating character, in its episodic occurrence and in the absence of any detectable disturbance of the ninth nerve function.

### The Vagus (Tenth Cranial) Nerve

The motor part of the vagus nerve originates in the nucleus ambiguus of the medulla which it leaves in a series of rootlets adjacent to the glosso-pharyngeal nerve. It passes through the jugular foramen to the neck, chest and abdomen, supplying motor fibres to the soft palate, the pharynx and, via its recurrent laryngeal branch, to all the intrinsic muscles of the larynx.

The tenth nerve conveys sensory impulses from the dura mater of the floor of the posterior cranial fossa and from part of the external auditory meatus. These sensory fibres, after they enter the medulla, pass to the fifth nerve nucleus. Tactile impulses from the pharynx are also conveyed in the vagus to the fifth nerve nucleus. The vagus has extensive afferent and efferent connections with the heart, lungs and gut.

#### EXAMINATION

Clinical examination of the tenth cranial nerves includes close attention to the patient's speech. Lesions of the vagus nerve or its recurrent laryngeal branch may give rise to dysphonia; interruption of its motor fibres, by paralysing the palate, will give a nasal quality to the voice.

The soft palate should be inspected. In bilateral lesions of the tenth nerves the whole soft palate droops; in a unilateral palsy there will be drooping of one side of the soft palate, the uvula being deviated to the normal side. The patient should be asked to sustain phonation by uttering a prolonged 'Ah' and palatal movements should be observed whilst he does so. In bilateral palsies the palate will not elevate and in unilateral lesions one side of the palate remains immobile, and the uvula moves towards the normal side. Movement of the posterior pharyngeal wall should be observed during phonation. If one side is paralysed it tends to move laterally, like a curtain, towards the normal side. The palatal and pharyngeal reflexes should be examined (p. 272).

In the presence of dysphonia or whenever a lesion of the tenth nerve is suspected, the vocal cords should be inspected (p. 170).

#### INTERPRETATION

*Unilateral lesions* of the tenth cranial nerve occur at the base of the skull as a result of fractures, tumours or chronic basal meningitis, and the adjacent ninth and eleventh nerves are usually also implicated. Isolated lesions of the vagus nerve are uncommon but its *laryngeal branch* is often damaged in the neck by trauma or by malignant tumours. Abductor vocal cord palsy is often the earliest sign of recurrent laryngeal nerve palsy. Later the adductors are also affected and the cord lies in the midway position between abduction and adduction. In a unilateral palsy the voice is usually hoarse but the degree of dysphonia is variable since compensatory movements by the unaffected cord across the midline mitigates the disability. If the palsy is bilateral and partial the cords do not abduct on inspiration so giving rise to respiratory stridor. When there is complete interruption of both recurrent laryngeal nerves, the cords rest in the cadaveric position and cannot abduct or adduct. Phonation is thus impossible, and if the patient is asked to cough, he cannot build up intrathoracic pressure by closing the cords; he thus produces a 'bovine' cough which is a prolonged, low-pitched noise without the explosive quality of a normal cough. Isolated paralysis of the adductors of the cords is usually bilateral and of hysterical origin. The patient loses his voice but can talk in a whisper. There is no respiratory disturbance and the cough has its normal explosive quality, indicating that the adductors can in fact function normally.

*Bilateral tenth nerve lesions* are seen as part of true bulbar palsy and bilateral supranuclear affection of the structures innervated by the tenth nerve contribute to the picture of supranuclear bulbar palsy.

### The Spinal Accessory (Eleventh Cranial) Nerve

The major part of the eleventh cranial nerve derives from the anterior horns cells of the first to the fourth cervical segments. Fibres leave the lateral aspect of the cord and ascend, uniting as they course upwards with fibres from higher cervical segments. Eventually the spinal part of the nerve enters the skull through the foramen magnum. Within the skull the nerve is joined by its smaller cranial component which arises in the medulla. The two constituents separate as they leave the skull through the jugular foramen. The spinal accessory nerve again descends into the neck where it supplies the upper half of the trapezius and sternomastoid muscles. The lower half of trapezius obtains its nerve supply directly from the third and fourth cervical segments.

#### EXAMINATION

The eleventh cranial nerve is tested by examining the bulk and power of the sternomastoid and trapezius muscles. When testing the former it is useful, in the first instance, to examine both together by asking the patient to press his chin downwards against the resistance of the examiner's hand. Both sternomastoids will, in normal circumstances, then stand out and can be inspected and palpated. Differences in bulk can quickly be recognised by this technique. Each sternomastoid should afterwards be tested by asking the patient to turn his chin against resistance to each side in turn; there will be weakness on turning the head away from the side of a muscle whose strength is impaired.

When examining the upper fibres of the trapezius the patient, standing upright, should be inspected from behind. If there is wasting of the upper trapezius a flattening of the muscle on the side affected will be apparent. The vertebral border of the scapula will be displaced away from the spine in its upper part and towards the spine at its lower end. The whole arm droops and hence the finger tips on the involved side reach nearer the ground than do those on the normal side. The power of the trapezius should then be tested by asking the patient to shrug his shoulders against resistance.

## INTERPRETATION

*Involuntary movements* frequently implicate the sternomastoid muscles. Turning movements of the head due to contraction of one sternomastoid may occur as part of the picture of chorea or dystonia. Spasm of the sternomastoid may be a major feature of spasmodic torticollis but usually other nearby muscles also are involved in this condition which sometimes is due to disease of the basal ganglia and sometimes seems to be a psychogenic manifestation.

*Upper motor neurone lesions* produce only slight weakness of the sternomastoid muscles and cause little functional disability.

*Bilateral lower motor neurone* affections of the spinal accessory nerves may occur as part of the picture of true bulbar palsy. Marked weakness on the two sides is manifest by the head falling backwards. Bilateral wasting of the sternomastoid muscles is more often due to a myopathy such as dystrophia myotonica (p. 71) rather than a neural lesion. Myasthenia may cause intermittent weakness of both sternomastoids.

*Unilateral lower motor neurone* lesions of the eleventh nerve are uncommon and, in isolation, are rare. Lesions of the nerve at the jugular foramen by fractures of the skull, basal meningitis or tumours usually also implicate the ninth, tenth and twelfth nerves. Within the neck, trauma, particularly missile wounds, may damage the nerve.

## The Hypoglossal (Twelfth Cranial) Nerve

The hypoglossal nerve arises from its nucleus in the medulla which it leaves medial to the ninth, tenth and eleventh nerves. It then passes through the hypoglossal canal into the neck and on via the angle of the mandible to supply all the muscles of the tongue. Each twelfth nerve receives an upper motor neurone supply from the precentral gyri of both cerebral hemispheres.

## EXAMINATION

Inspection is the most important aspect of the examination of the tongue which should first be scrutinised as it lies on the floor of the widely opened mouth; it should then be protruded and again carefully inspected. Atrophy is usually easily recognised since it causes the tongue to become wrinkled and thinner. Spontaneous contractions (fasciculation) of the muscles may be apparent. They persist even when the tongue is at rest and may also be seen on its underside. Tremors usually are prominent when the tongue is protruded and are much less evident when the tongue lies relaxed in the mouth.

If there is unilateral weakness of the tongue, it deviates, on protrusion, towards the paralysed side, because of the action of the normal genioglossus. The patient should be asked to move the tongue in and out and from side to side, slowly and rapidly in turn. He should also be asked to press the tongue against the cheek whilst the examiner's fingers resist the movement by pressure on the outside of the cheek. If there is unilateral paresis there will be an impairment of the ability to move the tongue towards the normal side.

### INTERPRETATION

Involuntary movements of the tongue may occur. Rapid protrusion and retraction, called a 'trombone' tremor may be seen in Parkinsonism and occasionally in general paresis of the insane. Choreiform movements of the tongue may be a feature of Sydenham's or Huntington's chorea. Irregular and continual rotatory movements of the tongue may be induced by drugs, such as levodopa and the amphetamines.

Bilateral supranuclear lesions cause the tongue to assume a more conical form and its voluntary movements are sluggish. Bilateral upper motor neurone lesions are sometimes due to vascular lesions in both internal capsules and they may also result from the generalised degeneration of motor neurone disease. Such supranuclear lesions invariably affect others of the lower cranial nerves and usually implicate the fifth nerves as well. This produces the picture of supranuclear or pseudobulbar palsy, where dysarthria, dysphonia and dysphagia are accompanied by a spastic, immobile tongue and an abnormally brisk jaw jerk.

A lesion of one pyramidal tract above the medulla causes the protruded tongue to be deviated slightly towards the paralysed side. There is no accompanying weakness or fasciculation nor does the slight weakness produce any significant disability.

Bilateral lower motor neurone lesions are most commonly part of a true bulbar palsy and will be found in association with weakness of the other motor cranial nerves. Severe disability with dysarthria, dysphagia and dysphonia results. Bilateral wasting of the tongue accompanied by fasciculation is often observed in motor neurone disease and much less frequently may result from poliomyelitis, from tumours or vascular lesions in the medulla, or from syphilis.

Unilateral lesions of the twelfth nerve are uncommon but may arise occasionally from vascular disease in the medulla or from lesions at the base of the brain such as chronic syphilitic or tuberculous basal meningitis. Tumours arising in the post-nasal space may erode the skull base and implicate the twelfth nerve. Trauma may also damage the nerve and is particularly liable to do so after its exit from the hypoglossal canal. When the twelfth nerve is unilaterally involved by these processes there are usually attendant lesions of ninth, tenth and eleventh cranial nerves.

# THE MOTOR SYSTEM

At the bedside it is convenient to consider motor and sensory functions separately but precise, skilled, willed movements require an intact sensory system as well as a properly functioning motor apparatus. Normal motor activity may be disturbed by:

1. A loss of learned movement patterns. The organised sequences of motor activation which underlie voluntary actions may be impaired in the absence of paralysis. This is called dyspraxia or apraxia.
2. Paralysis or weakness.
3. Impairment of coordination.
4. Changes in tone.
5. Involuntary movements.

The examination of the motor system seeks to define which of these defects are present and, in conjunction with other signs such as the patient's gait and changes in reflexes, will enable the examiner to localise lesions of the motor system to the various pathways and levels of the central nervous system. The motor pathways are shown in Figure 61. Assessment of motor function includes detailed inspection, and examination of tone, power, coordination and fine movements. In some cases more specialised tests designed to reveal dyspraxia may also be employed.

## Inspection

The ability accurately to observe requires more than just seeing. It involves knowledge of likely deviations and of awareness of changes derived from previous experience. If the gait and other motor functions are carefully scrutinised by an informed clinician it is often possible, on inspection alone, to diagnose the nature of a patient's disabilities.

**Posture.** The posture of the patient should be noted. The distinctive hemiplegic picture resulting from intracranial lesions of the pyramidal pathways is the posture of *decorticate rigidity*; the affected arm is flexed and adducted across the chest with the leg on the same side stiffly extended. The features of *decerebrate rigidity* are extension of the neck, back and legs; the arms are internally rotated, adducted and extended except at the wrist where they are flexed. Such a posture immediately suggests the presence of a lesion of the motor pathways in the mid-brain. Flexion at neck, hip, knee and elbow presents a posture characteristic of Parkinsonism. A patient suffering from this disease when lying may hold his head above the pillow for long periods.

**Muscle Wasting.** After an overall examination of posture the examiner should inspect the shape and bulk of the patient's musculature. Differences in bulk between corresponding muscles on the two sides of the body are valuable clues to the presence of wasting or atrophy but it is important to remember that in patients who do heavy manual work the dominant arm and hand often show disproportionate muscle hypertrophy. This is illustrated by the marked increase in size of muscles in the racket arms of professional tennis players.

K

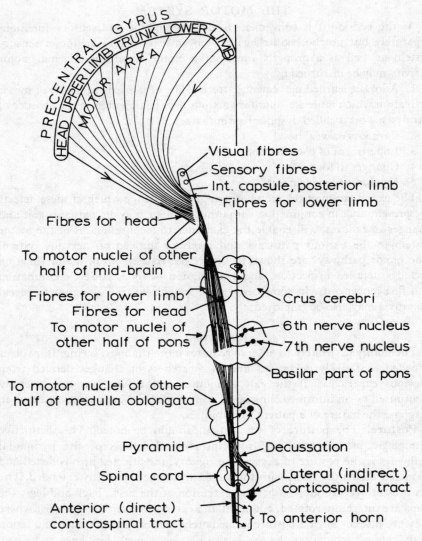

Fig. 61    The Motor Pathways.

The assessment of wasting should include comparisons of the relative affection of proximal and distal parts of limbs. In most instances muscle wasting is more easily and more certainly detected by visual inspection than with a tape measure.

**Fasciculation.** In wasting muscles it is often possible to see fasciculation. This is produced by the spontaneous contractions of large groups of muscle fibres or of whole motor units. It is usually visible through the skin. The contractions usually occur sporadically and successively involve different parts of the muscle. The movements are usually of fine amplitude. When seen it suggests a lower motor neurone lesion lying proximally near the anterior horn cells as in progressive muscular atrophy (motor neurone disease). It is not always present when there is denervation.

Sometimes fasciculations are seen in normal people. In such instances the movements are usually rather coarser and tend continually to affect the same area of muscle in the thighs or the thenar eminences after unwonted exercise. A similar phenomenon (myokymia) may cause spasmodic contractions of the orbicularis oculi, levator palpebrae superioris or other facial muscles. This is a benign condition commonly produced by fatigue and anxiety. Benign fasciculation and myokymia are particularly liable to arouse fears in medical students and doctors who may interpret them as having sinister significance. Their distribution, the absence of associated muscle wasting and their usually transient nature point to the absence of an organic lesion.

**Voluntary Movements.** Inspection will also reveal something of the precision, speed and quality of movements. Clumsy movements of the hands may imply incoordination or dyspraxia. Delay in initiation of movements and reduction in their amplitude once initiated will suggest extrapyramidal hypokinesis. The complete lack of use of one limb or one side of the body may indicate the presence of a hemiplegia.

**Involuntary Movements.** There should be a careful inspection and analysis of any involuntary movements, of which *tremors* are the commonest. They are defined as rhythmic movements resulting from alternating contraction and relaxation of groups of muscles. In the limbs, where they are usually seen, tremors produce oscillations about a joint or group of joints. When a tremor is observed its rate and amplitude should be estimated and the directions of movements analysed. The tremor most frequently seen is rapid and fine in amplitude and is an exaggeration of normal physiological tremor. All apparently smooth movements are underlain by a tremor whose rate is 10 per second. In normal circumstances this oscillation can be demonstrated only by utilising some form of amplification. If a large sheet of paper is laid over the out-stretched hand of a normal subject it will be seen that the edges of the paper are in continuous fine movement. If normal physiological tremor is increased in amplitude it becomes visible to the naked eye. This is the mode of production of the tremor seen so often in anxious patients, in alcoholics and in those who over-indulge in tea, coffee, tobacco and other drugs. A slow, coarse tremor is a cardinal feature of Parkinsonism and characteristically involves a beating of the thumb towards the index finger. In its fully developed form it is of 'pill-rolling' type when the thumb runs across the tips of all the fingers. Parkinsonism tremor can be reduced by asking the patient to carry out a voluntary movement.

*Myoclonus* is a term used to describe sudden shock-like contractions which involve one or more muscles or a whole limb. Myoclonic jerks may occur singly or repetitively. They are common in grand mal epilepsy but also are an uncommon manifestation of some widespread degenerative diseases of the brain.

*Choreiform movements* are irregular, jerky, semi-purposive and ill sustained. These involuntary movements tend to move from one part of the musculature to another in quick succession. This latter observation is important since it distinguishes choreiform movements from the much commoner *habit spasm* or *tic*. Tics are common and their forms vary widely in different individuals. Facial grimaces are frequently encountered. The tic of an individual is a repetitive, stereotyped movement; the same movement, even if complex, is repeated over and over again.

*Athetoid spasms* are slow writhing movements principally affecting the distal parts of limbs. Many extrapyramidal diseases lead to involuntary movements which are both choreiform and athetoid in type.

*Dystonic movements* (sometimes called torsion spasms) are similar to athetoid movements but tend to affect the proximal part of the limb or the trunk so that turning, twisting movements of the trunk or limbs occur.

Similar to choreiform movements but much greater in amplitude and more forceful are the movements of *hemiballismus*. There are violent flail-like, throwing movements of the limbs which, as the name implies, are usually unilateral. These tend to occur acutely as the result of vascular damage to the sub-thalamic nucleus.

*Spasmodic torticollis* is a common type of involuntary movement, resembles a tic and usually comprises repetitive, rotatory movements of the head and neck to one side, sometimes accompanied by extension of the neck at the same time.

Other involuntary movements, not easily categorised, may occur (p. 61). In each case the type of movement should be minutely observed and described.

## Palpation

Palpation of muscles is not of primary importance in the examination of the motor system but may sometimes give information of value. Palpation of the apparently large muscles in the Duchenne type of dystrophy reveals the doughy consistency of fatty infiltration (pseudo-hypertrophy) rather than the elastic feel of normal muscle tissue. Palpation is sometimes useful in confirming minor degrees of wasting suspected on inspection. If the bulk of a fully contracted muscle belly is palpated and compared to its fellow on the opposite side slight differences may be detected.

## Examination of Tone

Tone, for clinical purposes, may be defined as the resistance felt when a joint is moved passively. In normal people who are relaxed the manipulation of a joint evokes a slight, elastic resistance from the adjacent muscles. The degree of this tension can be gauged only by repeated examination of normal people.

There are certain essential prerequisites for the accurate assessment of muscle tone. The patient should lie supine with his head and neck resting in the neutral position, comfortably upon a pillow. Time must be spent, if necessary, in achieving the cooperation and relaxation of the patient. The elbow joint and the wrist, hip, knee and ankle should then be put through a full range of passive movements. The knee, for instance, should always be put into a position of full extension before it is flexed. Each of these joints should first be manipulated rapidly and then more slowly. It is a useful preliminary, having got the patient relaxed, to grasp the forearm and shake the upper limb gently. The resulting passive movements at the wrist joints can then be observed. This is a valuable way of checking that the patient is relaxed as well as providing information about the muscle tone around the wrist. A similar manoeuvre can be employed in the legs. The patient's leg, supported on the bed, should be grasped below the knee and the leg gently rocked from side to side. The evoked passive movements of the ankle are observed. Any local lesion such as arthritis should be excluded before ascribing neurological significance to increased resistance to joint movements. Tone may be increased (hypertonia) or decreased (hypotonia).

**Hypertonia.** Hypertonia is of two distinct types. The increase in tone which accompanies lesions of the pyramidal pathways is called spasticity. It is characterised by a rapid build-up in resistance during the first few degrees of passive movement and then, as the movement continues, there is a sudden lessening of resistance. This phenomenon is likened to the sensations encountered when opening a clasp knife and in shorthand terms is called "clasp-knife spasticity". This phenomenon is much more commonly and more easily detected in passive movements of the knee joint in pyramidal lesions than it is in the upper limbs. Rigidity is the term used to describe a resistance to passive movement which is sustained throughout the range of the movement. This phenomenon gives rise to sensations reminiscent of those produced by bending a lead pipe and occurs in diseases of the basal ganglia. It is variously referred to as lead-pipe, plastic or extra pyramidal rigidity. When tremor is superimposed on to rigidity the resistance to passive movement is jerkily increased as if a ratchet were slipping over the teeth of a cog. This is called cogwheel rigidity and is commonly seen in Parkinsonism. Extrapyramidal and cogwheel rigidity are most easily detected at the wrist when relatively slow manipulation is employed.

**Hypotonia.** This is usually harder to assess than an increase in tone. Decreased resistance to passive movement is difficult to distinguish from good relaxation. A more useful sign of hypotonia in the arms is a change in posture. When a patient suffering from rheumatic chorea (which is attended by hypotonia) is asked to stretch out his hands and spread his fingers it will be found that the wrists are flexed and the metacarpophalangeal joints are hyperextended giving rise to the so-called 'dinner fork' deformity.

**Associated Features.** Tone can often be difficult to evalute. Some help in its assessment may be obtained by comparing one side with the other. In many cases alterations in tone achieve clinical significance only because there are associated features such as clonus and increased tendon reflexes.

CLONUS. This is the term applied to a rhythmic series of involuntary muscular contractions evoked by a sudden passive stretch of muscle. A few beats of clonus are commonly elicited in nervous patients, especially in the calf, and such a finding may or may not be significant. Sustained clonus, i.e. contractions which continue as long as stretch is applied, reflects exaggerated tendon reflexes as a result of damage to the pyramidal pathway and is a 'hard' neurological sign. Clonus is most commonly evoked at the knee and ankle joints. Patellar clonus is elicited by sharply pushing the patella towards the

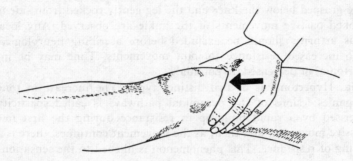

FIG. 62　Testing for Knee Clonus.

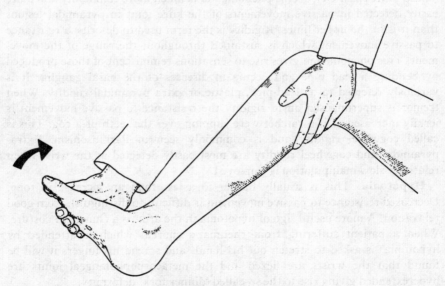

FIG. 63　Testing for Ankle Clonus.

foot whilst the patient lies supine and relaxed with his knee extended and supported by the bed as illustrated in Figures 62 and 63. Clonus at the ankle is produced by a brisk dorsiflexion of the foot with the leg in the position shown in Figure 63.

### Power

There are two methods by which muscle power can be tested. The patient may be asked to contract a group of muscles as powerfully as he can, and thus move a joint and then maintain the deviated position of the joint whilst the examiner tries to restore the part to its original position. This is called *isometric testing*. Alternatively the patient may be asked to put a joint through a full range of movement using maximal power whilst the examiner opposes the movement trying to prevent its accomplishment. This is *isotonic testing*. Both methods are effective; many clinicians employ either technique at will. To detect minor degrees of weakness isotonic testing is more sensitive than the isometric method. Any variability and undue fatiguability of muscle power should be noted.

The testing of power should not degenerate into an unseemly trial of strength between the patient and the examiner. The temptation to display one's virility by using excessive force should be resisted; the examiner should be aware of similar irrational ambitions on the part of patients, some of whom may take pleasure attempting to hurt or humiliate him by pushing him off balance. The alert examiner will be aware of this and easily avoid it by suddenly withdrawing his resistance.

*Major Movements.* In most instances it is necessary only to test the power of movements of major joints. It is recommended that a regular routine be followed; thus first the power of flexion and extension of the neck should be tested; abduction and adduction, flexion and extension of the shoulders should be examined. Flexion and extension at the elbow, flexion, extension and pronation of the wrist, pronation of the forearm, abduction and adduction of the fingers, the power of opposition of thumb and little finger and the power of the hand grip should be assessed.

Trunk muscles should be tested by examining the power of flexion and extension and of lateral flexion of the trunk against gravity and against resistance. The muscles of the anterior abdominal wall may best be examined by asking the supine patient to raise his head from the pillow against resistance. Whilst the patient performs this manoeuvre the abdominal muscles should be observed and palpated. If upper or lower segments of the rectus abdominis are weak, the umbilicus will be drawn away from the weakened muscles.

In the lower limbs, flexion, extension, abduction and adduction of the hips, flexion and extension of the knees, dorsiflexion and plantar flexion, inversion and eversion of the ankles and flexion and extension of all the toes should be tested.

**Individual Muscles.** If there is localised weakness or wasting a more detailed examination of appropriate individual muscles should be made. The evaluation of muscle power should be recorded quantitatively using the grading recommended by the Medical Research Council, viz..

0—No active contraction

1—Visible palpable contraction without active movement

2—Movement which is possible with gravity eliminated

3—Movement which is possible against gravity

4—Movement which is possible against gravity plus resistance but which is weaker than normal

5—Normal power

The methods by which the actions of individual muscles are tested, details of motor nerve distribution and the segmental derivation of nerves needs to be known. These details are graphically set out in the Medical Research Council publication *Aids to the Investigation of Peripheral Nerve Injuries* (H.M.S.O.), and it is recommended that this booklet be purchased and until familiarity is achieved it should be constantly available for reference.

**Significance of Loss of Power.** Weakness may result from generalised loss of muscle tissue associated with some systemic or metabolic diseases. Myopathic weakness is often most evident in the proximal limb musculature. Myasthenia gravis produces loss of power which fluctuates in severity and which can be improved by the intravenous injection of edrophonium. Weakness due to lower motor neurone lesions is attended by wasting of muscles. The pattern of weakness produced by lower motor neurone lesions may conform to the distribution of one or more peripheral nerves or of motor roots. Systematised affection of lower motor neurones as in motor neurone disease tends to produce weakness which is initially distal and is usually symmetrical.

Damage to upper motor neurones causes weakness of movements not of individual muscles. Pyramidal lesions tend to affect whole limbs. Paresis of one limb (monoplegia) results from a lesion affecting upper motor neurones near the motor cortex since they are here spread over a wide area (Figure 61). A hemiplegia is commonly caused by interruption of the pyramidal tract in the opposite internal capsule where the fibres are closely packed together and all are damaged by quite a small lesion. Paraparesis, weakness of both legs, is usually caused by lesions of both pyramidal pathways in the spinal cord. Tetraplegia refers to paralysis of all four limbs and is produced by high spinal cord lesions.

The examination of motor power should assess the presence and severity of weakness but it is equally important to define its distribution as this provides clues to the site of the causative lesion.

## Coordination

The smooth and accurate performance of purposeful movements requires intact sensory and motor functions as well as efficient control by higher centres. Any lesion which causes weakness may be accompanied by clumsiness but incoordination is particularly prominent in sensory and cerebellar ataxia.

**Sensory Ataxia.** This results from defective proprioception and can to some extent be mitigated by visual control of movements. It is, therefore, exacerbated when the eyes are closed.

**Cerebellar Ataxia.** The posterior lobe of the cerebellum functions as a feed-back centre. The progress of a limb in motion is monitored by proprioceptive information fed to the cerebellum. Through its connections with the motor cortex the cerebellum causes adjustments to be made in patterns of motor activation so that the limb's movements are accurately and smoothly aimed. When this guidance system is disturbed movements err in direction and velocity. The inco-ordination thus produced, cerebellar ataxia, is not susceptible to visual compensation.

**Testing Coordination.** A most useful test of coordination in the arm is the *finger-nose test*. The patient is asked to hold his arm outstretched and then to touch the tip of his nose with the tip of his index finger. A variation on this test which renders it more sensitive requires the patient to touch first the tip of his own nose and then the end of the examiner's index finger held at arm's length away from the patient. The sensitivity of this test may still further be increased if the examiner moves his index finger from place to place whilst the patient's finger is en route to it. An alternative manoeuvre is the *finger-to-finger test* in which the patient is asked to extend and abduct the arms fully and then to bring the tips of the index fingers through a wide circle to the midline where they are brought into approximation with each other. They should not touch but should be held separated by about a quarter of an inch. Whilst the patient performs these various actions the smoothness and accuracy of movements is observed. The patient with sensory ataxia may perform these acts smoothly when the eyes are open but his performance will markedly deteriorate when he closes his eyes due to loss of awareness of the position of his limbs in space. If cerebellar ataxia is present movements are clumsy and jerky (dyssynergia). The patient may overshoot the target (dysmetria). *Intention tremor* is most characteristic of damage to the posterior lobe of the cerebellum. Here the patient's hand is steady at rest but develops a tremor of increasing amplitude as it approaches its target.

In the lower limb the patient is asked to perform the *heel-knee test* by placing one heel on the opposite knee and then sliding the heel accurately down the front of the shin to the ankle and back again. This test too can be made more sensitive by first making the patient raise his leg to touch the examiner's index finger with his great toe before proceeding to perform the heel-knee test as outlined above.

Rapid alternating movements are rendered irregular in force and rhythm by cerebellar disorders. They may be tested by asking the patient quickly to pronate and supinate the forearms or to slap the palm of the examiner's hand repeatedly with the front and back of his own hand. This sequence is performed several times in quick succession. Impairment of rapid alternating movements is called *dysdiadokokinesis*. Patients vary widely in their abilities to perform such movements. Labourers tend to perform less well than those whose jobs require manual dexterity. Most people perform the tests more precisely and rapidly with the dominant hand and some are very clumsy indeed when using the other hand.

### Assessment of Fine Movements

The examination of the motor system should include an assessment of the patient's capacity to carry out small, precise, coordinated finger movements. Such movements are usually the earliest to be affected by lesions of upper motor neurones and are the last to recover therefrom. The hypokinesis associated with diseases of the basal ganglia is often most easily and earliest detected by slowing and poverty of fine finger movements; as already outlined one of the signs of cerebellar defect is the inability to make rapid movements of the hands.

The most useful and the simplest of the various tests of fine movements is to ask patients, as rapidly as possible, with each hand in turn to make 'piano-playing' individual finger movements. A supplementary test consists of rapidly touching the tips of the little, ring, middle and index fingers successively with the tip of the thumb of the same hand.

In addition to these formal tests one should always observe the patient carrying out those mundane, everyday activities which demand precise coordination of finger movements, such as fastening buttons, tying ties and shoe laces.

### Testing for Dyspraxia and Apraxia

Difficulty in the performance of fine movements may have been noted despite the fact that formal examination has revealed no evidence of incoordination or weakness or sensory defect. This would suggest that the patient has difficulty in formulating and synthesising movement patterns, i.e. that he suffers from dyspraxia. If this suspicion is aroused it should be explored by asking the patient to carry out specific tasks. He should be asked to pick up small objects from a table, to wind his watch, and to simulate throwing a ball, combing his hair and putting on his spectacles. He should be required to cut a piece of paper with scissors, to tie a knot in a piece of string, and to fold a piece of paper and place it in an envelope.

These simple tests may be supplemented by asking the patient to draw geometrical figures such as a square or a triangle and to construct similar figures from matchsticks.

The patient's writing should be examined. Dyspractic patients write slowly and with difficulty. The formation of letters may be incomplete and their size variable and what is written rarely keeps to the horizontal.

Suspected dyspraxia may sometimes be confirmed as patients dress for they may attempt to put their coat on back to front or in extreme instances try to put their trousers on their arms. Bilateral dyspraxia may arise from a lesion in the parietal lobe of the dominant hemisphere. A lesion in the non-dominant parietal lobe may give rise to dyspraxia confined to the non-dominant arm and hand. Very often dyspraxia will be associated with other signs of cortical disturbance such as agnosia (p. 297) or dysphasia (p. 238) which will aid in the localisation of the lesion. The bizarre nature of dyspractic disturbances may sometimes lead the unwary to make a diagnosis of hysteria.

## Summary of Examination of the Motor System

The examiner should develop an approach which will enable him to elicit the information outlined above with economy of effort and the minimum of duplication of tests. A useful preliminary to the examination of the motor system is to ask the patient to hold his arms out straight with the fingers spread, first with his eyes open and then maintain this position with his eyes closed. Observation of this very simple manoeuvre will often give information which will direct the emphasis of the rest of the examination. Involuntary movements of the arms will be apparent. Abnormal postures may be seen. If one arm tends slowly to drift downwards this will be an indication of paresis of that arm. Intention tremor revealed during the initial examination of the arms may indicate the need to examine other cerebellar functions with care.

In general the scheme for examination of motor function will be applied first to the upper limbs and then repeated in the lower limbs.

Inspection should take note of posture, of wasting and its distribution, of the presence or absence of fasciculation and of voluntary movements. Tone should be assessed by passive movement of all joints of the relaxed patient. Attempts should be made to elicit clonus at knee and ankle. Power in muscle groups should be tested and if necessary it should be evaluated in individual muscles. Coordination and fine movements should be examined and in appropriate instances specialised tests should be set the patient to explore the possibility of dyspraxia.

## Interpretation of Abnormalities of Motor Function

Examination of motor functions will determine which of the five modes of disturbance considered on page 277 are operative. The next stage in analysis is to decide where the lesion is situated. Motor function may be disrupted at any of seven levels, viz.:

**1. The highest level.** Here ideas of movement are formulated and movement patterns are elaborated and stored so that they can be placed at the disposal of the executive motor system. Parts of the cortex of the frontal and parietal lobes are especially concerned with this level of motor activity whose derangement causes apraxia or dyspraxia.

**2. The level of the upper motor neurone** This comprises a motor system which originates in cortical neurones whose axonal prolongations run downwards to establish connections with the contralateral motor cranial nerves and through the pyramidal tracts with the lower motor neurones on the opposite side of the spinal cord (Fig. 61). Interruption of this system anywhere along its extensive course causes paralysis of movement and an increase of tone accompanied by clonus. Attendant reflex changes are discussed on pages 302 to 305.

**3. The level of the lower motor neurone.** This provides a link between the higher motor pathways and the final effector apparatus where axons of the anterior horn cells terminate as part of the neuromuscular junctions. Dissolution at this level causes weakness and wasting of those muscles innervated by the damaged lower motor neurones.

**4. The level of the neuromuscular junction.** This constitutes a communication between the neural motor pathway and the muscle. The electrical impulses carried along the lower motor neurone evoke the release from the neural termination of a transmitting substance, acetylcholine, which causes depolarisation of the muscle membrane. Interference with the chemical transmitter's role causes a variable weakness of muscle, usually unaccompanied by wasting.

**5. The muscular level.** This is the terminal and effector part of the motor pathway. Depolarisation of muscle, biochemically initiated, spreads electrically and causes the muscle fibres to shorten or contract. Impairment of this process leads to weakness which is usually attended by loss and atrophy of fibres.

**6. The cerebellar level.** This influences the direct motor circuit. It takes part in a feedback system, processing information about the state of motor activity and by modifying cortical activity adjusts the rate and direction of movements and provides a stable postural base for movements. Disruption at this level does not lead to weakness but to incoordinate, imprecise movements which sometimes are associated with hypotonia.

**7. The extrapyramidal level.** This comprises a complex lattice work of fibres and interspersed nuclear masses running from the cortex to the brain stem whence descending motor fibres run downwards into the cord to influence lower motor neurone activity. Impairment at this level causes not paralysis but a delay in initiation and a poverty of movement, attended by involuntary movements and alterations in tone.

To localise the level of motor dysfunction supplementary evidence about, particularly, reflex function may be required and the process of final synthesis occurs when the whole examination of the nervous system is completed (p. 315).

## THE SENSORY SYSTEM

The testing of sensation is considerably simplified for the clinician if he pays attention to the patient's symptoms and is aware of the basic physiological and anatomical substrates of the sensory pathways. For clinical purposes sensation is divided into (1) superficial modalities comprising touch, pain and temperature (exteroception), (2) deep sensations concerned with muscle and joint (or position) sense and deep pressure (proprioception), (3) visceral sensations largely served by the autonomic nervous system (interoception), and senses such as smell, sound and taste providing information about the distant environment (distance reception). Information from all the active sensory pathways is correlated, integrated and interpreted in the cerebral cortex.

There is still a divergence of opinion as to whether the different modalities of sensation are subserved by specialised end organs or by end organs which are flexible and which respond to different types of energy. Touch end organs are distributed in a punctate manner over the skin and are activated by pressure which distorts or deforms them. Pain may arise superficially in the skin, from deep structures such as muscles or tendons or from viscera. Pain endings have the capacity to respond to high intensity stimuli of any nature, such as extremes of heat and cold which, in common, are potentially damaging to the tissues. Sherrington referred to pain as a nociceptive mechanism, sensitive to noxious agents. Deep pressure and deep pain are probably subserved by end organs similar to those of pain in the skin.

Clinically it is customary to refer to temperature sensation but it seems clear that there are discrete receptors distributed in a punctate manner over the skin, some of which respond to heat and others which respond to a fall in temperature.

Proprioceptive function comprises two components. The first concerns the appreciation of passive movement, and the second an apprehension of the position of body parts after movement.

Vibration sense is a term in common usage but it refers not to a specific sensory modality but rather to discernment of repeated patterns of pressure mediated by end organs in the skin as well as in deeper structures. Vibration is felt particularly well through bone which probably serves merely to amplify the stimulus. Vibration sense is the perception of a temporal dispersion of touch and pressure and is analogous to the appreciation of flicker by the visual system.

Sensations of touch, pressure and position are carried in the peripheral nerve in relatively large, fast-conducting afferent fibres. Pain is conducted in two types of fibre, transmitting impulses at different speeds and serving different types of pain sensation.

**Sensory Pathways.** The cells of origin of peripheral sensory fibres lie in the dorsal root ganglia whence proximal processes enter the spinal cord via the posterior spinal nerve roots. On entering the cord the fibres separate into two groups which then travel in the spinal cord by two distinct pathways (Fig. 64). Some of the fibres which subserve the sensations of touch and light pressure and all of those subserving joint position sense and perhaps all concerned with vibration sense, ascend in the posterior columns to the gracile and cuneate nuclei at the lower end of the medulla. Here second order

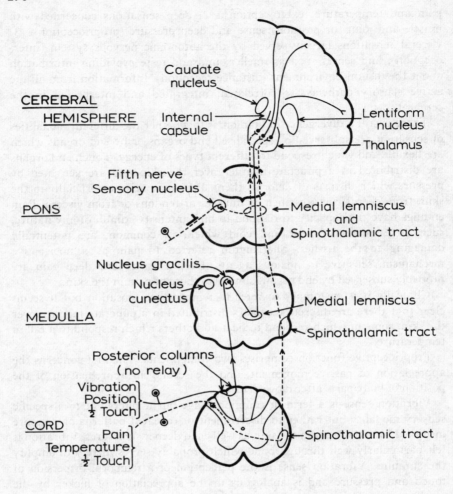

FIG. 64   The Main Sensory Pathways.

neurones arise; their fibres decussate and pass upwards through the medial lemniscus to the ventral nucleus of the thalamus.

Fibres which transmit pain and temperature sensation and some of those subserving touch, synapse in the posterior horn, in the cord, near to their point of entry. Thence fibres from second order neurones, cross to the opposite side and ascend in the lateral spinothalamic tract. This tract preserves its laminated structure in its passage upwards through the cord. Those fibres from the lowest segments lie outermost in the tract whilst those arising from more proximal segments lie nearer the centre of the cord (Fig. 65). Those fibres concerned with touch which cross within the cord lie

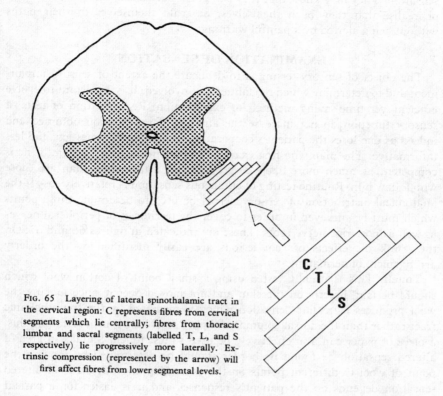

FIG. 65 Layering of lateral spinothalmic tract in the cervical region: C represents fibres from cervical segments which lie centrally; fibres from thoracic lumbar and sacral segments (labelled T, L, and S respectively) lie progressively more laterally. Extrinsic compression (represented by the arrow) will first affect fibres from lower segmental levels.

anteriorly in the anterior spinothalmic tract. The spinothalamic pathways run to the ventral nucleus of the thalamus. From the thalamus third order neurones pass to the sensory cortex.

**Symptoms.** The most frequent sensory symptoms are pain, numbness and altered sensation or paraesthesiae. Pain due to neural lesions is often described as burning or stabbing. Patients usually describe impairment or loss of sensation as numbness. Paraesthesiae may also be referred to as numbness or as 'pins and needles' by the patient but sometimes the altered or perverted sensation may be more imaginatively interpreted by him as a feeling of, for instance, wet sand on the limbs or a feeling of hot water running down the skin. In many instances patients who complain of pain or paraesthesiae or numbness will be able to delineate the distribution of their sensory symptoms fairly precisely and hence guide the examiner to the areas which need careful examination.

Patients usually are aware of any significant reduction of temperature sensation. They may know that they can grasp hot objects without discomfort or realise that they burn themselves, or scald themselves in their baths without being alerted by a painful warning.

## EXAMINATION OF SENSATION

The object of sensory testing is to delineate the extent of sensory impairment and to determine which modalities are involved. It is important to evolve efficient yet time-saving methods of examination. Reduplication of tests of sensory function do not increase the amount of information obtained and indeed as one loses the patient's cooperation, repetition becomes less and less informative. The man who first examines a patient's sensory system, if he is competent, is much more likely to get accurate information than are those who follow him. Routine testing of cutaneous sensation is relatively easy if the anatomical distribution of sensory nerves be used to determine those points which must be surveyed in order to cover the territories of peripheral nerves as well as posterior nerve roots. These are indicated in figures 66 and 67. On the trunk the effects of root lesions are easily identified by the orderly arrangement of dermatomes.

**Touch.** This is usually tested using a small point of cotton wool which should be laid directly on the skin and not moved over it since moving the wool produces a tickling sensation which is mediated by the spinothalamic tract rather than the dorsal columns. A light camel hair brush, or failing this, a piece of paper can also effectively be used to test touch. Should an area of altered sensation be found its border should be determined by moving the point of wool to different points on the skin. Mapping out areas of altered sensation depends on the patient's responses and it is easier for a patient quickly to detect enhancement of a sensation rather than its diminution. The stimulus should, therefore, be moved from a region of diminished sensation towards normally sensitive areas. The boundaries of the abnormality should be plotted and if necessary marked on the skin. In the less common circumstance when sensation in an affected area is abnormally heightened, the stimulus should be moved from the normal into the hypersensitive area.

**Pain and temperature sensations.** These are tested respectively by pin prick and by hot and cold water contained in tubes. The pin should be used gently. The patient should be asked what he feels when pricked. He should not be asked directly if he feels the pin because he may well feel the touch of the pin point even when pain sensation is impaired. It should, therefore, be established that he feels the sharp or painful sensation of the pin point. He should be asked, with the eyes closed, to distinguish between stimulation with the point and the head of the pin answering respectively 'sharp' or 'blunt'. He should also be asked to comment on any heightening or lessening of pain he feels as the pin is moved along the limb or along the trunk at the points indicated in Figures 66 and 67. Hot and cold tubes should be applied in random sequence to the skin; the patient with his eyes closed attempts to

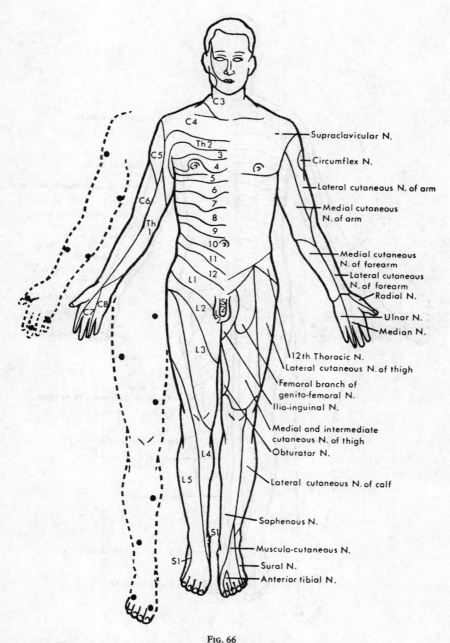

**Supraclavicular N.**
**Circumflex N.**
**Lateral cutaneous N. of arm**
**Medial cutaneous N. of arm**
**Medial cutaneous N. of forearm**
**Lateral cutaneous N. of forearm**
**Radial N.**
**Ulnar N.**
**Median N.**
**12th Thoracic N.**
**Lateral cutaneous N. of thigh**
**Femoral branch of genito-femoral N.**
**Ilio-inguinal N.**
**Medial and intermediate cutaneous N. of thigh**
**Obturator N.**
**Lateral cutaneous N. of calf**
**Saphenous N.**
**Musculo-cutaneous N.**
**Sural N.**
**Anterior tibial N.**

FIG. 66

Segmental and Peripheral Nerve innervation and Points for Testing Cutaneous Sensation of Limbs (Anterior). By applying stimuli at the points marked within the dotted outline, both the dermatomal and main peripheral nerve distribution are covered simultaneously.

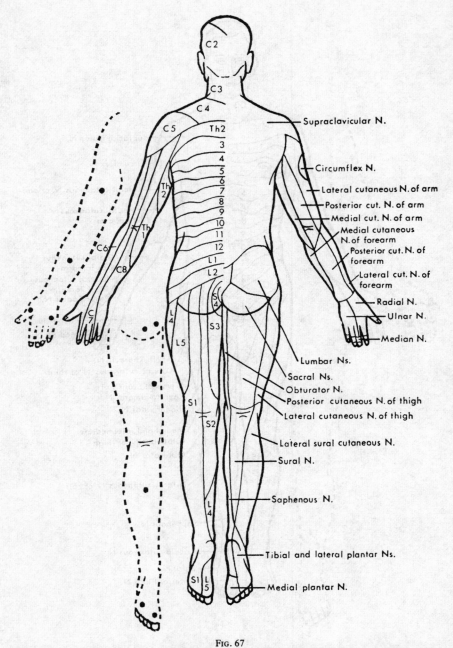

Fig. 67

Segmental and Peripheral Nerve Innervation and Points for Testing Cutaneous Sensation of Limbs (Posterior). By applying stimuli at the points marked within the dotted outline, both the dermatomal and main peripheral nerve distribution are covered simultaneously.

distinguish between them. It is necessary to preface the testing of temperature sensation by a careful explanation of what is required. In practice it is tested only in special circumstances as, for example, if there is reason to suspect dissociated anaesthesia (p. 300).

**Deep pain.** This is tested by firm squeezing over the muscles and tendons. The patient is asked to indicate when the pressure becomes painful and the examiner gauges whether the force applied would be painful in normal people.

**Joint position sense.** This is tested by passive movements. When impaired the distal parts of the limbs are almost always first affected and it is customary to test position sense first at the terminal interphalangeal joint of the great toe. The proximal phalanx is fixed by grasping it firmly in the finger and thumb of the examiner's left hand. The thumb and forefinger of the right hand grip the terminal phalanx on its lateral borders. The distal phalanx is then extended or flexed gently and the patient is asked to close his eyes and then indicate the direction of movement. It is important that several random movements be made before assuming that the patient's sensation is intact. Many patients even when they are unaware of the direction of movement will guess and answer 'up' or 'down' and obviously on any given occasion the patient has a fifty per cent chance of being right. The test, therefore, should be meticulously appraised. If the sensation of passive movement is only moderately impaired, the patient may be aware that movement has taken place but will be unable correctly to assess the direction of movement. When there is gross diminution the movement itself may be undetected. If position sense is normal at the periphery of a limb it is unnecessary to test more proximal joints. However, if there is impairment of joint position sense peripherally then similar tests should be employed at the ankle and knee. A similar process of testing may be adopted in the upper limbs. The terminal interphalangeal joint of the index finger is first examined and if indicated the proximal joints are studied. It is rare for gross impairment of position sense to be manifest at the hip or shoulder joints.

Concomitant signs of diminished position sense should be assessed. A deterioration in the performance of the finger-nose test (p. 285) when the patient's eyes are closed indicates impaired postural sensibility in the arms. When position sense in an arm is markedly impaired involuntary movements occur in the limb when the patient holds it outstretched with his eyes closed. The movements thus produced may closely resemble athetosis but may be differentiated therefrom by their amelioration when the patient opens his eyes and can then visually control the arm's posture.

*Rombergism* may be observed. To demonstrate this phenomenon the patient stands upright with his feet together, arms outstretched and eyes closed. If there is loss of postural sensation the patient rocks and sways. Unfortunately many normal people who are suggestible and apprehensive may exhibit similar instability under the test conditions and importance should not be attached to Romberg's sign unless it be accompanied by demonstrable loss of joint position sense in the limbs. In contrast it is significant if symptoms suggestive of Rombergism are volunteered by the patient. He may state that when he closes his eyes whilst washing his face he pitches forward against the washbasin or that he is very unsteady when he walks in the dark. Such symptoms strongly suggest marked diminution of position sense.

**Vibration sense.** This also is usually first impaired at the periphery of limbs. The base of a vibrating tuning fork, ideally a weighty one, with a frequency of 128 cycles per second, is placed on the dorsum of the terminal phalanx. It should carefully be explained to the patient that it is the sensation of vibration not cold or touch which he is trying to detect. The test may be made more objective and sensitive; a careful explanation and a demonstration of the vibratory sensation is given to the patient. He is then asked to close his eyes and the tuning fork, sometimes vibrating and sometimes still, is placed against the dorsum of the toe. The reliability of the patient's responses can thus be gauged. Minor degrees of impairment may then be detected if the examiner uses his own appreciation of the fork's vibration as a yardstick against which to measure the patient's responses. Should vibration sense be lost or impaired distally then the tuning fork should be moved proximally in order to establish the level at which it is normally appreciated. Because of the amplification of the vibrating stimulus afforded by bone it is customary to apply the fork to bony prominences; after the dorsum of the terminal phalanx it is placed successively over lateral malleolus, the upper part of the tibia, the iliac crests and if necessary over the costal margin. Similarly in the arm one may proceed from the terminal parts of the fingers to the wrist and the elbow.

**Barber's Chair Sign.** A distinctive sensory sign may sometimes be provoked by flexing the patient's neck. The patient should be asked rapidly to touch his chest with his chin and to relate any sensations thus evoked. Patients may describe an intense tingling, commonly likened to an electric shock, radiating down the arms, along the spine or down the legs when the head is bent forward. An account of this phenomenon may be volunteered by the patient in his history. This idiosyncratic feature was first described by Babinski who correctly attributed it to disruption of the sensory pathways in the mid-cervical region of the spinal cord. Later Lhermitte ascribed it to disseminated sclerosis. It most commonly occurs in sufferers from disseminated sclerosis but it is sometimes a feature of cervical spondylosis, syringomyelia or vitamin $B_{12}$ deficiency or indeed of any lesion in the cervical cord. This sign thus has fairly precise anatomical, not pathological, significance.

### Examination of Cortical Sensory Functions

Lesions of the sensory cortex impair the discriminative aspects of sensation. Accurate localisation of stimuli, and the assessment of shape, weight, size and texture of objects are the functions of this highest sensory level. The cortex receives information transmitted by the afferent pathways, integrates and correlates the several sensory impressions and interprets them in the light of previous experience. If there is peripheral disruption of the conducting pathways then the tests of the highest sensory level are invalidated. The patient must be able to understand what is required of him during testing and be able to communicate his responses. Intact basic sensations and adequate intellectual and language functions are therefore essential prerequisites for the study of cortical sensory performance.

A number of clinical tests are commonly employed:

**Two point discrimination.** This tests the ability to distinguish the contact of two separate points applied simultaneously to the skin. Special dividers, calibrated to show the amount of separation of their blunted points, are used for this test. The object is to determine the minimum distance of separation at which two points are identified as two distinct stimuli. Over the finger pulps two points separated by only 2 to 3 mm are normally so recognised. In the legs a separation of 50 to 100 mm is required before two discrete stimuli are appreciated and the test is seldom employed there. One or both points of a pair of dividers, opened to varying widths, should be applied randomly over the skin of the fingers, the patient, whose eyes are closed, being asked to say if he feels one or two points after each stimulation. It is abnormal if the two points need to be separated by more than 5 mm before they are distinguished over the finger pulps.

**Point localisation.** This tests the ability of the patient accurately to localise the point touched with the head of a pin or orange stick when his eyes are closed. He then opens his eyes and then puts his finger on the stimulated site. Localisation is more precise at the periphery of limbs than in the proximal parts thereof.

**Stereognosis.** This tests the ability to identify objects by palpation and requires not only intact peripheral sensation but the evocation in the cortex of the constellation of ideas and memories necessary for recognition. Suitable common objects such as a coin, a key, a pen, or a wallet are placed in the patient's hand whilst his eyes are closed. He is asked carefully to palpate the object with his fingers and then to identify it.

**Identification of textures.** This depends on the same mechanism as does stereognosis. A piece of paper, cloth, wood or metal is placed in the patient's hands and he is asked to identify the nature of the substance from its feel.

**Graphaesthesia.** This tests the ability to recognise numbers traced by a blunt object on the palm of the hand and, although normally accurate to a surprising degree, is impaired or lost in lesions of the sensory cortex.

**Sensory extinction.** This tests perception of stimuli at corresponding sites on both sides of the body. It is first necessary to demonstrate that a stimulus, either touch or pin prick, is felt when separately applied to an appropriate point on each side. If like stimuli are delivered, bilaterally and simultaneously, the stimulus may be perceived by the patient only on one side. The test should be repeated several times, the patient's eyes being closed throughout, in order to confirm that the responses are consistent. The stimulus is extinguished, or suppressed on the side opposite that of a lesion in the sensory cortex. This phenomenon is also known as *perceptual rivalry*. It must be re-emphasised that this test is applicable only if cutaneous sensations are preserved on both sides of the body.

### Interpretation of Sensory Abnormalities

It may sometimes be difficult to decide whether there is significant sensory loss  The intensity of successive stimuli such as pinprick will vary slightly since they are applied by the examiner who cannot deliver identical pressures repeatedly. Some meticulous and obsessional patients will detect and report such minimal variations and thus tend to confuse the examiner. Superficial sensation tends to be blunted over the thickened, hard skin of the hands of manual workers, and may appear to be heightened over the face or trunk. Some patients can easily be conditioned to recognise altered sensation in various areas. One half of the body or the distal parts of limbs are particularly liable to be implicated in this spurious sensory diminution which sometimes results from previous inept examinations of sensation.

Diminution of vibration sense at and below the ankles is a frequent finding in normal elderly people. The perception of deep pain sensation depends partly on the pressure applied to deep tissues by the examiner and partly on the readiness of the patient to interpret his feelings as painful. Evaluation of abnormalities of this modality is, therefore, difficult. Marked diminution or absence of deep pain, as in tabes dorsalis, can usually be recognised. Excessively tender calf muscles in vitamin B deficiency can also usually be validated by comparison with the patient's responses to similar degrees of pressure applied over the thighs or upper arms. Apparent diminution or heightening of deep pain sensation when of minor degree should not be given undue significance.

There are no easy rules whose application will enable the examiner infallibly to distinguish significant from spurious sensory signs but, in general, organic alterations of sensation are consistent and reproducible in their nature, degree and extent if they are diligently and competently sought. The history will help to avoid some of the difficulties. Virtually all patients of normal intelligence who have any considerable alteration of superficial sensation will volunteer an account of sensory symptoms. The finding of extensive or severe sensory loss in the absence of such symptoms should always cause the examiner sceptically to review the signs. Close observation of the patient's reactions will often help to confirm his spoken interpretations. When the pricking of a pin crosses the boundary between a cutaneous area wherein pain is diminished to one of normal pain appreciation the transition is usually accompanied by a facial grimace or a withdrawal movement of a limb. Such involuntary responses are strong evidence of organic sensory affection.

Once the extent and nature of sensory loss has been determined with confidence the localisation of lesions is comparatively simple.

**Peripheral Nerves.** Lesions of individual peripheral nerves or sensory nerve roots commonly give rise to subjective feelings of numbness and to diminution of all sensory modalities in their defined areas of distribution (Figs 66 and 67). Less commonly, partial lesions of peripheral nerves give rise to pain of a burning, exquisitely unpleasant quality. It is thought that this type of pain is mediated through the slower conducting, smaller pain fibres (p. 289). It is called 'delayed' or 'second' pain to distinguish it from the 'normal', 'first' or 'bright' pain which is conducted at faster rates in the larger pain fibres. This peculiarly unpleasant pain (causalgia) is liable to occur in the region supplied by nerves which have been damaged, but not completely disrupted, by trauma. The median and sciatic nerves are vulnerable to this type of reaction. Causalgia is accompanied by diminished sensation in the cutaneous area of the nerve involved and the skin itself may become thin, red and hairless.

Generalised polyneuropathies uncommonly give rise to similarly un-pleasant pain in those few instances when smaller pain fibres are relatively spared by pathological processes which damage the larger ones as in the '*burning feet syndrome*' sometimes caused by prolonged vitamin B defici-encies. Much more commonly generalised polyneuropathies cause numbness or paraesthesiae. The subjective and objective sensory features then affect the distal parts of limbs and usually involve the legs before the arms. Superficial sensory loss in a polyneuropathy is found over the distal parts of the extremities and extends along the limbs to a level which is uniform around their whole circumference. This is the 'stocking' and 'glove' type of sensory disturbance. Deep sensation, such as proprioception and vibration are usually little affected in polyneuropathy. If they are significantly impaired in associa-tion with glove and stocking anaesthesia it suggests that the causal lesion is diffusely damaging the cells in the dorsal root ganglia, or that there is a concurrent affection of the dorsal columns.

**Spinal Cord.** Sensation may be disturbed in several ways by lesions involving the spinal cord. Tumours which compress the cord may also impinge on an adjacent sensory root and hence give rise to diminution of all modalities in the corresponding dermatome. Sensory fibres may be damaged in the dorsal root entry zone, and lesions here also cause sensory loss in segmental dermatomes. The spinal sensory tracts may be interrupted and the level reflected in a loss of sensation at and below the segmental level of the lesion in the cord.

When the spinothalamic pathway is disrupted there will be a diminution of pain and temperature sensation below the level of the lesion and on the opposite side of the body. The upper border of this impairment will not necessarily correspond to the segmental level of the lesion because of the laminated structure of the tract (p. 291). In the cervical region, for instance, the fibres from cervical segments lie in the innermost part of the lateral spinothalamic tract. Fibres from thoracic, lumbar and sacral segments lie in bands, successively more laterally (Fig. 65). An extrinsic lesion such as a tumour which compresses the cord first affects the outermost layer of fibres, i.e. those from the sacral region and then progressively damages fibres from higher segments. Thus the upper level of sensory loss may correspond to a segmental dermatome lying well below the cord segment which is the site of damage. Intrinsic lesions often initially damage those fibres which have just entered the tract and spare, for a time at least, fibres from lower levels. The 'saddle' area of the buttocks, comprising the lower sacral dermatomes would be the last to be affected by a central cord lesion spreading centrifugally in the cervical region. Such topographical considerations help in the clinical differentiation between intramedullary tumours, which are rarely removable, and extramedullary tumours which may be curable.

Spinal cord lesions may cause loss of one modality of sensation in an area wherein other modalities are preserved. This is called 'dissociated' sensory loss. Most commonly pain and temperature sensations are lost whilst touch, vibration and position senses are intact. This pattern results from lesions which interrupt the lateral spinothalamic system but do not impinge on the dorsal columns. Dissociated anaesthesia is found in cases of syringomyelia but may also result from other processes, such as a tumour, damaging the central or lateral parts of the spinal cord.

**Intracranial lesions.** Within the *lower brain stem* lesions may give rise to impairment of pain and temperature on the ipsilateral side of the face and on the contralateral side of the body (sometimes called alternating analgesia).

*Above the pontine level* the spinothalamic tract and the medial lemniscus lie close together and are often damaged together. Lesions here which cause sensory impairment affect all modalities on the face, as well as on the body, on the side opposite the lesion. A hemianaesthesia involving the face and body is often due to interruption of the closely-packed sensory radiations in the contralateral *internal capsule*.

Lesions of the *thalamus* may give rise to spontaneous, intense, burning pain on the contralateral side, associated with diminution to touch over the same area. Pain can be provoked on the affected side of the body only by a painful stimulus of greater than normal intensity, i.e. the threshold for painful stimuli is raised. Pain, when thus evoked, has an ill-localised, particularly unpleasant quality.

Damage to the *sensory cortex* does not impair perception of pain, temperature and touch but causes a loss of discriminatory and correlative sensory appreciation.

## EXAMINATION OF THE REFLEXES

A neurological reflex depends on an arc which consists of an afferent pathway triggered by stimulating a receptor, an efferent system which activates an effector organ and a communication between these two components. Since a reflex response to an appropriate stimulus is involuntary, disturbances of reflexes afford objective signs of neural function. Some of the reflexes subserved by cranial nerves such as the corneal reflex and jaw jerk are

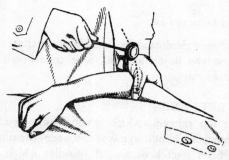

FIG. 68   Eliciting the Biceps Jerk, – C.5 (C.6).

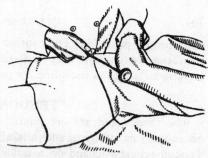

FIG. 69   Eliciting the Triceps Jerk, – C.6, C.7.

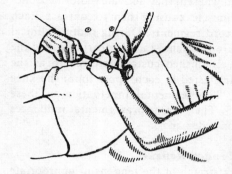

FIG. 70   Eliciting the Supinator Jerk, – (C.5), C.6.

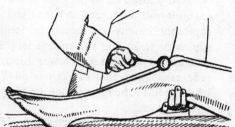

FIG. 71   Eliciting the Knee Jerk (*N.B.* the legs must not be in contact with each other), – L.3, L.4.

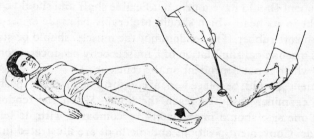

FIG. 72   Eliciting the Ankle Jerk of Recumbent Patient, – L.5, S.1.

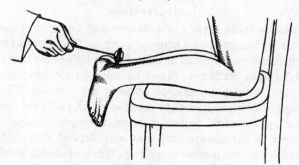

FIG. 73   Alternative Method of Eliciting the Ankle Jerk, – L.5, S.1.

described on page 262. The routine neurological examination should include elicitation of tendon (deep) reflexes in the limbs and of some superficial (cutaneous) reflexes, including the plantar responses.

## TENDON REFLEXES

The tendon reflexes are phasic stretch reflexes, which involve only two neurones, one afferent and one efferent with one synapse between them. Tendon reflexes depend on a sudden brief stretch of muscle spindles which evokes from them a synchronous afferent discharge. A volley of sensory impulses is conducted to the spinal cord wherein they activate motor neurones whose axons run back to the stretched muscles causing them to contract. Each reflex is subserved by its own spinal cord segments. During routine clinical examination the biceps jerk, the jerk from brachio-radialis (earlier called the supinator longus and hence by long established custom referred to as the supinator jerk) and the triceps jerk are tested in each upper limb; the knee and ankle jerks in the lower limbs. The segmental innervation of these reflexes is illustrated in Figures 68–73. There are suprasegmental influences which modify the function of the tendon reflex arc.

### Elicitation of Tendon Reflexes

These reflexes are evoked by a brisk stretch of the tendons of appropriate muscles, and this is most efficiently done by a tap from a tendon hammer. This instrument should have a firm but flexible shaft and should contain most of its weight in its head which should preferably be made of metal and well padded with soft rubber. The tendon, not the muscle, should be struck by the hammer as mechanical stimulation of a muscle belly produces a contraction of the muscle which is not dependent on the reflex arc.

The patient should be placed in a comfortable, relaxed position which allows the examiner easily to reach the limbs. When the tendon jerks are tested, the one side should immediately be compared with its fellow on the opposite side. Convenient positions and methods are illustrated in Figures 68 to 73.

### Interpretation

A normal tendon reflex results in a sudden displacement of part of a limb which then rapidly returns to its original position. The normal amplitude of such movements may be increased or decreased or there may be no movement. **Increased Tendon Reflexes.** Many patients, particularly when they are paying their first visit to a clinic or hospital are anxious. This tension is reflected in slight contractions of their muscles which facilitate tendon reflexes which become brisker than usual. A decision about whether reflexes are abnormally brisk is not always easy and may depend upon other evidence such as asymmetry or the plantar responses. When assessing a reflex response other muscles in the limb, as well as the one stimulated, should be observed.

When tendon reflexes are pathologically exaggerated there is often a spread of the evoked contractions beyond the muscle stimulated, as, for example, the finger flexion which often accompanies biceps and supinator jerks when they are pathologically exaggerated.

*The finger flexion jerk* may help to confirm the presence of significant hyperreflexia. The tips of the examiner's middle and index fingers are placed across the palmar surfaces of the proximal phalanges of the patient's relaxed fingers; the examiner then taps his own fingers lightly. A slight flexion often occurs normally but a very brisk contraction suggests hyperreflexia.

*Hoffman's sign* is another manifestation of hyperreflexia. It is elicited by first flexing the distal interphalangeal joint of the patient's middle finger and then flicking the terminal phalanx into extension. When tendon reflexes are hyperactive the thumb quickly flexes in response to this manoeuvre. Minimal flexion of the thumb may sometimes be evoked in normal people, particularly if they are apprehensive. If Hoffman's sign is unilaterally positive, it is a very strong indication of a significant increase in tendon reflexes on that side.

**Diminished or Absent Tendon Reflexes.** It should be emphasised that a few normal people have tendon reflexes which are difficult to obtain. Some patients who regularly take hypnotic or anticonvulsant drugs show a generalised reduction in the amplitude of their tendon reflexes. The significance of depressed tendon reflexes needs to be appraised by a comparison between the responses obtained on the two sides and between the amplitude of the jerks in the arms and those in the legs. If normally brisk contractions are seen in the arms and very poor responses are evoked at knee and ankles then it is probable that the latter findings are pathological.

In rare instances all the tendon reflexes may be absent in people who have no neurological disease. Usually, however, absence of one or more tendon jerks denotes a neural lesion. When no response is obtained after a routine tendon tap, the absence of the reflex should be confirmed by *'reinforcing'* the jerk. Tendon reflexes are increased in amplitude (i.e. potentiated or reinforced) by forcible contraction of muscles remote from those being tested. To reinforce the knee and ankle jerks the patient may be asked forcibly to clench his hands. An alternative procedure requires the patient to hook the fingers of his hands together and then forcibly to attempt to pull one away from the other without disengaging the fingers (Fig. 74).

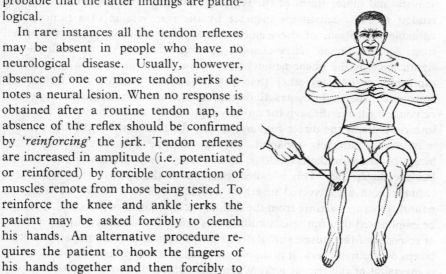

FIG. 74 Reinforcement in Eliciting the Knee Jerk.

Reinforcement of the reflexes in the upper limbs may best be obtained by asking the patient to clench his jaws or to push his knees hard together. It is important to remember that the phenomenon of reinforcement lasts for less than a second. The patient should, therefore, be told to perform the appropriate manoeuvre (previously demonstrated to him) almost synchronously with the examiner's tap of the tendon.

SITE OF LESION. When tendon reflexes are absent or pathologically diminished the next stage of the interpretation is to localise where the reflex arcs are damaged or interrupted. Lesions of muscle, myoneural junction, peripheral nerve or spinal cord might cause loss of reflexes. It is an important clinical observation that tendon reflexes disappear very late in the course of diseases which primarily affect muscle (i.e. myopathies). Whilst there are muscle spindles to respond to stretch and whilst the neural arc is intact, surviving muscle fibres continue to contract even when there is marked muscle wasting and weakness. By contrast lesions which damage peripheral nerves cause very early loss of tendon reflexes. As outlined above the reflex response depends on a synchronous volley of afferent impulses and a synchronous motor neurone discharge. Even minor dysfunctions of peripheral nerves cause either or both afferent or efferent impulses to become asynchronous and the tendon reflex is consequently lost.

Myasthenic disturbance at the neuromuscular junction usually causes no change in tendon reflexes though they may occasionally be temporarily diminished during periods of profound myasthenic weakness.

*Lesions within the spinal canal* may interrupt the connections between the sensory and motor limbs of the reflex arc and cause loss of reflexes. Absent tendon reflexes, caused for instance by the compression of a tumour, are valuable indications of the segmental level of a lesion involving the spinal cord. An uncommon reflex change, but one which is of precise localising significance, is the phenomenon of *inversion*. The transmission of a tendon tap stretches muscles other than that directly stimulated. In normal circumstances the slight contractions thus evoked are submerged by the major response mediated through the monosynaptic reflex arc. If, however, the arc is interrupted and the direct response is lost, the contractions in other muscles may become clinically apparent. This is sometimes seen after stretch of the biceps or brachioradialis tendons; no response is seen in the stretched muscle but the fingers flex. This is called inversion of the biceps or supinator jerk (usually both are involved together) and it is due to a lesion involving the neural structures arising from the fifth cervical segment of the cord. It should be emphasised that in these circumstances finger flexion occurs in the absence of response of the muscle stimulated. When finger flexion accompanies a brisk biceps or supinator jerk, it is simply an index of hyperreflexia. Less often seen is inversion of the triceps jerk. When this occurs, due to a lesion of the C.7 spinal segmental structures, tapping the tendon of triceps produces no contraction therein but causes a contraction of the biceps.

**Other abnormalities of tendon reflexes.** In uncomplicated and isolated cerebellar lesions the tendon reflexes are described as pendular; the limb oscillates several times after the initial jerk, before settling again to its original position. This phenomenon is most easily detected in the knee jerk when the patient is seated on the edge of a bed with his feet swinging freely off the ground (Fig. 74). It occurs rarely and is not a sign of great clinical value.

Occasionally one will observe a fairly brisk contraction of a muscle in response to a tendon tap followed by very slow relaxation. This delayed relaxation, most often seen at the ankle, is a consistent and reliable sign of hypothyroidism.

## SUPERFICIAL REFLEXES

These consist of muscular contractions evoked by cutaneous stimulation. The plantar response is the best known and most important.

**Plantar Response.** In normal people stimulation of the lateral border of the sole of the foot causes plantar flexion of the great toe and usually of the other toes. The stimulus should not cause injury but it should be of noxious character since this is a nociceptive reflex. However it should be remembered that the sole can be very sensitive. A blunted point such as the end of a car key produces an appropriate stimulus. A pin may be used but needs skilful handling to avoid lacerating the skin. The patient should lie supine with his legs extended. The stimulating point should be drawn along the lateral border of the foot from the heel towards the little toe (Fig. 75). This type of plantar stimulation in pathological circumstances gives rise to extension (dorsiflexion) of the great toe at the metatarsophalangeal joint. This is the sign described by Babinski who used a goose quill for its elicitation; it is often referred to by his name. The plantar response should, however, be described as 'flexor' when down going, or as 'extensor' when there is dorsiflexion since the use of Babinski's name often gives rise to the solecism of a 'flexor' Babinski response and to the ambiguity of an 'absent' Babinski response. Dorsiflexion

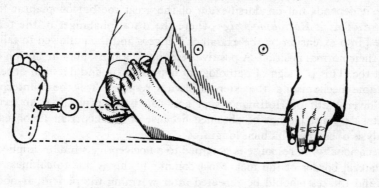

FIG. 75 Eliciting the Plantar Reflex.

of the great toe in response to plantar stimulation is often accompanied by other abnormal phenomena. There may be a sluggish spreading or 'fanning' of the other four toes. Sometimes an extensor plantar response is attended by simultaneous reflex contraction of the flexor muscles of the hip, knee and ankle. This is called the withdrawal response of which dorsiflexion of the great toe is a fragmentary manifestation.

INTERPRETATION. There has for many years been extensive investigation into this reflex which is generally accepted as the most significant clinical neurological sign. Doubt has been cast on the precise physiological significance of an extensor plantar response and particularly on the pathways which subserve it. These physiological debates are of interest but they do not detract from the clinical value of the sign. For practical purposes an extensor plantar response indicates a lesion of the complex upper motor neurone system which runs from the motor cortex down to the spinal cord and which is called the pyramidal pathway. It has been averred that in some instances damage to this fibre system does not result in an extensor plantar response, and that occasionally an extensor plantar response is observed in the absence of damage to this system. However, such instances are rare, and ill understood and there is no reason to abandon the clinical interpretation which regards the extensor plantar response as pathognomonic of a pyramidal lesion. Deductions made on this basis have proved themselves empirically over many decades.

The plantar reflex is normally evoked by stimulation of the sole in the area supplied by the first sacral sensory root. In cases wherein there are widespread and severe lesions of the corticospinal pathways the reflexogenic zone may be greatly enlarged. An extensor plantar response may then be produced by a number of techniques. Rubbing over the crest of the tibia, squeezing the Achilles tendon or a tap over the lateral malleolus may each induce dorsiflexion of the great toe. These signs have eponyms attached to them but are of little clinical importance since when they are obtainable the routine method of scraping the foot invariably elicits a significant response. One accessory sign of damage to the pyramidal pathways may sometimes be useful since it depends not on dorsiflexion of the great toe but on plantar flexion thereof. This is *Rossolimo's sign* where the distal phalanges of the toes are flicked into extension by the examiner's fingers and then allowed to fall back into their normal position. A positive response is a brisk plantar flexion of the great toe. This is a sign of pathological hyperreflexia and does not depend on the same mechanism as the extensor plantar response. It is the counterpart in the lower limbs of Hoffman's sign and can be helpful when an extensor plantar response cannot be obtained because of a concurrent lesion causing paralysis of extensor hallucis longus.

Occasionally no response is obtained to a nociceptive stimulus applied over the lateral border of the foot. Most commonly this is due to coldness of the feet and the test should be repeated after warming the patient. If no reflex movement is elicited despite warming there may be an impairment of cutaneous sensibility over the S.1 distribution or there may be paralysis of the long flexors or extensors of the great toe. The plantar response may be absent immediately after a complete transection of the spinal cord during the phase of spinal shock.

**The abdominal reflexes.** Normally a contraction of the muscles of the anterior abdominal wall is provoked when the skin of the abdomen is stroked or scratched. These responses are polysynaptic nociceptive reflexes. The patient should lie warm and relaxed in a supine position with a low pillow supporting his head. It is common to test four abdominal quadrants whose cutaneous nerves derive from the eighth to twelfth thoracic spinal segments. Upper and lower quadrants on each side are stimu-lated by drawing a pin towards the midline, parallel respectively with the costal margins and with the inguinal ligaments (Fig. 76). A pin is the implement which most effectively elicits abdominal reflexes but it should be used with care. It should be drawn lightly over the abdominal wall at an acute angle to the skin. If the pin be held vertically it frequently cuts the skin; there is never a need to penetrate the skin when testing the abdominal reflexes. If heavier pressure needs to be applied it is best to use instead a key or the shaft of the tendon hammer.

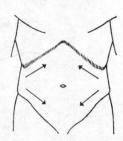

Fig. 76 Sites of Stimuli for Eliciting the Abdominal Reflexes.

INTERPRETATION. In most people the muscles under-lying the area stimulated will contract briskly. However when the abdominal wall is lax in women who have borne many children and in obese patients the reflexes may be absent without there being any associated neural lesion. The abdominal reflexes may occasionally be lost because of impaired pain sensa-tion in the skin or because of lower motor neurone lesions affecting the abdominal musculature. In most instances absence of responses in a young relaxed patient with good abdominal muscles strongly suggests an upper motor neurone lesion. The reflexes may be lost on one or both sides, reflecting unilateral or bilateral pyramidal tract involvement. While loss of abdominal reflexes is by no means invariable in pyramidal lesions, when disseminated sclerosis damages pyramidal pathways, the abdominal reflexes are consistently absent. Their loss is often a very early manifestation of upper motor neurone disruption in this disease. In pyramidal lesions due to motor neurone disease the abdominal reflexes are usually preserved. These empirical observations are sometimes useful in differential diagnosis, but they are not immutable laws and undue weight should not be attached to them. The pathophysiology underlying the differing vulnerability of the abdominal reflexes in different diseases is ill understood. Loss of abdominal cutaneous reflexes probably results only if other pathways, as well as the pyramidal tracts, are interrupted and such widespread lesions are liable to occur in disseminated sclerosis.

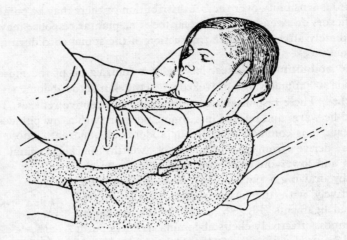

FIG. 77    Testing for Meningeal Irritation (Neck rigidity).

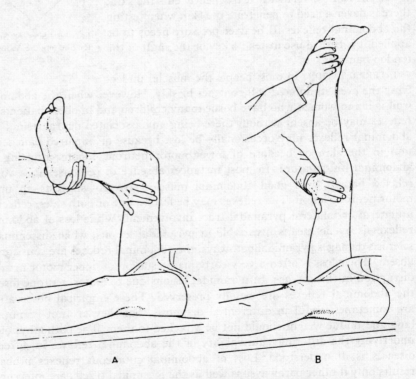

A                                                                              B

FIG. 78    Testing for Meningeal Irritation (Kernig's test).

**The cremasteric reflexes.** These are sometimes tested in male patients. Stroking or scratching the inner aspect of the upper part of thigh normally provokes an elevation of the testis on the same side. This reflex response may be lost as a result of an upper motor neurone lesion.

## MISCELLANEOUS TESTS

Under this heading are included those tests which, although not carried out routinely, are often indicated and may yield most important information in special circumstances.

### Signs of Meningeal Irritation

Inflammation of the meninges due to infection or blood in the subarachnoid space evokes a reflex spasm in the paravertebral muscles. In the cervical region this manifests itself by *neck rigidity* which impedes passive flexion of the neck. In any patient in whom meningitis or subarachnoid haemorrhage is a possibility neck flexion should be tested (Fig. 77). The neck initially should be slowly flexed but in the early stages of a meningeal reaction spasm may be more easily demonstrated if the neck is flexed abruptly. Normally the chin can be made to touch the chest without causing discomfort.

Meningeal irritation causing spasm in the lumbar region can be demonstrated by passive movements of the lower limbs (*Kernig's sign*). The patient lies supine with one leg extended; the leg to be tested is flexed at the hip and knee. Whilst the hip joint remains flexed the knee is extended as shown in Fig. 78. When there is meningeal irritation involving the posterior roots in the lumbar area it will be impossible fully to extend the knee because of spasm in the hamstring muscles.

### Signs of Nerve Root Irritation

When lumbar and sacral nerve roots are pressed upon by a prolapsed intervertebral disc, stretching of the sciatic nerve or the femoral nerve may give rise to pain. These nerve stretching tests are described on page 347.

### Signs of Tetany

In tetany a low serum calcium (or ionised calcium) causes an increased excitability of nerves, and painful muscle cramps result. *Carpopedal spasm* is the characteristic finding. The hands spontaneously take up the position known as the *main d'accoucheur,* in which there is opposition of the thumb, extension of the interphalangeal and flexion of the metacarpophalangeal joints. In latent tetany the same position can be induced within four minutes by inflation of the sphygmomanometer cuff to a level above the systolic blood pressure—*Trousseau's sign* (Fig. 79). A tap over the facial nerve in front of the ear provokes a brisk momentary contraction of the facial muscles, pulling the mouth to that side in latent tetany, but also in some normal subjects—*Chvostek's sign.*

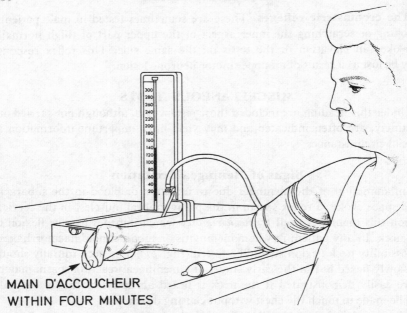

MAIN D'ACCOUCHEUR
WITHIN FOUR MINUTES

FIG. 79    Testing for Latent Tetany (Trousseau's sign).

## Signs Elicited by Palpation, Percussion and Auscultation

Palpation of the skull and of the spinous processes occasionally reveals local destructive lesions due to tumours or irregularities due to trauma. Percussion may elicit localised tenderness in the spinous processes overlying an epidural abscess.

Pulsation in the carotid arteries in the neck should be palpated and any asymmetry noted. The juxtaposition of the internal and external carotid arteries means that major lesions in the former may be disguised by normal pulsation in the latter. Auscultation of the neck may reveal a bruit due to stenosis in a carotid, vertebral or subclavian artery. To be significant such a murmur should be localised and not one conducted from the heart. Bruits may arise in internal or external carotids either on the side of a stenotic lesion or on the side opposite the narrowing because of increased flow in the other carotid system. Palpable or audible changes in the neck vessels may suggest a vascular cause for an intracranial lesion but precise anatomical interpretation of such abnormalities is often impossible.

A bruit which is audible over the skull or over the spine may on rare occasions be a most valuable sign. Aneurysms, particularly arteriovenous malformations, may produce murmurs which can be heard over the skull vault, or orbit, or, very rarely, over the spine. When clinical features suggest the presence of an arteriovenous anomaly a careful search for such bruits should be made in quiet surroundings.

# FURTHER INVESTIGATIONS

The clinical examination of the nervous system is an integral part of the general medical examination. Similarly, neurological investigations cannot be considered in isolation. In some instances a blood count which reveals a macrocytic anaemia may implicate vitamin $B_{12}$ deficiency as the cause of spinal cord lesions. A leukaemic blood picture or a diabetic glucose tolerance test may suggest the aetiology of varied neurological pictures. These examples could be multiplied. They emphasise the frequent need to utilise supplementary tests other than those which directly explore the central nervous system in order to evaluate neurological problems.

The intelligent selection of appropriate investigations is based on the clinical picture and should always take account of the discomforts and dangers attendant upon the investigative techniques. In a few cases extreme clinical urgency will demand that the definitive test, even if painful, be performed immediately. In most instances it is wise to instigate those investigations which are least disturbing and only later to proceed to uncomfortable or hazardous tests.

Some tests which are frequently indicated do no more than refine and supplement clinical examination. Slit lamp examination of the eyes may reveal a brownish band at the limbus characteristic of Wilson's disease (p. 75), and this technique will define the punctate cataracts of dystrophia myotonica. Audiometry, caloric testing and electronystagmography yield valuable information in cases of vertigo.

## Radiological Examination

Plain radiographs are important preliminary investigations in almost all neurological problems. A chest radiograph may reveal a bronchial carcinoma and hence explain a wide variety of metastatic and non-metastatic neural complications. Plain radiographs of the skull are indicated when the clinical picture is suggestive of an intracranial lesion. They may show erosions caused by tumours; thickening of the vault of the skull may be provoked by a subjacent meningioma. Lesions such as gliomas, tuberculomas and arteriovenous malformations may be delineated by abnormal calcification. Radiographs of the spine should be performed whenever a lesion of the cord or nerve roots is suspected. The vertebral bodies, the pedicles and the disc spaces may display abnormalities which would localise the site and suggest the cause of compression of the spinal cord. More complex radiological investigation is discussed on page 314.

## Serological Tests for Syphilis

In all patients who suffer from neurological disabilities of uncertain origin serological tests for syphilis should be performed on the blood.

## Examination of the Cerebrospinal Fluid (CSF)

Examination of the CSF is frequently necessary in the investigation of patients with neurological disease but it should not be done without good reason. It is usually unnecessary to perform a lumbar puncture when clinical signs and straight X-rays have already revealed a cerebral tumour. Lumbar puncture should never be performed if there is evidence of raised intracranial pressure.

Normally the CSF pressure is less than 150 mm of fluid; it contains less than 5 cells per cmm, 20 to 50 mg of protein per 100 ml, and 40 to 80 mg of glucose per 100 ml. An increase in the cell count may be found when an infective process affects the central nervous system.

A large number of polymorphonuclear leucocytes is found in bacterial meningitis and in the early stages of tuberculous and viral meningitis. A lymphocytosis may be due to viral meningitis or encephalitis, to neuro-syphilis or tuberculous meningitis; an increase in lymphocytes sometimes occurs in disseminated sclerosis. A rise in the protein concentration in the CSF is the commonest abnormal finding but is non-specific. Very high values are found when a spinal tumour blocks the subarachnoid space. A marked rise in protein is also associated with spinal neurofibromas and with the Guillain-Barré type of polyneuropathy. The proportion of gamma globulin in CSF protein is now usually estimated. Normally 5–15 per cent of the total protein content is gamma globulin. A rise in this fraction above 30 per cent is most often found in patients suffering from disseminated sclerosis, neurosyphilis or a connective tissue disorder. An indirect index of this variation in CSF protein pattern is given by the Lange curve or colloidal gold reaction.

A rise in the glucose content of the CSF merely reflects the hyperglycaemia of diabetes. Low levels are usually due to meningitis; the most marked falls are found in pyogenic meningitis. Low glucose levels, may rarely be due to infiltration of the subarachnoid space by malignant cells.

## Investigation in relation to site of lesion

The choice of more sophisticated and specific investigations is determined by the site of neurological lesions.

## Muscles and Peripheral Nerves

The investigation of primary diseases of muscle may require extensive biochemical testing. Of general applicability is the estimation of serum enzymes such as aldolase, lactic dehydrogenase and, most specifically, creatine phosphokinase whose concentrations reflect the rate and extent of muscle fibre disintegration.

Peripheral nerve disorders may also require a range of biochemical investigations such as vitamin assays, renal function tests and glucose tolerance tests.

In the investigation of diseases of peripheral nerve and muscular disorders, electrodiagnostic techniques are useful. *Electromyography* records muscle action potentials, using a needle electrode and an oscilloscope display system. This procedure will demonstrate denervation and differentiate neural from myopathic lesions. The estimation of conduction velocity in nerve trunks will gauge the extent of dysfunction in neuropathies and will define the site of localised compressions of peripheral nerves, as in the carpal tunnel.

### SPINAL CORD

Systematised lesions of the spinal cord need to be biochemically investigated. Localised damage to the spinal cord often requires investigation by *myelography*. In this radiological procedure a radio opaque dye is introduced into the subarachnoid space via a lumbar puncture needle. The dye is then manoeuvred along the spinal canal, by tilting the patient. Deformation of the column of dye will reveal compressive lesions and suggest their nature. This procedure is uncomfortable and sometimes painful root irritation ensues. It should be performed only when the clinical signs indicate the possibility of a lesion of the spinal cord curable by surgery.

### INTRACRANIAL DISEASE

A wide variety of techniques is available for investigation of intracranial lesions; harmless tests should be employed first.

*The electroencephalogram (EEG).* This records the electrical potentials of the brain after they are attenuated by passing through the skull and scalp. Potential changes are recorded simultaneously over several areas. Intracranial disease may cause normal electrical rhythms to be suppressed or more commonly, abnormal wave forms may be engendered. Such abnormalities may be generalised or localised. EEG abnormalities are more marked with acute lesions such as cerebral abscess than with slowly progressive or chronic lesions. Lesions within the substance of the brain such as gliomas produce more marked and earlier abnormalities than lesions such as meningiomas or angiomas lying outside the brain tissue. The EEG is more precise in its definition of lesions lying in the cerebral hemispheres than it is in lesions lying within the posterior fossa. The EEG will often reveal epileptic discharges but it alone cannot make a diagnosis of epilepsy.

*Echoencephalography.* This uses the reflection of a beam of ultrasound from mid line structures of the brain in order to demonstrate shifts of the cerebral hemispheres. Thus it can be used to demonstrate a unilateral space occupying lesion. It is a quick, painless technique which can be performed at the bedside and is now a routine investigation of those patients who may have such lesions as cerebral tumour or subdural haemorrhage.

*Radio-active cerebral scanning.* This is also an innocuous and useful investigation. An injected radio isotope (such as technetium) is often taken up differentially by diseased intracranial tissue compared to normal brain substance. Differing intensities of radio activities are recorded through the skull and abnormal areas mapped. In this way tumours, particularly meningiomas, can be localised.

*Computerised transverse axial scanning.* The E.M:I. scanner provides a new method of investigation which depends on the rates at which X-rays are transmitted through structures of different density. Readings are taken of the rate of transmissions directed through the skull at a multitude of angles and from these data the densities of the intra-cranial contents are computed. Pictures of the structure of the brain and the ventricles can be constructed and examined in much the same way as conventional radiographs. Lesions such as haematomas, infarctions, abscesses and tumours can be delineated because of the alterations they produce in the density of the intra-cranial contents. The technique is atraumatic, accurate and sensitive and the patient is exposed to less radiation than that required for a conventional skull radiograph. It may be performed on out-patients and should reduce the need for contrast radiography.

*Intracranial contrast radiography.* This is often required but should never lightly be undertaken. In *carotid arteriography* a radio opaque medium is injected percutaneously under local or general anaesthetic into the common carotid artery and films of the opacified cerebral vessels are taken in rapid succession. A similar technique is employed, though less frequently, to display the vertebral and basilar arteries. Cerebral angiography demonstrates occlusions or stenosis of the vessels as well as abnormalities such as aneurysms. Space occupying lesions of moderate size displace the arteries and veins. Angiography is the appropriate investigation when clinical signs point to a lesion in one cerebral hemisphere. It is not without danger, particularly in cerebrovascular disease.

*Pneumo-encephalography.* This outlines the ventricular system. 15 mls. of air introduced into the lumbar subarachnoid space through a needle, rises into the basal cisterns and into the ventricles, and is manipulated so that the ventricles are outlined. This technique may show displacement due to a tumour or dilatation due to obstructive hydrocephalus or cerebral atrophy. Pneumo-encephalography is safe only if intracranial pressure is normal but it causes severe headache for several days afterwards in most patients.

*Ventriculography.* This is the only safe contrast study in those patients who have raised intracranial pressure due to a posterior fossa tumour. Radio opaque dye is introduced into one lateral ventricle by a needle which is passed through a burr hole in the skull. The dye passes downwards into the 'narrows' of the third and fourth ventricles and the aqueduct. Obstruction or displacement of these structures will reveal the site of a tumour. Ventriculography is a major procedure and should be performed only when the suspicion of a posterior fossa tumour is high and when neurosurgical facilities are immediately available.

# THE METHODS IN PRACTICE

## THE DIAGNOSTIC PROCESS

The completion of the neurological examination is followed by the correlation and interpretation of all the available information in order to reach a diagnosis. This must be based on logical thought processes. There are a number of shorthand formulae in neurology as for instance the equation of dissociated anaesthesia with a diagnosis of syringomyelia, the attribution of bilateral clawing of hands and feet to peroneal muscular atrophy, the diagnosis of motor neurone disease because of obvious fasciculation and the labelling of any episode of weakness or paraesthesiae in a young adult as disseminated sclerosis. There is, of course, an expression of meretricious statistical probability in each of these assertions; diagnoses based on them will often be correct. But they are shibboleths. A quick gamble, even at favourable odds, is not a sound prelude to the best possible management of a patient. The diagnostic formulation should comprise a careful and orderly assessment of the nature of the patient's dysfunction. The neural systems and pathways damaged are then adduced. Next the distribution of lesions is defined. Finally the most likely pathological diagnosis is inferred. In other words what is disturbed, where and why?

## 1.   DISTURBANCE OF FUNCTION

The patient complains of the end results of disordered physiological functions whose nature is reflected in the abnormal signs revealed during the examination. This process is exemplified in the analysis of motor disturbances on pages 287 and 288. The signs found are correlated by the clinician so that the neural structures disrupted can be identified. The combination of signs attributable to lesions of different parts and paths of the nervous system need to be understood and memorised.

*Upper motor neurone (pyramidal tract) lesions.* These cause (1) weakness or paralysis of movement; (2) increase of tone of 'clasp-knife' type; (3) increased amplitude of tendon reflexes; (4) diminution of abdominal reflexes; (5) an extensor plantar response.

*Lower motor neurone lesions.* These give rise to (1) weakness or paralysis of muscles; (2) wasting of muscles; (3) there may be fasciculation in the involved muscles; (4) if many muscles in a limb are wasted, tone will be reduced therein; (5) if the affected muscles subserve tendon reflexes, these will be diminished or absent.

*Cerebellar lesions.* Damage to the posterior lobe of the cerebellum or of its connections with the brain stem are accompanied by (1) ataxia of gait; (2) intention tremor of limbs; (3) jerking nystagmus; (4) dysarthria of staccato or scanning type; (5) dysmetria and past pointing; (6) impaired alternating movements; (7) hypotonia and pendular tendon reflexes; (8) occasionally, smooth movements may be broken up into their constituent parts producing jerking, marionette-like, decomposition of movements.

*Generalised polyneuropathies.* These often cause (1) diminution of superficial sensation affecting the distal aspect of limbs over 'stocking' and 'glove' distributions; (2) wasting and weakness of distal limb musculature; (3) early loss of tendon reflexes.

*Spinal or cranial nerve damage.* This results in combinations of signs which depend on the area of supply to the individual nerves.

*Muscles.* Primary affections of muscle fibres lead to wasting and weakness of muscles usually (but not invariably) in the proximal parts of limbs. Fatty infiltration of muscle may cause an apparent increase in size of the affected muscles. Reflexes are preserved until muscle wasting is very marked.

*Sensory tracts.* Interruption of *dorsal columns* causes (1) ataxia of gait and limb movements aggravated by eye closure; (2) impaired position sense; (3) diminished appreciation of vibration. Lesions of the *spinothalamic* system cause impairment of pain and temperature sensation.

It is emphasised that these combinations of signs are those of fully developed pictures. Every abnormality is not to be expected in every case and the clinician must be prepared to deduce that a tract has been damaged when incomplete patterns of signs have been demonstrated.

## 2.  DISTRIBUTION OF LESIONS

The identification of damaged neural structures is followed by the definition of the site or sites of their involvement. All the observed signs may be due to a localised lesion affecting adjacent structures.

*Single lesions.* Impairment of specialised functions of the *cerebral cortex* result in dementia, dysphasia, apraxia, astereognosis and other forms of agnosia. Upper motor neurone lesions at the cortical level cause signs similar to those due to interruption of the pyramidal tract at more caudal sites but since the upper motor neurones are spread over a wide area in the cortex, lesions here typically affect only part of the opposite side of the body. A paresis confined to one limb (monoplegia) or to one side of the face is likelier than a hemiplegia. Bilateral pyramidal signs result from solitary cortical lesions only in the rare instance of a parasagittal affection. Lesions here, such as a meningioma, may impinge on both hemispheres on the neurones which lie close together on each side of the sagittal plane and which supply the legs. The demonstration of cortical abnormalities will often enable the extent of a lesion to be mapped out fairly precisely.

Localisation within the *cerebral hemispheres* is helped if a pattern of visual deficit has been elucidated; thus an upper quadrantic homonymous hemianopia points to a lesion in the temporal lobe on the side opposite the field defect (Fig. 49, p. 246).

A profound hemiplegia equally affecting face, arm and leg, associated with loss of sensation of all modalities on the paralysed side suggests a lesion affecting the *internal capsule* where the pyramidal and sensory pathways are packed closely together.

Lesions of the *brain stem* are characterised by ipsilateral impairment of one or more cranial nerves with concurrent contralateral affection of one or more long tracts usually the pyramidal pathway. Which cranial nerves are implicated will depend on which part of the brain stem is affected. A midbrain lesion is suggested if there is a third nerve palsy on one side and signs of upper motor neurone involvement on the other. Pontine damage is indicated by sixth and seventh nerve signs accompanied by contralateral pyramidal signs. Occasionally other tracts such as the spinothalamic pathway are interrupted. Lesions of the pons often give rise to ataxic nystagmus (p. 259).

*Spinal cord damage* is localised by correlating motor, sensory and reflex changes.

Upper motor neurone signs arising from cord lesions are often, but by no means always, bilateral. The location of the site of pyramidal tract lesions can be made only very roughly on the basis of upper motor neurone signs alone; if they are present in the arms then the lesion must be above the fifth cervical segment; if the abdominal reflexes are all lost then a segment above the eighth thoracic must be implicated; signs in the legs indicate a lesion above the conus medullaris.

The site of pyramidal tract damage is localised much more precisely if the offending lesion also involves the anterior horn cells or motor roots. Lower motor neurone signs, with wasting in a segmental distribution define the cord lesion accurately. Sensory signs may help to delineate the position of cord lesions; thus impairment of sensation over a segmental dermatome will indicate the level of a lesion on occasion. Interruption of sensory tracts may give rise to a level of sensory loss which sometimes corresponds to the site of the spinal lesion but often extends only to a more caudal level (p. 299). Spinal cord lesions disrupt reflex arcs and loss of tendon reflexes will reflect the segments which have been damaged.

Often the segmental level and the cross sectional areas of a spinal cord lesion may be gauged. In a hemisection of the cord below the lesion and on the ipsilateral side there will be found (1) upper motor neurone signs, (2) impaired position and vibration senses, (3) signs of vasomotor disturbance. On the contralateral side there will be reduced sensation to pain and temperature. This composite picture is called the *Brown-Séquard syndrome*.

**Multiple Lesions.** The analysis of a patient's signs may show that they cannot be explained on the basis of a single lesion. Two or more separated, *discrete lesions* may be defined, as for instance when lesions in optic nerves are found concurrently with evidence of spinal cord damage in multiple sclerosis.

*Lesions may be systematised,* i.e. similar types of fibres or cells may be affected in different parts of the nervous system. A symmetrical polyneuropathy is a systematised affection of peripheral nerves. Damage may be confined to groups of upper and lower motor neurones as in motor neurone disease or to dorsal root ganglion cells as in one form of carcinomatous neuropathy. Spinal tracts may be selectively damaged, singly or in combination as when dorsal and lateral columns are disrupted by vitamin $B_{12}$ deficiency.

*Diffuse damage* may be demonstrated when disorders affect wide areas of grey and white matter traversing structural and functional boundaries. Thus syphilitic disease may cause a generalised loss of cortical neurones; may interrupt the central prolongations of dorsal root ganglion cells and hence cause wasting of the dorsal columns; may damage the pyramidal and extrapyramidal motor systems; and may cause transverse cord lesions and cranial nerve palsies. All of these disturbances do not present concurrently but combinations of several such lesions are commonly found in the same patient. Repetitive head injuries also cause randomised, diffuse cerebral affection which results in the dementia, cerbellar ataxia and Parkinsonism of the 'punch-drunk' state. The recognition of the patterns of neural lesions, whether single or multiple and, if multiple, whether discrete, systematised or diffuse, provides part of the information needed to make the final aetiological and pathological diagnosis.

## 3. PATHOLOGICAL DIAGNOSIS

The most efficient prediction of the pathological process requires the integration of all the information gained from the patient's history, the general medical examination, and the neurological examination.

In the first instance the course of the development of the illness is reviewed and interpreted in order to estimate the general nature of the neural lesion. More specific clues to aetiology may be contained in the history. The story of an antecedent head injury in an elderly patient with a progressive intracranial lesion may suggest the likelihood of a subdural haematoma. A previous history of gonorrhoea or of a primary chancre may point to a diagnosis of neurosyphilis. A family history of epilepsy, muscle disease or ataxia may clarify the nature of a patient's illness. Circumstantial evidence from the general medical examination may indicate that the neural lesion is due to the same process which involves other systems. Thus evidence of peripheral vascular disease or of a cardiac arrhythmia might imply that a cerebral lesion was of vascular nature. Clinical evidence of anaemia and a smooth tongue would implicate $B_{12}$ deficiency as the likely cause of a myelopathy.

Finally the nature and distribution of neurological signs might inferentially suggest the probabilities of some causal lesions and help to exclude others. If a patient has signs of intracranial damage together with papilloedema then a space occupying lesion, such as a tumour, is likely. The reflex changes of the Argyll Robertson pupil have been found occasionally in patients with midbrain encephalitis or tumours, but their presence, in company with neurological deficit of almost any type, should suggest syphilis as the probable diagnosis. Patients with marked neurological abnormalities, particularly drowsiness and nystagmus, which disappear after a period in hospital may well be suffering from intoxication by either alcohol or drugs.

If the patient with neurological disease is approached in this manner it is often possible to make a firm diagnosis on clinical grounds alone. On those occasions when the information is insufficient for a confident inference to be drawn the probable causes may be deduced and a rational scheme of investigation can be designed. Many neurological investigations cause discomfort and some are hazardous and they should be performed only if they are essential in order to define potentially curable lesions. There is no justification for subjecting patients to angiography or air encephalography as a substitute for an adequate clinical examination.

The clinical examination of the nervous system is a medical technique of precision and elegance which can provide a recurrent intellectual stimulus to the clinician and more importantly it is an essential prerequisite to the proper and efficient management of patients.

## SUMMARY OF EXAMINATION OF THE NERVOUS SYSTEM

**Intellect, Speech, Gait**

**Cranial Nerves**   1. Sense of smell. 2. Ophthalmoscopy; visual acuity and fields. 3, 4, 6. Inspection, esp. lids and pupils; pupillary reflexes; ocular movements; nystagmus. 5. Facial sensation; corneal reflex; muscles of mastication; jaw jerk. 7. Facial movements; taste anterior $\frac{2}{3}$ tongue. 8. Hearing. 9. Sensation posterior $\frac{1}{3}$ tongue; gag reflex. 10. Phonation; movement of palate and pharynx. 11. Sternomastoid and trapezius muscles. 12. Inspection of tongue and its movements.

**Motor System.** Inspection of muscles; involuntary movements; tone; clonus; power; co-ordination; fine movements; dyspraxia.

**Sensory System.** Touch; pain; temperature; position and vibration senses; cortical sensory function.

**Reflexes.** Tendon and superficial.

**Supplementary Tests.** e.g. Tests for meningeal or nerve root irritation or tetany.

# CHAPTER 9
# The Locomotor System

'And so, from hour to hour, we ripe and ripe,
And then, from hour to hour, we rot and rot;
And thereby hangs a tale.'

SHAKESPEARE

Examination of the locomotor system is often only a part of the assessment of a patient with other complaints. Approached in this way it is not difficult to confirm that all is well. It is necessary only to determine that normal posture and a full painless controlled range of active movements are present. An awareness that posture and the normal range of movement change throughout life is an important point, well taken by Touchstone in *As You Like It*. However, where the general examination reveals an abnormality or when the patient's symptoms suggest involvement of the locomotor system, a more detailed study of the affected area is required. In the first part of this chapter a simple but comprehensive method is set out which can be incorporated with the routine physical examination. This is designed to achieve a rapid assessment of the patient, indicating which region or regions require more detailed review should any abnormality be found.

The second part of the chapter begins with a section dealing with pain in relation to the locomotor system. Thereafter the detailed examination of the various regions is presented. In each instance introductory sections deal with the essential anatomical and pathological features and how these influence the history-taking and the methods of examination. The junior student should initially limit his study to the first part, and thereafter refer to the relevant section of Part II as specific problems arise.

## Part I
## GENERAL EXAMINATION

In the history pain predominates and should be analysed as described on page 29 and correlated with the pain patterns encountered in the locomotor system (p. 331). To do this it is helpful to take the patient through a typical day and note how his symptoms are affected by rest and activity and what factors aggravate or relieve them (p. 331). In this way a typical pattern often emerges.

The ideal arrangement for examination is that the patient is observed as he walks into the consulting-room, thus allowing an early assessment of posture and gait. Good lighting and adequate space are essential. The examination couch should not lie alongside a wall. It must be accessible from both sides and there must be no obstacle preventing a full range of movements of the patient's limbs.

## Posture

For adequate assessment the patient should be able to stand and walk. Where this is not possible some idea of the posture can be gained by examination of the patient in the supine and prone positions. Normal posture varies from age to age, passing through a cycle of change (Fig. 80). *In utero*, and for a short time after birth, there is a generalised dorsal convexity of the spine, or kyphosis. When the child holds up its head the cervical spine develops a curve convex ventrally—a lordosis. When the child begins to walk, a second lordosis develops in the lumbar region, often of an exaggerated amount, and the legs remain flexed and abducted at the hips and flexed at the knees. Only in the juvenile and young adult does the typical human erect posture pertain, but pregnancy or adiposity again exaggerates the lumbar lordosis. Thereafter the lumbar discs degenerate and the lumbar lordosis is

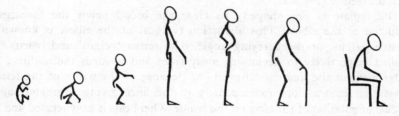

FIG. 80    The Seven Ages of Man.    Posture changes.

lost; the flexion of the hips dating from the previous era is unmasked and with sticks a second quadruped stage is reached. The cervical discs degenerate further and, finally, the general kyphosis of the foetus is reproduced in the wheelchair. In prehistory the cycle was often completed by burial in the womb posture of the foetus.

Thus variations in the curves of the spine are to be expected throughout life. When exaggerated, or when angular rather than curved, they become abnormal. An angular kyphosis, usually the result of destruction of the vertebral bodies over a short length of the spine, is known as a gibbus.

Viewed from in front or behind, the pelvis should be level, the iliac crests being on the same horizontal plane, and the spine in a vertical line. Lateral curvature is always abnormal and is known as scoliosis. In the cervical region it is termed torticollis, or wry-neck. Scoliosis may be due to faulty posture and be correctable, it may be due to protective spasm where a painful lesion is present, or it may be due to structural changes and be permanent. These can be differentiated by asking the patient to bend forwards keeping the legs straight. A postural scoliosis will then be corrected; scoliosis due to a painful condition will be associated with limited flexion to a greater or lesser degree; a curve due to a painless structural lesion will persist even on flexion, and a hump will be revealed on the convex side of the curve. This is because lateral curvature is accompanied by rotation of the vertebrae at the apex of the curve (p. 344 ).

The posture of the limbs varies in the sexes when seen from in front. In the male the shape is of an inverted triangle. The arms hang straight from the shoulders. The pelvis is narrow so the femora do not have to converge sharply to allow the tibiae to be parallel and together (Fig. 81).

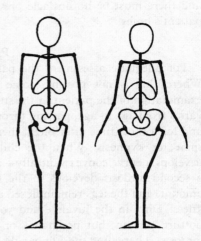

FIG. 81  Skeletal Differences in Male and Female.

The female is pear-shaped. To clear the broad pelvis the forearm is abducted at the elbow. This abduction (valgus) at the elbow is known as cubitus valgus, or the carrying angle. The terms 'valgus' and 'varus' are applied respectively to deviations away from and towards the midline, the body being in the anatomical position. Because of the width of the female pelvis the femora slope more acutely to the knee giving a greater, again valgus, angulation of the tibia on the femur. Where this is exaggerated and the tibiae no longer lie parallel it is known as genu valgum, or knock-knee deformity. Where the reverse angulation, or varus, is present the tibia is adducted on the femur and the deformity of genu varum, or bow-leg deformity, is produced.

## Gait

The normal human gait is a complex phenomenon in which movement occurs in several joints simultaneously in three dimensions. Biped gait would be expected to result in abrupt oscillation of the body up and down and from side to side. It is converted into an even undulation of small amplitude, at least in the male, by movements occurring between the spine and pelvis, at the hip, knee and ankle. Interference with the proper action of one of these components can usually be compensated by extra movement at the others and might be overlooked unless the patient is examined wearing little clothing. Interference with more than one results in an obvious limp.

Although there are great variations in normal gait and in the degree of abnormality of abnormal gaits, the latter can first be divided into two types—those that are painful and those that are not.

**Painful Gait.** The rhythm more than the contour of the gait is disturbed. The patient takes weight off the painful members as quickly as possible and the timing is dot-dash, dot-dash, painful-normal, painful-normal. When pain is severe the limb, flexed at hip, knee and ankle, is put delicately to the ground and the patient hops quickly on to the sound leg. The painful region is supported by one hand, if it is within reach, and the other arm is outstretched as a counter-balance. At the other extreme the only sign may be a shortening of the stride on the affected side.

**Painless Gaits.** The contour rather than the rhythm of the gait is abnormal. The different varieties can be classified as follows:

1. Osteogenic—due to shortening or deformity of bone.
2. Arthrogenic—due to joint stiffness, laxity or deformity.
3. Myogenic—due to weakness of muscle.
4. Neurogenic—due to organic disorder of the nervous system.
5. Psychogenic—due to functional disorder of the nervous system.
6. Prosthetic—due to wearing an artificial limb.

**Osteogenic Gait.** When the patient is clothed and wearing special footwear there may be little or no evident disturbance of gait, but when he is stripped for examination no difficulty should be encountered in detecting the cause of the abnormal gait.

**Arthrogenic Gait.** Complete loss of movement, ankylosis, of the hip or ankle, when not accompanied by deformity, results in very little disturbance of gait and may pass unnoticed in the clothed patient. In the common deformity of fixed flexion of the hip the gluteal region becomes prominent as the leg extends, and the gait is awkward. If the hip has an abduction deformity, an unsightly gait results as the leg has to swing out and round at each pace. When the hip is fixed in a few degrees of flexion and neutral abduction–adduction, the contour of the gait is little disturbed and the patient can climb and descend stairs in a normal manner.

The effect of a stiff knee is immediately obvious and the patient has to mount stairs one step at a time with the sound leg leading, and descend with the stiff leg leading.

A stiff ankle or foot, if not accompanied by deformity, causes little interference with the normal gait. If the foot is plantar flexed, in equinus (p. 364), the gait will resemble that of a 'drop foot' (p. 243).

**Myogenic Gait.** The effect of muscle weakness will depend on its site and degree, e.g. in pseudo-hypertrophic muscular dystrophy or as a result of myopathy in severe osteomalacia in the elderly, there is the characteristic waddling gait due to involvement of the gluteal muscles (p. 324).

**Neurogenic Gait.** SPASTIC PARALYSIS. The scissor gait is typical of the 'spastic' patient whose brain has been severely damaged from birth. The arms are adducted at the shoulder and flexed at the elbow and wrist. The posture is stooping with the legs flexed and adducted at the hips and flexed at the knee and ankle. The patient hitches each knee round and past its neighbour with a jerk, scraping the plantar flexed foot along the ground. In the mildly affected patient the only noticeable abnormality will be the curious impression that the patient is wearing heavy boots which he finds difficult to raise off the ground at the beginning of each step.

The gaits of patients suffering from hemiparesis or paraplegia are described on page 243.

FLACCID PARALYSIS. In contrast to the gaits of an ankylosed hip or foot the corresponding gaits in muscle paralysis are very obvious. Paralysis of the muscles controlling the knee, however, can be compensated by the hip and calf muscles and there may be no limp.

1. *Hip*. If the abductors of the hip are paralysed, the pelvis cannot be held level when the weight is on the affected limb. The pelvis tilts towards the opposite side and to counteract this the patient has to lean the trunk towards the affected side (Fig. 106, p. 356). This gives the impression of the patient lurching or dipping towards the paralysed side. A similar gait is seen in congenital dislocation of the hip. When both limbs are involved a waddling gait results.

2. *Knee*. If the extensors of the hip and the calf muscles are functioning, paralysis of the muscles controlling the knee will not result in a limp as the joint can be locked in full extension by the action of either when taking the body weight. If the hip extensors are also weak, the patient may push back on the thigh at each step with his hand to lock the knee in extension. If in addition the calf muscles are weak the patient will be unable to walk without a supporting caliper.

3. *Ankle and Foot*. Paralysis of the dorsiflexors of the foot results in the so-called 'drop-foot' gait (p. 243). When the foot and ankle flexor muscles are paralysed the gait lacks 'spring' and the so-called 'peg-leg' gait results.

CEREBELLAR AND EXTRA PYRAMIDAL LESIONS. The characteristic gaits from these causes are described on page 244.

**Psychogenic Gait.** Hysteria may be suspected if the gait is bizarre or if the patient appears to be strangely unmoved by the disability. The malingerer, on the other hand, is more likely to mimic a painful gait but usually fails to achieve the typical rhythm. He tends to linger on the painful member and creates an impression of great agony while doing so.

**Prosthetic Gait.** Clothed, a patient with a 'below-knee' prosthesis is difficult to detect. With an 'above-knee' prosthesis the patient hitches the whole leg forwards, snapping the knee into extension and bringing the foot heavily to the ground. The most characteristic feature may be the sound of the artificial leg striking the ground or the creaking of the supporting straps and hinges.

## Routine **Examination of the Limbs** and Spine

The examination follows the usual sequence of inspection and palpation. Note is taken of any deformity, swelling, discolouration or muscle wasting. Active movements are performed and compared with those of the normal limb, or with the expected range of a patient of a similar age if both sides are affected.

Palpation confirms the findings on inspection and detects any tenderness, changes in skin temperature, and abnormalities in the pulses. Active movements are repeated while the joints are palpated to detect crepitus or clicks. Passive movements may then be assessed and compared with the active range.

**Upper Limbs.** These are inspected particularly for joint swelling, deformity and muscle wasting. Thereafter the range of movement of each joint is assessed.

SHOULDER. The patient is asked to raise the arms forwards to the fullest extent and should be able to do so to the vertical. He is asked to touch the back of the neck and then bring the arms down to touch the small of the back keeping the arms in the coronal plane as they descend. Any limitation of movement or painful arc of movement is noted. If the total range is limited, the examiner should stand behind the patient, immobilise the scapula with one hand and ask the patient to repeat the shoulder movements. The relative contributions of gleno-humeral and scapulothoracic movements will then be apparent. Normally each should provide about half the total range.

ELBOW. The patient is instructed to bend and straighten both elbows simultaneously, limitation in this range being revealed by comparison of one with the other side. The patient then pronates and supinates the forearms as demonstrated by the doctor. At the same time the elbow must be kept at the patient's side to prevent movement at the shoulder. Deformity or limitation of movement indicates the need for careful palpation of the joint.

WRIST. After inspection the patient is asked to put the hands in the position of prayer and then lower the hands, keeping the palms together. This demonstrates the extreme of dorsiflexion. The backs of the hands are then placed together and the arms raised to demonstrate the extreme of flexion, the two sides being compared. If these movements are normal, others need not be checked.

HAND. The hands should be inspected for deformity, skin colour and muscle wasting. Hand movements are normal if the patient can fully extend and 'spread' the fingers and then fully flex them to form a closed fist with the thumb over the fingers so that the thumb nail is seen in full view from the palmar aspect and not side on, as in adduction of the thumb (Fig. 92, p. 336 .

**Spine.** Any deformity or abnormality of posture will be noted on inspection. The patient is asked to touch each shoulder with his chin and then with each ear. Up to the third decade at least, both should be possible. The patient is then asked to touch his toes without bending his knees. The level to which he can reach is noted and whether this movement is achieved by a smooth general flexion of the spine. Protective spasm or structural change will be unmasked.

**Lower Limbs.** The patient stands with his feet parallel and about six inches apart. The pelvis should then be 'level', the iliac crests being in the same horizontal plane. Viewed from in front, any genu valgum or varum or deformity of the ankle or foot is noted. Particular note is made of the arch of the foot. This examination is repeated from behind and the posture of the heels assessed; they should lie vertically but will be adducted (varus) in club foot and pes cavus, or abducted (valgus) in some forms of flat feet. The patient is now asked to stand on tip toe, do a full knee bend, and finally, without support, stand on each leg in turn while bending the other knee to a right angle (Trendelenburg sign, p. 356). Failure to achieve the first, second or third of these manoeuvres indicates the need for further examination of the leg and ankle (p. 363), the knee (p. 357) or the hip (p. 350) respectively.

The patient now lies supine on the examination couch and is asked to bend each knee and hip to the maximum. He then grasps each knee with both hands and pulls it as firmly as possible against the abdomen. The range of movement in knee and hip is noted and also whether the other leg is raised off the couch at the same time (Thomas test, p. 353).

Examination of the hip is completed by rolling the leg as it rests on the couch into internal and external rotation. If the range is equal on both sides and normal for the patient's age (p. 354), all other movements are likely to be normal. If not, the hip must be more fully examined (p. 351). The knee is inspected to exclude swelling of the joint or wasting of the thigh muscles, especially if any limitation of active movement was noted in the previous manoeuvre. If an abnormality is found, a full examination of the joint is required (p. 357). The ankles and feet are again examined and particular note made of deformity and mobility of the ankle, also comparing on the two sides the subtalar and mid-tarsal joints (p. 367).

The patient turns over to lie prone and his agility while completing this movement is noted. The contour of the spine is again examined by inspection and palpation. The strength of the back muscles is tested by asking the patient to raise the head and shoulders off the bed without using the hands.

## Measuring and Recording the Movement of Joints

Direct measurements of the movement of the spine is difficult. Indirect methods, however, can be objective and useful and are described with the examination of the components of the spine.

Movements of the joints of the limbs can be measured directly and objectively recorded by the use of a goniometer. Such records are useful, while descriptions of movements as good, fair or bad are useless. There are various

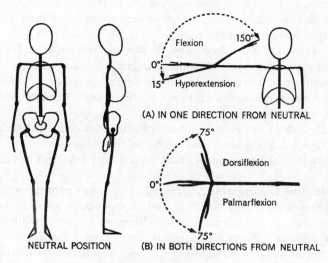

Flexion
150°
0°
15° Hyperextension
(A) IN ONE DIRECTION FROM NEUTRAL

75°
Dorsiflexion
0°
Palmarflexion
75°
NEUTRAL POSITION   (B) IN BOTH DIRECTIONS FROM NEUTRAL

FIG. 82   Measuring Movements of Joints.

methods of recording the range of movement, but the Neutral Zero Method is recommended as it is simple and generally accepted.

In this method all the joints are considered to be in neutral position when the body is in the classical anatomical position, with two exceptions. Firstly, the hands are flat against the thighs in the sagittal and not the coronal plane. Secondly, the feet are at right angles to the leg in the sagittal plane, not plantar flexed (Fig. 82).

In certain joints, such as the elbow and knee, movement can normally occur only in one direction from neutral, e.g. flexion 0° to 150° or extension 150° to 0°. Extension past 0° normally does not occur and is therefore referred to as hyperextension 0° to ?°. In other joints, such as the wrist and ankle, movement normally occurs in both directions from zero and is defined as palmar or plantar flexion 0° to ?°, and dorsiflexion or extension 0° to ?° (Fig. 82). Finally, certain joints such as the shoulders and hips allow movement in all directions from neutral. Such movements are defined as flexion, extension, abduction and adduction, all from neutral. Combined they result in circumduction.

Both the active and the passive movements are measured and separately recorded if they differ. Where limitation of movement is present it is best described by the arc of movement present. For example, if a patient lacks 30° of extension of the elbow and can flex to 90° from there, his range of movement is described as flexion 30° to 90°.

## The Interpretation of Abnormal Joint Movement

The movements of a joint can be restricted or increased by changes in the bone, cartilage, synovial membrane, capsule, ligaments, muscles, and related nerves. By the systematic examination of each structure in turn, the cause of the abnormal movement can be found.

**Bone, Articular Cartilage and Synovial Membrane.** Inflammatory change, whether traumatic, rheumatic, degenerative, or infective in nature, causes diminished movement in all directions (Fig. 83). The degree of limitation corresponds to the acuteness of the process. Tenderness, if present, is general over all the joint.

Complete lack of movement accompanied by pain is due to acute infection or recent trauma. These are differentiated by the history.

Complete lack of movement without pain means ankylosis or fusion of the joint.

**Capsule and Ligaments.** A strained or sprained capsule or ligament is painful when stretched by active or passive movement towards the opposite side of the joint, and movements in this direction are restricted by protective spasm of muscles. Movement towards the strained ligament relieves the painful tension and is not limited (Fig. 84). Tenderness is localised to the sprained area. An effusion may be present as the capsule is intact.

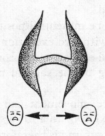 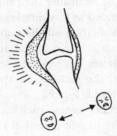

FIG. 83   Inflammation of a Joint.          FIG. 84   Sprain of Capsule or Ligament.

A ruptured ligament is initially painful on movement towards the opposite side of the joint. This movement is excessive in degree. Movement towards the same side 'closes' the joint and relieves pain. Any fluid in the joint escapes and causes swelling and bruising over the ruptured ligament (Fig. 85).

**Intra-articular Structures.** A structure, such as a torn semilunar cartilage, displaced in a joint is compressed by movement towards it. Pain is localised over the structure and that movement is restricted. Movement away from the object is not painful or reduced. An effusion is usually present in the joint (Fig. 86).

**Muscle.** *Painful Lesion in Muscle.* Active contraction, even when no movement takes place, causes pain. Active movement involving the muscle causes pain and is restricted. Passive movement in the same direction relaxes the muscle, relieves pain, and is not restricted to the same extent.

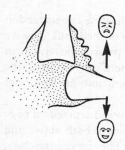

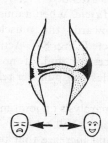

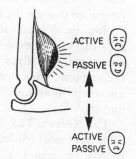

FIG. 85   Rupture of Capsule or Ligament.

FIG. 86   Rupture of Semilunar Cartilage.

FIG. 87   Painful Lesion in a Muscle.

Both active and passive movements in the opposite direction cause pain and are therefore restricted (Fig. 87).

Pain arising in a strained ligament can be differentiated from pain arising in a muscle close to the joint by making the suspected muscle contract without movement of the joint (isometric contraction). This will cause pain if the muscle, not the ligament, is the cause. For example, in tennis elbow passive extension of the elbow is painful but this stretches both the capsule of the elbow and the extensor muscle origin. The patient now clenches the fist without moving his elbow—thus contracting the extensor muscles, and pain results, localised to the extensor origin, proving that this is the source of the pain.

When examining a muscle which acts over two joints, the same principles apply. When movement at one joint influences the range of movement at a neighbouring joint, derangement of such a muscle is suspected. For example, if there is fixed equinus or flexion of the ankle joint when the knee is extended, this could be due to changes in the ankle joint itself or to contracture of the gastrocnemius muscle or soleus muscle. Flexion of the knee relaxes the

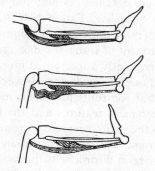

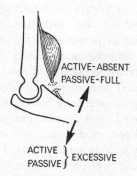

FIG. 88   Lesion of Gastrocnemius Muscle.

FIG. 89   Rupture of a Muscle.

gastrocnemius muscle and has no effect on the soleus muscle or the ankle joint. If dorsiflexion is now possible, the gastrocnemius muscle must have prevented it when the knee was extended (Fig. 88).

*Rupture or Paralysis of a Muscle.* When a muscle is paralysed or its tendon divided, active movement towards the muscle is abolished but passive movement, initially, is unaffected (Fig. 89). Active and passive movement in the opposite direction is excessive and, if no treatment is initiated, the uncontrolled antagonist muscles will pull the related joint into an abnormal posture.

**The Nerves.** The effect of paralysis on joint movement is discussed on page 323. Abnormal tension on a nerve will result in limitation of both active and passive movement which would increase that tension. The nerve stretching tests described on page 347 illustrate how such limitation of movement in the case of a prolapsed lumbar intervertebral disc can be differentiated from that caused by joint or muscle lesions.

## Part II

## REGIONAL EXAMINATION

'Another man, Adwyne by name, in the town of Dunwych, that dwelled on the sea-shore, was so contracted that he could not use the free office of hand or foot. His legs were cleaving to the hinder part of his thighs so that he could not walk, and his hands were turned backward. Nothing could be done by them The extremities of his fingers were so rigorously contracted in the sinews that he could not put meat to his mouth In this grievous sickness he passed his young age.'
ANON [Quoted from Griffith, E F. 1951 *Doctors by Themselves.* London. Cassell.]

The above quotation, the earliest recorded account of the admission of a patient to St. Bartholomew's Hospital, was written in the twelfth century and is a graphic but extreme example of the complexities which may occur in the locomotor system in neglected patients. A very detailed examination may be required for the elucidation of each local disability. Expert help is often required as is indicated by the large numbers of patients attending orthopaedic and rheumatic clinics. While the treatment of traumatic damage from the increasing number of road accidents is frequently a specialised procedure, the initial assessment may have to be carried out by any doctor. However, the undergraduate need not be overawed by what confronts him if his methods are based on an understanding of the anatomical features and the pathological conditions commonly encountered in the various regions. A competent history will do much to clarify the problem and as the interpretation of the significance of pain is of particular importance in disorders of the locomotor system this is considered before the examination of the individual regions.

# PAIN PATTERNS IN LOCOMOTOR DISORDERS

Pain, the cardinal symptom of lesions involving the locomotor system, often has a characteristic pattern in time or in relation to certain activities. This is frequently so clear that the diagnosis can be made from the history alone, and indeed must be when the clinical signs are few or absent, as may occur, for example, in the carpal tunnel syndrome.

The pattern of a patient's complaints can be delineated by taking him through a typical day. The following questions cover most activities without suggesting any replies. How do you feel on rising and dressing? How long can you remain comfortably on your feet? How far can you walk? (It is useful to refer to a well-known local thoroughfare to estimate distance. In Edinburgh we are fortunate in having Princes Street as our 'measured mile'.) How long can you sit in comfort? How do you feel at the end of the day? How do you sleep? What makes the pain worse? What makes the pain better?

This routine also gives an estimate of the patient's abilities which can be compared with the findings at a later date. When organic disease is present a consistent story unfolds in contrast to the vague indifference of the hysteric and the aggressive resentment of the malingerer who fears too detailed interrogation.

The following notes provide a guide to the characteristic features of pain encountered in the locomotor system.

### TRAUMATIC LESIONS

**Sprained Ligaments.** After the initial acute phase when pain may be severe and constant, pain occurs only with movement which stretches the damaged structure and is relieved when the ligament is relaxed.

**Chronic Strain of Ligaments.** In weight-bearing ligaments, in the back or the foot for example, the patient is most comfortable when rising in the morning. As the day goes on the supporting muscles tire and an aching pain develops which is relieved by rest.

**Fracture.** The student must be familiar with all the signs and symptoms of a fracture but only three are present in all fractures—pain, local tenderness, and interference with function to a greater or lesser degree. Crepitus must never be elicited in the conscious patient. Pain occurs on any movement if the fracture is not impacted.

### INFLAMMATION

**Acute Lesions.** The pain steadily increases, even at rest, is throbbing in character, and the patient becomes ill and febrile, especially if there is formation of pus and the building up of tension in a structure such as a joint or the bone marrow. Remissions of pain and fever occur if pus escapes. When a joint is involved, all movement is inhibited by protective spasm of the controlling muscles. Any attempted movement, active or passive, causes pain. If the patient sleeps deeply, this spasm may relax and the patient wakens with a characteristic cry as some movement occurs causing pain. When there is infection in bone near a joint, movement of that joint may be inhibited by spasm. Gentle examination, however, will demonstrate that a small range of movement is present. In infants, localising signs are less easy to discover but immobility of the affected part is commonly present, often accompanied by irritability, crying and vomiting.

**Chronic Lesions.** The features are similar but more prolonged than in acute inflammation and the local and general reactions are less severe. Some movement will still be possible in an early low grade infection of a joint. In rheumatoid arthritis pain and stiffness are characteristically worse in the morning. The patient may take several hours to 'get going'.

## NEOPLASTIC LESIONS

**Benign Tumours.** With the possible exception of osteoid osteoma, such tumours do not cause pain unless by pressure on neighbouring structures.

**Malignant Tumours.** Pain is not an invariable feature but, when present, is not related to any special activity and is not relieved by rest. A pathological fracture may occur as a result of minor trauma and cause sudden acute pain.

## DEGENERATIVE LESIONS

**Osteoarthrosis.** This term, indicative of 'wear and tear' is more accurate than *'osteoarthritis'* which infers inflammation. Joints so affected are stiff and difficult to move after disuse, but move more freely with use. Thus pain and stiffness after rest, relieved by activity but recurring as the patient tires, are characteristic of osteoarthrosis. This pain is often not immediately relieved by rest and the patient may have difficulty in settling comfortably.

**Prolapsed Invertebral Disc.** The pattern of pain here may be spread over years. Before the acute episode there is frequently a period of odd aches and pains, often accepted by the patient as a normal reaction to his activities. An acute episode occurs when bending or lifting, or on the day following such activities, or with no discernible cause. The pain subsides with rest, but may take several weeks to disappear. Thereafter periods of comfort are interspersed with major or minor episodes of pain. Gradually this characteristically episodic pattern merges into the osteoarthritic pattern described above.

**Ischaemia.** Intermittent claudication is described on page 140.

# THE UPPER LIMB

### The Forearm, Wrist and Hand

The hand, compared to the foot, has retained a simple form which, with opposition of the thumb, enables it to create and use tools. Its sensibility is the best substitute for the eyes of the blind or of the normal person in the dark. Finally, it aids communication between individuals by signs or the use of appropriate tools.

The hand is not a common site of congenital deformity. It seldom shows signs of wear and tear, with the exception of osteoarthrosis in the distal interphalangeal joints of the fingers, Heberden's nodes (p. 70), and in the carpo-metacarpal joint of the thumb, especially in the female. It is, however, a common site for rheumatoid change, involving tendons and joints, particularly the metacarpo-phalangeal, proximal interphalangeal, and wrist joints.

The hand's function depends on mobility and the smooth gliding of part on part, tendon in sheath. This makes it liable to a special group of friction syndromes involving its tendons—tenosynovitis. The hands are unusually liable to injury, for obvious reasons. So intimate is the relationship of the skin, bones, joints, tendons, nerves and vessels that it is seldom that injury involves a single structure. Because the hand is constantly contaminated by the environment, open injuries often become infected. Once established, infection may spread in the natural tissue spaces in the hand or along its tendon sheaths.

## ANATOMICAL FEATURES

**Rotation of the Forearm.** This movement depends on the integrity of the superior and inferior radio-ulnar joints and on the concavity of the volar aspects of the shafts of the radius and ulna. In pronation these two concavities fit into one another. Rotation will be limited if this curve is distorted, as may occur after a fracture.

**Joints.** The interphalangeal joints allow only flexion and extension; the metacarpo-phalangeal joints in addition to flexion and extension allow abduction and adduction, but only when extended. The wrist joint allows flexion and extension, radial and ulnar deviation, and circumduction.

**Muscles.** The muscles in the forearm are the powerhouse of the hand and wrist. Without the help of the intrinsic muscles of the hand, however, neither a proper grip nor fine movements are possible. If the intrinsic muscles are paralysed the long muscles acting alone cause clawing of the fingers. Such a hand is useful only as a paperweight or a hook.

**The Deep Fascia and Skin.** In the palm both structures are thickened and bound together at the skin creases. On the dorsum the skin and the deep fascia are thin and elastic. Because of these differences any generalised swelling of the hand will be more evident on the dorsum. The skin has a very abundant nerve and blood supply on both aspects of the hand.

**Nerve Supply.** The radial, ulnar and median nerves are all implicated in the proper functioning of the hand.

The *radial nerve* supplies the wrist and finger extensors and an insignificant area of sensation on the dorsum of the index metacarpal. Damage to the nerve is liable to occur in the spiral groove on the shaft of the humerus, resulting in a 'drop wrist' deformity. The grip is considerably weakened because the flexors now have no antagonist to steady the wrist.

The *ulnar nerve* supplies sensation on the ulnar border of the hand. Its motor contribution is most important in the hand, where it supplies all the small muscles except the short flexor, abductor, and opponens of the thumb, and the lumbrical to the index and sometimes the middle finger. The nerve may be damaged at the elbow or the wrist, resulting in the clawhand deformity. The ring and little fingers are clawed, and wasting of the muscles between the metacarpals is most evident in the cleft between the index and thumb. The clawing—extension at the metacarpo-phalangeal joint and flexion at the interphalangeal joints—is the result of the unopposed action of the long flexors and extensors.

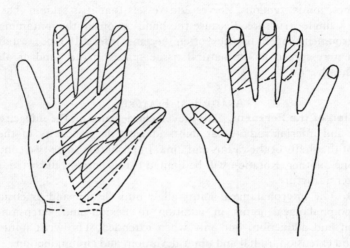

Fig. 90    The Use of Diagrams in Case Recording.
Area of anaesthesia in a patient with a lesion of the right median nerve.

The *median nerve* supplies the main bulk of the flexor muscles in the forearm and the small muscles of the thumb, as well as the lumbrical to the index and middle fingers. The common site of damage is at the wrist, causing paralysis of the muscles supplied in the hand. The muscles of the thenar eminence waste and the thumb falls into the flat, ape-like or simian deformity. Although this interferes significantly with hand function, the most disabling component of the injury is loss of sensation on the volar aspect of the thumb, index and middle fingers (Fig. 90). It is from this area that so much information is received about the environment. Activities such as dressing and sorting change in the pocket can no longer be performed unless under direct vision.

Variations in the distribution of the nerve supply, particularly between median and ulnar, are very common in the hand.

## EXAMINATION OF THE FOREARM, WRIST AND HAND

The extensive range of information which can be obtained from critical inspection of the hands is described on pages 67 to 70. Note should be made of the posture, deformity, nutrition and, most important in the hand, of any scars, wounds or contractures. Diagrams showing scars, amputated portions, or other deformities make an accurate and easily understood record (Fig. 91). The hand distal to any wound must be carefully examined. An apparently trivial laceration may involve tendons, nerves or joints. Some authorities consider the thumb, others the index finger, as the first digit. In order to avoid confusion, therefore, the digits must never be numbered but must be specified

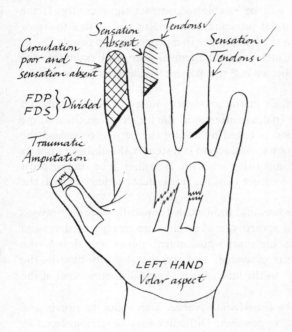

FIG. 91   THE USE OF DIAGRAMS IN CASE RECORDING.

This diagram summarises at a glance the following mass of information:

1. Traumatic amputation obliquely through the distal phalanx of the thumb.

2. Deep laceration of the index finger over the middle phalanx running obliquely from the radial side to the ulnar side of the finger. The digital nerves, arteries and both flexor tendons have been divided.

3. Deep laceration of the middle finger obliquely over the radial aspect of the middle phalanx. The digital nerve on the radial aspect has been divided. The tendons are intact.

4. Superficial laceration of ring finger over the ulnar aspect of the proximal phalanx without damage to tendons or nerves.

5. Closed fracture of the metacarpal of the middle finger obliquely through the mid-shaft with displacement.

6. Closed fracture of the metacarpal of the ring finger transversely through the mid-shaft without displacement.

by name—thumb, index, middle, ring, and little finger. This may be tedious, but it will reduce the risk of the wrong finger being treated, or even amputated.

The colour, texture and temperature of the skin, and the condition of the nails, are noted and the peripheral pulses are examined. Sensation is tested and local tenderness or signs of inflammation sought.

ASSESSMENT OF HAND FUNCTION. This involves examination of the active and passive movements of the wrist and digits. Where movement is limited, it is assessed as described on page 327 and the cause is located. A long time may be required to complete the examination of the whole hand and record the findings.

The integrity of individual tendons is tested by observing if their normal action is present.

*Flexor digitorum profundus* flexes the proximal and the distal interphalangeal joints. It is the only muscle which flexes the distal interphalangeal joints and its action is therefore tested by flexion of this joint while the finger is held in extension at the proximal joint and in flexion at the metacarpophalangeal joint.

*Flexor digitorum sublimis* flexes the proximal interphalangeal joints. When testing this tendon the action of profundus can be eliminated by extending all the fingers not being examined. The flexor profundus has a muscle belly common to all the fingers; if three of the fingers are extended, the muscle controlling the fourth finger will be unable to contract significantly. If the finger then flexes at the proximal interphalangeal joint this is due to flexor sublimis. The only exception is the little finger in a proportion of people.

*The lumbricals* flex at the metacarpo-phalangeal joint and extend at the interphalangeal joints. Test by asking the patient to do this following the example of the examiner.

*Interossei* assist the lumbricals in the movement noted above, and abduct (dorsal interossei) and adduct (palmar interossei) the fingers from the midline of the middle finger. Abduction is tested by asking the patient to spread the extended fingers against resistance. Adduction is tested by the ability to hold a card between the fingers in competition with the examiner. The fingers must be in extension, and in order to ensure this, the test is best carried out with the hand on a flat surface.

The intrinsic muscles, interossei and lumbricals frequently become fibrosed and contracted in rheumatoid arthritis, and produce an exaggerated version of their normal action. The metacarpo-phalangeal joints are flexed, the proximal interphalangeal joints extended, and the distal joints flexed—the so-called swan neck deformity. In the later stages of this disease several of the joints may become dislocated.

*Thenar Muscles supplied by the Median Nerve.* The abductor brevis and opponens combine to produce opposition. Difficulty may be encountered in differentiating between true opposition and adduction which is produced by the ulnar supplied adductor pollicis. Observe the nail of the thumb from the palmar aspect. On adduction (ulnar nerve) it is seen in side view. In opposition it has rotated and is now in full view (Fig. 92).

*Thenar Muscles supplied by the Ulnar Nerve.* Paralysis of adductor pollicis is accompanied by muscle wasting in the palm between the thumb and the index finger. The patient is asked to hold a thin book between the radial side of the clenched fingers and the extended thumb. When the adductor is not functioning

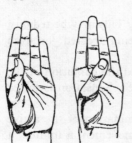

Fig. 92 Adduction and Opposition of the Thumb.

the thumb cannot be held extended and flexion at the metacarpo-phalangeal and interphalangeal joints occurs. This is because the adductor cannot hold the head of the metacarpal against the index finger (Fig. 93).

*Extensor Tendons.* Assessment of paralysis is not difficult, but these tendons are liable to rupture at any of three sites. (1) Separation may occur from the distal phlanx with or without a fragment of bone. This results in mallet finger deformity. (2) The central slip of the extensor which inserts to the bone of the middle phalanx may rupture, producing the 'boutonnier' deformity as the lateral portions slip to each side of the finger. The proximal interphalangeal is then flexed and the distal joint extended. (3) The extensor pollicis longus occasionally ruptures at the wrist after a Colles' fracture, or in rheumatoid arthritis, causing the equivalent of a mallet finger.

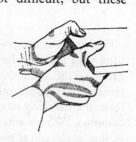

FIG. 93   Normal and Paralysed Adductor Pollicis.

## Special Tests.

1. FRACTURED SCAPHOID. In recent injuries pain is caused on attempting to grip powerfully, and tenderness is accurately localised to the anatomical snuff box. Repeated radiological examination may be required to confirm the diagnosis.

2. TRIGGER FINGER AND THUMB. Flexion is not limited, but extension of the inter-phalangeal joints is, until straightening of the finger suddenly occurs, accompanied by a click felt over the thickened part of the flexor sheath at the level of the metacarpal head. In babies the condition is often not noticed until extension at the inter-phalangeal joints is permanently limited. The thumb is most frequently involved at this age, but the thickened flexor sheath is easily palpable over the metacarpal head.

### The Elbow

Congenital abnormalities are not commonly found in the humerus but this bone is not infrequently the site of acute osteomyelitis in the young. Fractures occur at all ages, and the intimate relationship of the humerus with three nerves—the circumflex at its neck, the radial in the mid-shaft and the ulnar at the elbow—may result in injury to these nerves. Fracture at the supra-condylar level may damage the brachial artery and cause ischaemic changes in the flexor muscles in the forearm (Volkmann's ischaemic contracture).

The elbow is not a common site of congenital deformity or degenerative change, but next to the knee it is the most frequent site of osteochondritis dissecans. The reaction of the elbow to trauma is unpredictable. Minor trauma may be followed by complete stiffness, whereas gross disorganisation of the joint may be compatible with excellent function. One stiff elbow, provided it is not too extended, is not a great handicap, but stiffness of both elbows causes severe disability. Patients with rheumatoid arthritis use the elbows to prop themselves up in bed and the resultant trauma is a factor in the production of the nodules which are frequently found over the upper posterior aspect of the ulna in these circumstances.

## ANATOMICAL FEATURES

The joint is composed of two parts, that between the humerus, radius and ulna, and the superior radio-ulnar joint. The former allows flexion through a range of 150°, and the latter allows rotation of the wrist through 180°. In the female, in the anatomical position, the forearm is abducted on the humerus to form the carrying angle, cubitus valgus and some degree of hyperextension is common. Where this angle is increased, by fracture of the capitellum for example, the ulnar nerve becomes stretched and its function may be impaired.

The joint between the humerus, radius and ulna is stable, and is not dislocated easily. The head of the radius, however, particularly in children, may dislocate, but this causes surprisingly few symptoms.

## EXAMINATION OF THE ELBOW

Most of the examination can be performed without touching the patient, but merely by observing the limb and its movements.

**Inspection.** With both arms exposed, deformity is detected by inspecting the elbow from behind with the arm flexed and extended. The relationship of the olecranon and the lateral and medial epicondyles in the abnormal joint is compared with that of the normal side. The hollow over the head of the radius is filled in when an effusion is present. A flexion deformity cannot be easily differentiated from a valgus deformity. By the same token, the degree of valgus or varus cannot be accurately measured with the elbow even slightly flexed.

**Palpation.** This is conducted for bony contour, local tenderness, or signs of inflammation. In tennis elbow tenderness is well localised in the region of the lateral epicondyle at the extensor origin. Pain is reproduced by gripping, by resisted extension of the wrist, and by passive extension of the elbow while the forearm is pronated and the wrist flexed. The patient can lift objects with the hand supine, but experiences pain when lifting the same object with the hand pronated. An effusion in the joint is most easily felt over the head of the radius on the postero-lateral aspect of the joint. Here the head of the radius lies almost subcutaneously and is easily palpated if the forearm is rotated at the same time. Loose bodies are seldom palpable as they tend to collect in the coronoid and olecranon fossae which are covered by muscle. The ulnar nerve is palpated and compared with the normal side to determine any enlargement, tenderness or excessive mobility.

**Movement.** The patient should move both arms at the same time, when the range of each will be compared. The patient is then asked to flex the elbow to a right angle and keep the elbow touching his side while supinating and pronating both hands. Care must be taken to ensure that the elbow is kept to the side when measuring pronation because the movement can be simulated very easily by abduction at the shoulder.

**Tests of Stability.** The collateral ligaments can be tested only when the elbow is fully extended.

**Ulnar Nerve.** The ulnar nerve is involved so readily in elbow lesions that the muscles and areas of sensation which it serves are routinely examined.

## The Shoulder

The alignment of the upper limb has changed little from that of the reptile. Most of man's activities involve the use of the hands within an oval limited above and below by the orifices of the alimentary tract, sideways by little more than the breadth of the shoulders, and the extent of his reach forwards. The emphasis is on mobility rather than stability, despite which congenital dislocation of the shoulder is virtually unknown. In the young adult dislocation readily occurs following injury and thereafter the tendency to recurrent dislocation is very great. In the older patient the joint has a marked tendency to become stiff, because of little understood changes in the soft tissues of the shoulder. Whatever the cause, this condition, conveniently and graphically described as 'frozen shoulder', is so common from early middle age onwards that it must be kept in mind when examining a patient suffering from any painful condition from the neck to the finger-tips. The shoulder will stiffen if movement of the joint is not maintained because of pain in the neck or arm, after myocardial infarction or following a hemiplegia. In contrast to the frozen shoulder, osteoarthrosis and inflammatory lesions are relatively uncommon in the shoulder region.

### ANATOMICAL FEATURES

**Movements.** Movement of the shoulder is a complicated synthesis of motion at four joints. The gleno-humeral and scapulothoracic joints each account for about half of the total range, and it is important to measure the contribution made by each. Movement at the acromio-clavicular joint is not important and at the sterno-clavicular joint only little more so.

Rather than define the range of movement and try to explain the complex relationship between rotation, flexion and abduction, the reader is invited to demonstrate these movements to himself. The range of movement varies with the rotation of the arm. This can be demonstrated with the elbow flexed to a right angle and the forearm acting as an indicator of rotation. Abduction can proceed only a little beyond 90° with the arm in neutral rotation. If the arm is externally rotated, full abduction is possible. In full internal rotation almost no abduction is possible. When limitation of movement is present, the gleno-humeral and scapulo-thoracic contributions must be separated. This is achieved by holding the inferior angle of the scapula with one hand and abducting the arm with the other (Fig. 94).

Rotation can be measured again by using the forearm as an indicator. With

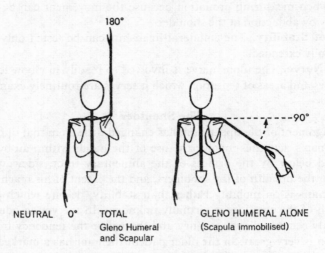

FIG. 94    Movements at the Shoulder Joint.

the arm by the side in neutral rotation and the elbow flexed to 90°, the forearm will be directed medially by some 20° and not in the sagittal plane; 90° of rotation should be possible from this position in both directions. The forearm cannot quite reach the coronal plane in external rotation, but the patient should be able to touch the small of his back in internal rotation. With the arm in full external rotation and the elbow flexed at 90°, abduction of the shoulder will bring the hand up to the back of the neck. A reasonably accurate measurement of full rotation, therefore, is the ability to touch the small of the back and the back of the neck.

**Rotator Cuff.** This term is applied to the fused tendons of supraspinatus, infraspinatus and teres minor. These, with the tendon of subscapularis, form a hood-like structure covering the head of the humerus, holding it into the socket of the glenoid and initiating gleno-humeral abduction. This structure, and especially the supraspinatus tendon, is the most common site of pathological change in the shoulder. When swollen and tender it affects the movement of the shoulder in a characteristic way. As abduction proceeds the swollen portion becomes compressed under the acromion and causes pain. Once it has passed this point painless movement is continued. Patients very quickly learn to avoid this by externally rotating the humerus as abduction proceeds so that the tender area is not compressed under the acromion.

When rupture of the rotator cuff occurs, attempts to abduct the shoulder produce only a shrugging of the shoulder as a whole, the arm barely leaving the side. The deltoid can only pull the humerus in its own axis up against the acromion. If, however, the humerus is passively abducted to 45°, the deltoid can now abduct the rest of the way. Patients learn trick movements to compensate for loss of the initial abduction by passively swinging the arm from the side and 'catching' it with the deltoid to complete abduction. Soon after injury when the shoulder is painful it is impossible to tell whether abduction is inhibited by pain or prevented by rupture of the rotator cuff. Abolition of the pain by injection of local anaesthetic resolves the problem as the patient can then initiate abduction if the cuff is intact.

The long head of the biceps may be involved in lesions of the rotator cuff. This lesion is suspected when resisted flexion of the elbow causes pain in the shoulder.

**Nerve Supply.** The spinal segments which supply the shoulder girdle contribute to the phrenic nerve. In painful lesions affecting areas subserved by the phrenic nerve, such as the diaphragm, pain may be referred to the tip of the shoulder in the area of C4, owing to the fact that the greater part of the phrenic nerve is derived from this root.

### POINTS IN THE HISTORY

Lesions in the neck, lung, pericardium and the pleura and peritoneum covering the central parts of the diaphragm may cause pain in the shoulder. Theoretically this should cause little difficulty because no limitation of movement or other abnormality should be found on examination of the shoulder. However, this reasoning may be confounded by the tendency of the shoulder in the elderly to become stiff when immobilised by pain from other sites. Painful lesions in the root of the neck, and the most sinister is an apical bronchial carcinoma, tend to cause pain radiating down the inner side of the arm.

Occasionally ischaemic lesions of the heart cause shoulder pain, but the clinical features of the pain, especially if it is induced by exercise which does not involve the use of the arms, should resolve any doubt about its true origin. Phrenic pain is referred to the tip of the shoulder and may be aggravated by deep breathing. True shoulder pain tends to radiate to the insertion of the deltoid muscle and seldom extends beyond the elbow. When a calcified deposit in the rotator cuff ruptures into the sub-acromial bursa the pain is so severe that immediate operation may be required for its relief.

### EXAMINATION OF THE SHOULDER

**Inspection.** When only one shoulder is affected much may be learned by simple inspection and comparison with the normal side.

Anterior dislocation of the sterno-clavicular joint is not uncommon and except in the early stages after injury, does not interfere with shoulder movement. The deformity caused by the prominent medial end of the clavicle is easily seen or palpated. Posterior dislocation is less common and is usually accompanied by severe pain and commanding symptoms, including difficulty in swallowing and extreme pain on lifting the head when supine. The deformity, however, especially in the early stages when accompanied by swelling, is not obvious even on radiological examination.

M

Fracture at the mid-shaft of the clavicle presents little difficulty in diagnosis. Dislocation of the acromio-clavicular joint may be confused with fracture at the lateral end of the clavicle; both cause a distinct 'step' between the acromion and the upwardly displaced clavicle or medial fragment. Neither injury causes much disturbance of shoulder function except in the early stages.

Anterior dislocation of the shoulder poses few diagnostic problems because the humerus displaces downwards as well as forwards. The normal smooth curved contour of the shoulder is replaced by the ugly angular projection of the acromion process of the scapula. Posterior dislocation is frequently not diagnosed immediately after injury, even with the help of radiological examination. A nearly normal contour of the shoulder is preserved because the head of the humerus displaces directly backwards and not downwards. If the patient is muscular, this and the swelling after an injury may be accepted as the reaction to a strain of the joint. Inferior dislocation is rare, the patient being in the sorry plight of not being able to bring the arm to the side. This 'I am a teapot' posture may amuse the onlooker, but it does not amuse the patient.

**Palpation.** Careful palpation may be required to confirm what is suspected on inspection. Local tenderness must be accurately defined, especially in lesions of the rotator cuff. This structure can be more fully explored if the patient clasps his hands behind his back during the examination. Occasionally, in a lean subject, a gap may be palpable where the rotator cuff has ruptured.

SCAPULAR MOVEMENTS. The ability to shrug the shoulders up, backwards and forwards is noted. Weakness of the serratus anterior will be made obvious if the patient raises the arms forwards to press against the wall with both hands. Where the muscle is weak, the medial border of the scapula projects backward, producing the so-called 'winging' of the scapula.

GLENO-HUMERAL MOVEMENTS. Standing behind the patient, the examiner steadies the scapula by grasping the inferior angle and then putting the shoulder through both active and passive movements.

TOTAL RANGE OF MOVEMENTS. The patient is asked to raise the arm forwards and upwards to the limit, and then to the same end point through abduction. Any painful arc of limitation of movement is noted.

ROTARY MOVEMENTS. By flexing the elbow to a right angle, the forearm acts as an indicator. The shoulder is externally and then internally rotated with the arm at the side. The easiest way to demonstrate a full range of rotation is to ask the patient to touch the back of the neck and the small of the back.

# THE SPINE

Before considering the cervical, thoracic and lumbar segments separately, it is worth again remarking on the posture of the spine as a whole. At all times the normal spine should present as a straight line viewed from the front or the rear. As seen from the side, posture varies with the patient's age, depending mainly on the state of the intervertebral discs after maturity.

## Cervical Spine

The cervical spine is the most mobile section of the vertebral column. While the posture changes steadily throughout life, the neck is seldom in the same position for any length of time, waking or sleeping. Degenerative changes are therefore common but are not necessarily accompanied by symptoms. This mobility is also a factor in the liability of this part of the spine to injury. Congenital deformity is not uncommon, but when present is easy to detect. Infection in the cervical vertebrae is rare in contrast to the soft tissues of the neck where enlarged lymph nodes are commonly found as a result of infection from the mouth or pharynx.

### ANATOMICAL FEATURES

In the cervical spine the transverse process projects laterally from the body of the vertebra, protecting the more easily crushed cancellous bone of the body in the event of injury. The facet joints, however, lie more horizontally than at other levels of the spine; thus forced flexion of the neck is unlikely to produce a crush fracture of the body, and more often results in forward dislocation of the upper vertebrae.

The vertebral canal is almost filled by the cervical enlargement of the spinal cord. The emerging cervical roots pass between the articular facets and the intervertebral disc. Prolapse laterally of a cervical disc may produce compression of these roots; a central prolapse may produce pressure on the cord itself. Osteophytic outgrowth from the vertebral body with or without similar change in the facet joint is a common cause of root irritation in the lower cervical region (cervical spondylosis).

Of the movements in the neck, rotation takes place mainly at the atlanto-axial joint, nodding of the head at the atlanto-occipital joint, and flexion-extension in the mid-cervical joints.

### EXAMINATION OF THE CERVICAL SPINE

Because of the intimate relationship of the bones, joints, blood vessels, spinal cord and nerve roots, a lesion of the cervical region may produce symptoms both locally and widely referred. Examination of the neck must therefore include a neurological examination of the upper limbs and elsewhere as indicated.

**Inspection.** Deformity is easily detected. Where a painful lesion is present, the gait is characteristic. The patient walks with care to avoid jarring the neck, moving the whole body to look to the side. The chin may be supported by the hand. Torticollis or wry-neck is the most common deformity and is emphasised on movement. If it has been present for several years asymmetry of the face will have developed.The patient is asked to touch each shoulder in turn with the chin and then the ear. Any limitation of active movement is noted and compared later with the passive range of movement.

**Palpation.** The bone contour is explored; in the root of the neck accessory ribs may be palpable or even visible. Local tenderness, skin temperature and the condition of the cervical lymph nodes are assessed, the latter with the neck slightly flexed. Movements are repeated while palpation continues, to detect crepitus. Passive movements are carried out if there is any impairment of range. An accessory rib may obliterate the radial pulse if traction is applied to the arm with it by the patient's side. Contraction of an abnormal scalenus anterior muscle may obliterate the radial pulse when the patient turns his head to the affected side and then takes and holds a deep breath (Fig. 27, p. 168).

The *foraminal compression test* is performed if a cervical disc lesion is suspected. The examiner's hands are placed on the patient's head, with the patient standing or sitting, and gentle downward pressure applied. If no pain is produced, the manœuvre is repeated with the neck flexed to either side, in forward flexion and in extension. The test confirms the presence of root compression if it causes the characteristic reference of pain.

### Thoracic Spine

This segment of the vertebral column is the least mobile, and throughout life maintains a kyphosis. In contrast with its immobility is its tendency to develop gross deformity whatever the cause—congenital, developmental, or a variety of disease processes.

Congenital lesions are not common, for at this level the neural canal and arch are closed at an early stage. Developmental lesions (e.g. epiphysitis), and infection commonly affect this segment. Tuberculosis infection usually involves several vertebral bodies and, before the introduction of specific chemotherapy, resulted in gross destruction of the bodies and an angular kyphosis or gibbus deformity. When idiopathic scoliosis or scoliosis secondary to poliomyelitis occurs at this level, the deformity may be very severe. The rotation element of scoliosis is best seen in the thoracic spine. At the apex of the lateral curve the vertebral bodies no longer face ventrally, but are directed towards the convex side of the curve. The ribs, instead of projecting laterally, are now, on the convex side of the curve, directed dorsally, becoming sharply angulated to cause a so-called razor-back deformity. This results in narrowing and distortion of the chest cage and may interfere with the action of the heart and lungs. Such patients experience little pain but have a limited expectation of life.

### ANATOMICAL FEATURES

The movements of the thoracic spine consist of flexion and extension and a slight degree of lateral flexion and rotation. The range of movement is small and difficult to measure on clinical examination. The movement of the ribs, however, is easily assessed and can be affected by disease of the spine, such as ankylosing spondylitis, which not only stiffens the spine but may also immobilise the ribs.

## SPECIAL POINTS IN THE HISTORY

Pain in the thoracic spine is less common than in either the cervical or lumbar spine. Disc lesions are infrequent, but can occur and be accompanied by girdle pain radiating into the chest and mimicking the pain of cardiac disease. In the younger patient infection of bone, pyogenic or tuberculous, has to be kept in mind although it is much less frequently encountered in Britain than formerly. In middle and old age pathological fracture associated with either osteoporosis or malignant disease is a common cause of pain.

## EXAMINATION OF THE THORACIC SPINE

**Inspection.** With the patient standing, the posture is inspected from the front, back and side, and any deformity noted. The ranges of movement on forward and lateral flexion and on extension are recorded. Particular note is taken of the effect movement has on any deformity present. If it is due to faulty posture, it will correct on forward flexion. If due to structural changes, it will be unaffected by movement. The movement of the chest on breathing is also examined.

**Palpation.** The bony contour is first examined and areas of tenderness defined. Where local tenderness is not immediately obvious, gentle percussion with the fist may elicit it.

## Lumbar Spine

This segment of the spine falls heir to many infirmities. The lumbosacral region is a common site for congenital anomalies which often cause no trouble. Trauma frequently results in damage at the upper end of the lumbar spine where the mobile lumbar segment joins the less mobile dorsal spine. Degenerative changes develop in the lower lumbar intervertebral discs in the third decade and osteoarthrosis changes in the facet joints by middle age.

Low backache or lumbago is encountered in almost every department of clinical practice and the cause may lie outside the locomotor system proper. Lesions in the lumbar spine may cause symptoms in the lower limbs, with or without accompanying back pain.

## ANATOMICAL FEATURES

In the adult the spinal cord ends at the level of the second lumbar vertebra. At the dorso-lumbar level, a common site for injury, the neural canal contains the spinal cord and lumbar nerve roots. Injury at this level may seriously damage the spinal cord, which will not recover, and nerve roots which may recover.

The transverse processes of the lumbar spine are analagous to the ribs and abnormalities are common at the upper end of the lumbar spine; vestigial ribs may be mistaken for a fracture on radiological examination. The sacrum is formed by the fusion of five segments of the spine. The last lumbar segment not uncommonly fuses partially or completely with the first sacral segment— sacralisation of the fifth lumbar vertebra. Conversely the first sacral segment may fail to fuse to the remainder of the sacrum—lumbarisation of the sacral segment. The two can be differentiated only by a count of the remaining segments of the spine.

The intervertebral disc consists of a tough outer ring of fibrous tissue, the annulus, and a central jelly-like nucleus with a very high water content. The depth of the disc varies during the day. A fit young adult may be about 2 cm shorter by the end of the day, due mainly to changes in the discs. By the third decade degenerative changes begin in the lower lumbar discs, setting the stage for disc lesions to follow. They take the form of tears of the annulus with or without extrusion of the nucleus and are accompanied by pain. The disc does not, however, slip in and out of place. Less dramatically, this degenerative change may result in permanent narrowing of the disc. The corresponding facet joints between the vertebrae develop osteoarthrosis. Such changes are 'normal' in most individuals by the fifth decade, but are not always accompanied by symptoms.

Pus from a chronic infection of the lumbar spine may collect in the sheath of the psoas muscle, forming a palpable tumour in the iliac fossa before tracking farther down the sheath of the muscle to present as a swelling or a sinus in the groin. Acute infection causes spasm of the muscle and flexion of the hip. Active flexion of the hip aggravates the pain and passive flexion relieves it. This contrasts both with infection in the hip where all movements are painful, and with a lesion causing tension of the femoral roots (p. 349) where active and passive flexion of the hip relieves pain.

## SPECIAL POINTS IN THE HISTORY

The mode of onset and the pattern of lumbar pain are particularly important. The acute pain of a disc protrusion comes on suddenly when bending or on the day after such activity. This so overshadows the occasional backaches to which the patient has become accustomed during the preceding period of disc degeneration that these are often not mentioned by the patient. Careful enquiry will reveal the pattern of minor backache, the acute episodes which settle with the rest, followed by further minor aches, acute episodes, or both. Disc lesions, therefore, cause episodic pain with periods of freedom from symptoms. Recurrences can very often be related to stooping or lifting. Osteoarthrosis in the lumbar region causes the usual pattern of pain and stiffness after rest relieved by acitivity and recurring when the patient tires.

Chronic ligamentous strain, in contrast to osteoarthrosis, causes pain at the end of the day with freedom from pain at the start of the day. Gluteal pain may occasionally be caused by ischaemia and then has the usual pattern of claudication.

Pain not relieved by rest suggests a more serious lesion, such as infection or spondylitis in the younger patient, and in the older groups primary or secondary malignant disease. Sacral pain may be due to pathological conditions in the pelvis, especially in the female. Coccygeal pain should not be regarded as a local phenomenon until a cause higher in the spine or in the pelvis has been excluded.

### EXAMINATION OF THE LUMBAR SPINE

**Inspection.** With the patient standing, the posture is observed from behind. The spine should be straight. The most common cause of deviation at this level is a lumbar disc lesion which causes the patient to list to one or other side. If the prolapse is lateral to the adjacent root the patient leans towards the opposite side and pain is aggravated by lateral flexion towards the same side as this pulls the root against the prolapse (Fig. 95). If the prolapse is medial to the root, in the 'axilla' between root and dura, the patient lists to the same side as the lesion. Therefore the direction to which the patient deviates depends on the relationship of the disc prolapse to the adjacent root and not on which side the disc prolapse occurs.

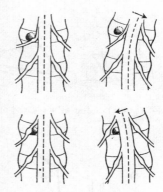

The patient is then inspected from the side and the presence, accentuation, absence or reversal of the normal lordosis noted. Where a painful lesion is present the lordosis is obliterated or even reversed. The patient is asked to bend forwards and to each side. The level reached and the influence of movement on the lumbar spine are noted. Finally the patient is viewed from in front.

FIG. 95 Deviation of Spine in Prolapsed Intervertebral Disc.

**Palpation.** This is performed with the patient supine and prone, and again the contour of the spine, the presence of tenderness, and the skin temperature are assessed. Examination of the abdomen, groins and breasts is followed by rectal examination if indicated.

SPURLING'S TEST. If firm pressure by the thumb is applied between the laminae over a prolapsed disc the pain will be aggravated and radiation of the pain produced. This may not happen immediately, and pressure may have to be maintained for some seconds. When negative, no tenderness or radiation of pain is caused by the test.

### Nerve Stretching Tests.

1. SCIATIC ROOTS. Usually the fifth lumbar or first sacral root is involved in a lumbo-sacral disc prolapse. Tension is put on these roots by flexing the hip with the knee straight, so-called *straight leg raising*. Normally 90° of flexion

at the hip should be possible. Where the root is stretched round or over a prolapsed disc, the same amount of straight leg raising will not be allowed (Fig. 96a & b). When the limit of straight leg raising has been achieved, further tension on the root is caused by dorsiflexing the ankle, so pulling the ultimate component of the sciatic nerve, the posterior tibial nerve, 'round' the ankle; if positive, the pain is aggravated and is felt in the back of the leg radiating into the lumbar region in some instances (Bragard sign, Fig. 96c). This test differentiates limitation of straight leg raising due to disc prolapse from that due to short hamstring muscles or a lesion in the hip.

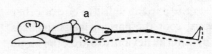
Neutral. Nerve roots slack.

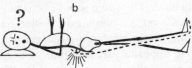
Straight leg raising limited by tension of root over prolapsed disc.

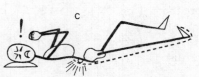
Tension increased by dorsiflexion of foot. (Bragard Test).

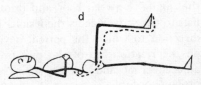
Root tension relieved by flexion at knee and ankle.

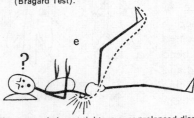
Knee extended, root tightens over prolapsed disc causing pain radiating to the back. (Lasegue Test)

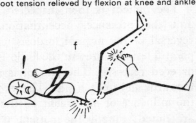
Pressure over centre of popliteal fossa bears on posterior tibial nerve which is 'bow stringing' across the fossa causing pain locally and radiation into back.

FIG. 96    Stretch Tests—Sciatic and Posterior Tibial Nerves.

2. POSTERIOR TIBIAL NERVE. This test is even more accurate and may be useful in diagnosing malingering (p. 370). Straight leg raising is performed as described above. At the limit the knee is flexed, reducing tension on the sciatic roots and the hamstrings. Unless the hip is stiff, further flexion at the hip will now be possible. Having achieved more flexion at the hip, the knee is again extended until pain is produced (Lasègue's sign, Fig. 96d & e). At this stage the posterior tibial nerve is stretched like a bowstring across the popliteal fossa. Firm pressure is applied with the ball of the thumb over the nerve in the popliteal fossa. If positive, pain radiates up as far as the lumbo-sacral region (Fig. 96f).

3. FEMORAL ROOTS. Disc prolapse at higher levels may involve the roots of the femoral nerve (L2, 3). The femoral nerve passes into the thigh in front of

the pubic ramus, and straight leg raising will relieve any tension on these roots. They are stretched by extending the hip with the knee flexed. This is done with the patient lying prone. Where there is a large disc prolapse or a painful flexion deformity of the hip, the patient may not be able to lie prone, but the test can then be performed with the patient lying on the unaffected side. In either case the knee is flexed. This may be enough to reproduce the pain and cause the patient to flex the hip to relieve the tension on the root. Where limitation of extension is due to changes in the hip, knee flexion should have no effect on the pain. If knee flexion alone causes no pain, the hip is extended with the knee still flexed. If the test is positive, it will cause pain radiating into the back (Fig. 97).

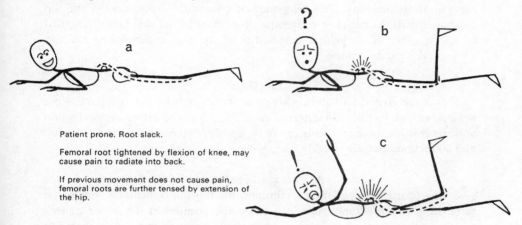

Patient prone. Root slack.

Femoral root tightened by flexion of knee, may cause pain to radiate into back.

If previous movement does not cause pain, femoral roots are further tensed by extension of the hip.

FIG. 97    Stretch Test—Femoral Nerve.

**Neurological Signs.** Detailed examination of sensation, motor function and reflexes is a most important part of the examination when nerve root involvement by a disorder of the lumbar spine is under consideration.

### Associated Joints.

1. SACRO-ILIAC JOINTS. The sacro-iliac joints are involved at an early stage in ankylosing spondylitis, but other lesions are uncommon. Movement of the sacro-iliac joint cannot be measured on clinical examination, but stress can be put on the joint by various manipulations. If these cause pain in the region of the joint, it may be considered as a source of the patient's symptoms.

Rotation of the sacro-iliac joint is achieved by first flexing the corresponding hip and knee, and then adducting the leg while preventing the whole trunk from rotating by holding the shoulder of the same side on the couch with the other hand. The sacro-iliac joint can also be subjected to stress by firm compression and distraction of the anterior superior iliac spines.

2. HIP JOINTS. Detailed examination is described on page 350. If a full and equal range of rotation is present, tested simply by 'rolling' the patient's legs

on the couch as he lies on his back, all other movements of the hip will be normal.

# THE LOWER LIMB

Before considering individual regions it is worth remembering that the posture of the legs varies throughout life, as does the posture in the spine. These changes do in some measure resemble the changes that have occurred in the evolution from the quadruped to the biped stance. The arm has not been subjected to similar change and is therefore a less common site of congenital abnormality. The frequency of congenital dislocation of the hip compared with the rarity of congenital dislocation of the shoulder is matched by the number of congenital deformities of the foot compared to the few congenital hand deformities.

## The Hip

This is the largest ball-and-socket joint and its posture changes from acute flexion with abduction and external rotation at birth to extension, adduction and neutral rotation in maturity. With ageing, extension, internal rotation and abduction decrease steadily.

### ANATOMICAL FEATURES

Owing to the depth of the acetabulum, the hip is a stable joint, but at the same time is remarkably mobile because the femur has developed a neck which is narrower than the maximum circumference of the head. In the adult the acetabulum faces outwards, downwards, and slightly backwards. The neck of the femur is set on the shaft at an angle of 130° and is directed forwards, anteverted, some 30°. The adult hip is most stable when the femur is extended. In the infant the acetabulum is directed forwards; the neck of the femur is set at a greater angle on the shaft and is directed at least 70° anteriorly. The infant's hip is therefore most stable when flexed and abducted and is in danger of dislocation if extended and adducted at this age. In contrast, the adult hip is most liable to dislocation when flexed and adducted, the posture adopted when sitting. This accounts for the increasing frequency of posterior dislocation in car accidents.

The femoral and obturator nerves supply sensory branches to the hip and the knee joint, explaining the frequent reference of pain to the knee from lesions of the hip joint.

**Movements.** As the hip is a ball-and-socket joint, flexion, extension, abduction, adduction, rotation and the combined movement of circumduction are possible. The actual range changes throughout life, as does the posture of the joint. As age increases, the first movements to decrease are extension and internal rotation, then abduction.

### SPECIAL POINTS IN THE HISTORY

Pain arising from the hip is most commonly situated in the groin, but may radiate down the thigh to the knee or be present in this joint alone. Any patient who cannot accurately localise pain in the knee should be suspected of having a disorder of the hip. Gluteal pain and pain down the back of the thigh suggest the spine as a source of the symptoms.

The patient's age and sex are important diagnostic guides because at certain ages each sex is particularly liable to characteristic disorders of the hip.

## Lesion Liability and Age

| | | |
|---|---|---|
| 0–1 years | Congenital dislocation of hip (C.D.H.) | Females > Males |
| 4–10 | Perthes' disease | Males > Females |
| | Infection, acute or chronic | Males = Females |
| | Traumatic synovitis | Males > Females |
| Puberty | Slipped upper femoral epiphysis | Males = Females |
| 20+ | Osteoarthrosis on previous damaged hip (Perthes', C.D.H.) | Males = Males |
| 45+ | Primary osteoarthritis | Females > Males |
| 50+ | Fractured neck of femur | Females > Males |
| | Trochanteric fractures | Females = Males |
| | Metastases; pathological fracture | Females = Males |

### EXAMINATION OF THE HIP

**The gait.** This should be observed with the patient lightly clad, otherwise the disability from a stiff hip may pass unnoticed. When adequate inspection is possible it is obvious that the pelvis moves with the leg in this condition. The gait of gluteal dysfunction, whatever the cause, has been described (p. 324).

**Posture.** If the hip is mobile and one leg is short, the pelvis tilts down towards the shortened side and a scoliosis develops, or the patient simply flexes the hip and knee of the longer leg (Fig. 98). A 'raise' under the short leg corrects the posture of the hips and the back. A series of wooden blocks, ranging from ½ cm. to 6 cm. in depth, is used to determine the comfortable amount of elevation required by a standing patient to compensate for shortening of a leg.

Fixed adduction of the hip causes

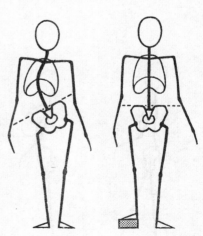

FIG. 98   Posture Changes in Short Leg.

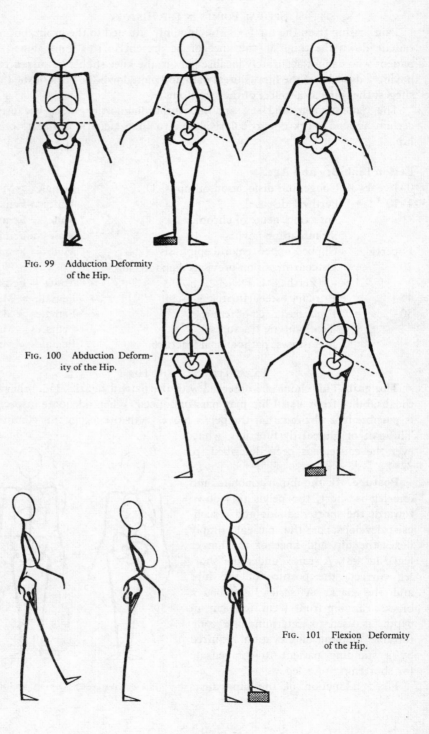

FIG. 99   Adduction Deformity
of the Hip.

FIG. 100   Abduction Deformity of the Hip.

FIG. 101   Flexion Deformity
of the Hip.

apparent shortening of the leg. Bending the other knee or using a raise on the affected side does not correct the scoliosis (Fig. 99).

A fixed abduction deformity causes apparent lengthening of the leg. The patient can adjust his posture by flexing the knee on the affected side and decreasing his lordosis, or by wearing a raise under the normal but apparently short limb, allowing a scoliosis to develop (Fig. 100).

A fixed flexion deformity will cause apparent shortening, but the patient will be able to compensate by increasing his lordosis and no scoliosis will occur. A raise under the affected leg will allow the spine to return to normal lordosis (Fig. 101). A single deformity seldom occurs. The most common combination is adduction and flexion of the hip.

**Inspection of the Supine Patient.** When the patient lies on the examination couch it is difficult to detect deformity of the hip, because the pelvis can tilt to compensate for a considerable malposition of the hip. The pelvis must first be positioned so that the iliac crests are on the same horizontal plane and at right angles to the spine. Any fixed abduction or adduction will immediately be revealed. A flexion deformity will be masked by the patient tilting the pelvis forwards, increasing the lumbar lordosis. The *Thomas test* consists of obliterating the lumbar lordosis by flexing the unaffected hip to its limit and then continuing flexion which straightens the lumbar spine. The affected leg will then be raised off the table, revealing the amount of flexion deformity present.

Inspection is completed by looking for swelling, signs of inflammation, muscle wasting or sinus formation. Although it is impossible to see distension of the hip joint when an effusion is present, the limb takes up the characteristic posture of slight flexion, abduction and external rotation. If an infective process has caused destructive changes in the joint, flexion, adduction and internal rotation will develop.

**Measurement of Leg Length.** Accurate measurement can be achieved only by special radiological techniques, but clinical examination gives a reasonable assessment of any discrepancy. Where a fixed deformity of the hip joint is present and the legs are brought parallel, the limbs will apparently be unequal in length as shown in Figure 102. The amount of *apparent shortening* is measured between a fixed point, the xiphoid process or the umbilicus, and the tip of the medial malleolus.

*True shortening* is measured from the anterior superior iliac spine to the medial malleolus (Fig. 103). The

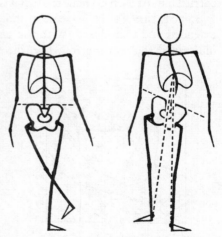

FIG. 102    Measurement of Apparent Shortening of the Leg.

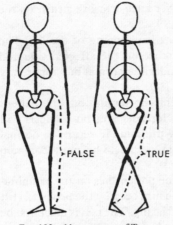

FIG. 103 Measurement of True Shortening of the Leg.

normal limb must be measured in a comparable position to the abnormal one, in respect of adduction or abduction, if reasonable accuracy is to be achieved.

Measurement of Bryant's triangle, Nelaton's line and Shoemaker's line are time-honoured exercises, designed to determine whether shortening occurs above or below the greater trochanter, but are not recommended.

**Palpation.** In adults it is difficult to detect anything other than gross swelling around the hip joint. Palpation can localise tenderness and so give some indication of the source of the symptoms.

### Measurement of Movement.

1. FLEXION. The pelvis must be immobilised in order to be certain that the movement being measured is that of the hip alone and not also of the pelvis on the spine. The iliac crest is stabilised with one hand while the other grasps the leg (Fig. 104a). The Thomas test is then carried out to see if any fixed flexion is present. This routine is performed first on the normal side and the range compared with the abnormal.

2. ABDUCTION AND ADDUCTION. Movement of the pelvis must again be eliminated. With the patient supine the examiner grasps the opposite iliac crest and lays that forearm across the pelvis to touch the anterior-superior iliac spine on the side nearest to himself (Fig. 104b). Abduction and adduction are then carried out. At each extreme the pelvis will be felt to turn with the limb.

3. ROTATION. This movement should be carried out with the hips first extended and then flexed. With the patient supine, and using the patellae as indicators, the legs are rolled on the couch and the range measured by the

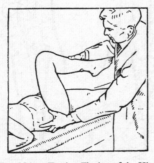

FIG. 104a  Testing Flexion of the Hip.

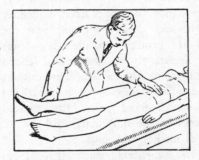

FIG. 104b  Testing Abduction of the Hip.

(From ADAMS, J. C. (1971). *Outline of Orthopaedics*, 7th ed. Edinburgh and London: Churchill Livingstone.)

excursion of the patellae or by the arc through which the toes rotate. A more accurate method is performed with the patient prone. The knees are flexed to a right angle and the tibiae then act as indicators of the arc of rotation. The range of rotation of the flexed hips is measured by flexing both the hip and the knee to a right angle as the patient lies supine. Again the tibiae act as indicators of the degree of rotation.

The accurate measurement of rotation is particularly important if slipping of the upper femoral epiphysis is suspected. An increase of external rotation at the expense of internal rotation is one of the earliest clinical findings. Conversely, a tendency to congenital dislocation is accompanied by more internal than external rotation.

**Tests of Stability of Hip.** This problem is encountered in congenital dislocation in infants, slipped epiphysis in adolescents, traumatic dislocations in adults, and fractures of the neck of the femur in the elderly.

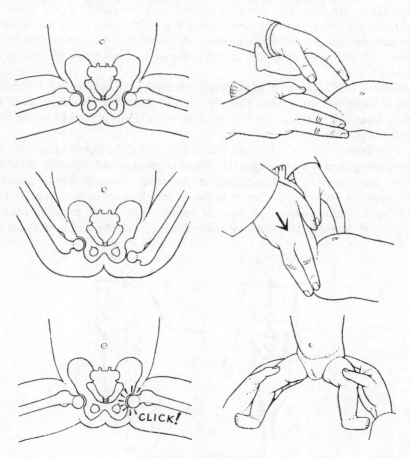

FIG. 105   Ortalani's Test.

IN INFANCY AND CHILDHOOD. Congenital dislocation of the hip must be diagnosed as soon as possible after birth, certainly many months before the child walks. Thus many of the classical signs are useless. The three most obvious features are:

1. Shortening and external rotation of the limb. The mother may remark that the child does not move the affected leg as much as the other.

2. Asymmetry of the thigh and buttock folds.

3. Limitation of abduction: 90° of abduction in each hip should be possible in an infant.

If any of these signs are present, Ortolani's test should be performed. This test is now carried out on newborn infants as a routine in many maternity units.

*Ortolani's Test* (Fig. 105). With the infant supine, the hips and knees are flexed to a right angle and the knees brought together. Pressing gently backwards the hips are slowly abducted and extended. If the hips are unstable, the first part of the manœuvre will push the head of the femur out of the acetabulum. As abduction proceeds the head of the femur will be felt to click back into place. This test is very accurate and can be performed on the newborn baby.

Testing for 'telescoping' of the limb depends on an established dislocation and is therefore a late sign. The term vividly describes the sensation of the limb apparently sinking into the trunk as it is thrust in the axis of the limb itself towards the trunk.

*Trendelenburg Sign.* This sign demonstrates that the hip abductors are not functioning, and is useful in the late stages of congenital dislocation of the hip when the patient is walking, and in assessing the disability in anterior poliomyelitis involving the lower limbs. When the normal subject stands on one leg the glutei contract so that the opposite side of the pelvis is tilted up slightly. If the patient stands on the affected leg when the actions of the glutei

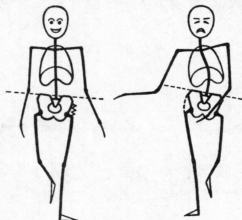

FIG. 106   Trendelenburg Sign.

are deficient, the opposite side of the pelvis will tilt downward and balance can be maintained only by leaning over towards the side of the lesion (Fig. 106). The test is performed with the patient's back to the examiner. The patient stands on the normal leg and flexes the knee of the other leg to a right angle. The pelvis remains level or tilts up slightly on the other side. The patient then stands on the abnormal leg and the pelvis tilts down on the opposite side. When walking, the patient compensates for the lack of abduction by leaning over to the affected side so that the centre of gravity is as nearly as possible over the hip. This causes the patient to dip, or lurch, towards the affected side.

IN PUBERTY AND IN ADULT LIFE. Instability associated with slipped upper femoral epiphysis (adolescent coxa vara), traumatic dislocation of the hip, and fracture in the region of the neck of the femur is apt to occur at a particular age and is associated with characteristic postures.

*Slipped Upper Femoral Epiphysis.* This occurs at puberty. The limb is externally rotated, adducted and shortened.

*Traumatic Dislocation.* This occurs in mature patients.

1. Posterior dislocation in which the limb is flexed, adducted and internally rotated is the more common.

2. In anterior dislocation the limb is flexed, abducted and externally rotated.

*Fracture in the Region of the Neck of the Femur.* The limb is externally rotated, adducted and shortened. This is the same deformity as in slipped epiphysis because the same mechanism is involved.

## The Knee

The knee is the largest joint in the body and it is particularly prone to injury by twisting owing to the fact that its stability through a range of movement of 150° is entirely dependent upon the control of muscles and ligaments. In addition, its exposed position renders it liable to direct injury. Repeated kneeling brings both a tendency to traumatic bursitis and a risk of direct infection of the joint by puncture wounds. Inflammation due to rheumatic fever and rheumatoid arthritis commonly involves the knee joint, but blood-borne infection is now rare in Britain. Over the years the stress of weight-bearing often leads to degenerative changes, especially in the obese. Serious congenital abnormalities are rare.

### ANATOMICAL FEATURES

The stability of the knee depends more on the related muscles and ligaments than on the shape of the bones. There is normally a degree of valgus, or abduction, of the tibia on the femur when the knee is fully extended. In this position, because of the shape of the condyles of the femur, the tibia externally rotates on the femur. This in turn causes the collateral ligaments and the anterior cruciate ligament to become stretched. In this situation the tibia is 'screwed home' on the femur and the joint is 'locked' in full extension and able to sustain the body weight with minimal muscle action. With a few degrees of flexion the external rotation is undone, and the ligaments are relaxed. It is now possible to abduct and rotate the tibia on the femur, or vice versa. When the ligaments are tight in full extension, they are particularly liable to injury.

The semilunar cartilages, attached by their periphery to the capsule, are relatively mobile structures. When the tibia is abducted, adducted, or rotated on the femur, the cartilage is sucked between the bones on the 'open' side of the joint. A sudden change of position then may trap the cartilage, which tears from its periphery. The torn portion, resembling a 'bucket handle', comes to lie between the condyles of the femur. The knee is then said to be locked because extension is obstructed to a varying degree, although flexion may be largely preserved. Occasionally one end of the bucket handle separates from its attachment and a 'parrot beak' tear results. This is liable to become caught momentarily between the tibia and femur. The patient is aware of a sensation of the knee being about to give way, or it may actually give way under his weight. This is in contrast to the 'locking' of a bucket handle tear. Both incidents are usually related to movement involving flexion and rotation while taking the body weight, for example changing direction when running or twisting round when kneeling.

The quadriceps is the most important group of muscles controlling the knee. When these muscles contract they tend to pull in a straight line from the greater trochanter to the tibial tubercle. Because of the normal valgus of the knee, this tends to displace the patella laterally. This tendency, however, is controlled by the action of the obliquely disposed vastus medialis muscle. The more valgus the knee, the greater the tendency to lateral displacement of the patella and the more important the action of the vastus medialis.

### Special Points Regarding the History and Examination

The anatomical features which have been discussed underline the importance of a detailed history of the mechanism of any injury of the knee. The menisci are liable to be torn by twisting injuries, though derangement of the medial meniscus is less common in the female. Possibly because of the greater valgus at the knee in the female, lateral dislocation of the patella with spontaneous reduction is not uncommon. The history will be identical with a medial cartilage injury. Sudden pain with the sensation of something giving way on the inner side of the joint is felt as the knee is bent with or without rotation. Inspection soon after this episode will settle the diagnosis. With both injuries bleeding occurs. With a cartilage injury it is confined within the joint and no bruising is seen. With dislocation of the patella, the retinaculae on the medial side are torn, blood escapes into the subcutaneous tissues, and bruising is visible.

A violent blow applied to one side of the knee in extension is liable to cause partial or complete rupture of the opposite collateral ligament. The quadriceps muscles react rapidly to injury, infection or lack of use by wasting and losing bulk. The knee itself reacts differently according to the degree of injury. Moderate violence, or slight violence often repeated, causes an effusion of varying degree. An effusion takes some hours or even a day to develop.

Severe violence results in bleeding into the joint which becomes distended with fluid—a haemarthrosis. The history is often the only means of differentiating between a large effusion and a haemarthrosis. An effusion takes some time to develop; a haemarthrosis develops rapidly. Aspiration of the joint settles the issue.

Very severe violence will rupture ligaments. Bleeding will occur, but, as the synovium as well as the capsule and ligament will be torn, the blood will escape from the joint and present as swelling and bruising about the damaged side of the joint; no fluid will be detected in the joint.

Osteoarthrosis is common in the knee, and the pain and stiffness after sitting may be described as 'locking' by the patient. This underlines the importance of finding out exactly what the patient means and of not accepting such terms uncritically.

Again it is worth remembering that pain in the region of the knee need not have its origin in this joint. Where pain arises in the knee itself, the patient can usually indicate its site accurately. When the patient points vaguely to the front of the lower thigh and knee, one should suspect that the hip is the source of the pain.

## EXAMINATION OF THE KNEE

**Inspection with Patient Erect.** The gait of a stiff knee is immediately evident and need not be described. Provided there is reasonable control of the hip or foot, a patient can walk even when all the controlling muscles of the knee are paralysed, because of the locking mechanism described above.

Abnormalities of posture are most evident when the patient stands. The most difficult problem is to determine when knock-knee, or genu valgum, becomes abnormal in degree in the two- to four-year-old child. The distance between the medial malleoli when the child stands with the feet parallel and the knees just touching is a useful measurement to record for comparison in the future. It is not possible to give an absolute figure for any particular age, but in the majority the deformity corrects spontaneously by the age of six to eight years. Over this age separation of the malleoli by more than 5 cm is a deformity which is unlikely to correct itself. Before delivering reassurance that spontaneous correction will occur, it is wise to inspect the mother's knees unobtrusively. Asymmetrical genu valgum is abnormal at any age.

**Inspection with Patient Supine.** Deformity can again be reviewed, and in particular the amount of genu valgum measured, as noted above. Wasting of the muscles and any swelling of the joint can now be more easily assessed.

**Palpation.** The bony contour is checked and signs of inflammation are sought. Muscle girth should be recorded in order to follow progress when wasting is present. The level above the patella at which this measurement is made should also be noted.

Tenderness must be accurately localised. The whole extent of both collateral ligaments and the joint line must be palpated. This latter cannot be localised accurately with the knee extended, but in flexion the joint line become visible in the thinner subject and is at least palpable in fat patients.

A *trace of effusion* can be detected only by the massage test. With the knee straight, any fluid in the antero-medial compartment of the knee is massaged up into the suprapatellar pouch. Then by pressure over the suprapatellar pouch and lateral compartment with the finger and thumb of the opposite hand the fluid is squeezed back into the antero-medial compartment. The normal depression medial to the patellar tendon is seen to bulge as the fluid accumulates there.

A *moderate effusion* gives rise to a *patellar tap*. With the knee straight the suprapatellar pouch is emptied by pressure with one hand, and the para-patellar compartment by pressure with the other hand, leaving the index finger free to elicit the tap. With this finger the patella is pressed sharply against the femur. If there is sufficient fluid to 'float' the patella off the femur it will be felt to tap against the femur.

A *large effusion* outlines the suprapatellar pouch as an inverted crescentic swelling immediately above the patella and a tap may be easily elicited. By squeezing this swelling while palpating on each side of the patella with the other hand an effusion can be differentiated from synovial thickening by the transmission of a fluid impulse from hand to hand when an effusion is present.

LOOSE BODIES. A very careful examination of the knee is required where there is a history of locking. If this symptom results from a particular movement, a meniscus injury should be suspected. When its occurrence is unpredictable, locking is likely to be due to loose bodies. A palpable loose body can move in all directions and usually disappears between the condyles of the femur. Thick patellar retinaculae may be mistaken for loose bodies as they roll under the examining finger. Their position and the fact that they can be moved from side to side and not up and down helps to identify them.

**Movements of the Knee.** The normal range in the adult is flexion 0 to 150°. In some subjects a few degrees of hyperextension are possible. This is found more frequently in females.

When fully extended no abduction, adduction or rotation of the tibia on the femur is possible. With only a few degrees of flexion, abduction, adduction and rotation through a small range are possible.

When only one knee appears to be affected the active range is examined first in the normal and then the abnormal joint. The passive range is then performed in the same order, and during this examination a hand is placed on the knee to detect the presence and character of crepitus. The site of any pain and its relationship to a particular arc of movement are noted. Care is taken to detect even a few degrees of limitation of extension. When a bucket handle cartilage tear is displaced, passive extension of the knee is blocked. The sensation is of pushing against a firm rubber stop, and the knee recoils as soon as pressure is released. The patient usually complains of pain at the site of the torn cartilage. This 'rubbery' block to extension can be mimicked by an effusion in the knee, but passive extension then does not cause the same localised pain.

The most accurate method of demonstrating a few degrees of loss of extension is to lie the patient prone with the legs projecting over the end of the examination couch, supported only by the thighs. The level of the heels can be compared as an indication of unequal extension of the knees.

**Tests of Stability.** To test the *collateral ligaments* the knee must be fully extended. The patient's ankle is held between the examiner's elbow and side, leaving both hands free to abduct and adduct the tibia on the femur while keeping the knee straight (Fig. 107). Normally no movement should be detected. Where a ligament is strained no movement occurs, but pain is localised over the damaged ligament when it is stretched. When a ligament is lax, the knee 'opens' when pushed from the opposite side and is felt to 'close' with a click when pressure is released.

The *cruciate ligaments* are tested with the knee flexed to a right angle. This position is maintained by the examiner sitting on the patient's foot (Fig. 108). The patient should be warned before doing this because the polite patient withdraws the foot, and the less polite complains. With both hands now free the examiner first checks by palpation that the hamstring muscles are relaxed; otherwise the test is invalid. To test the anterior cruciate the tibia is grasped just below the knee and is drawn forwards. To test the posterior cruciates this movement is reversed. Starting with the normal knee the degree of antero-posterior glide of the tibia is noted as the normal for that patient. Any

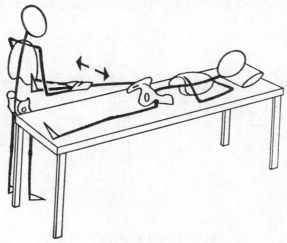

FIG. 107    Testing the Collateral Ligaments of the Knee.

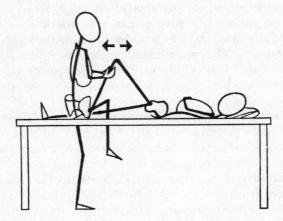

FIG. 108    Testing the Cruciate Ligaments of the Knee.

movement in excess of this in the suspect knee is abnormal. Excessive anterior 'glide' or 'draw' is due to laxity of the anterior cruciate, and posterior displacement is associated with laxity of the posterior cruciate ligament. Gross instability of a cruciate ligament is usually associated with laxity of one of the collateral ligaments and vice versa.

*The McMurray Test.* The object of this test of stability of the semilunar cartilages is to induce a torn cartilage to engage between the tibia and the femur by reproducing the mechanism which originally caused the displacement. When this happens, the patient experiences the typical symptoms and a palpable, and occasionally audible, 'click' or 'clunk' results. There is a risk that the examiner will lock the patient's knee and be unable thereafter to free it again.

The patient must be able to relax. To examine the right knee the examiner

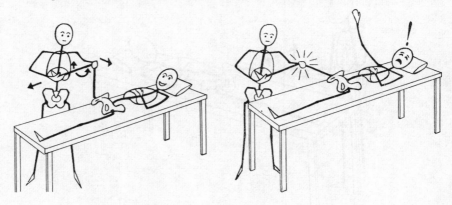

FIG. 109    The McMurray Test of the Semilunar Cartilages.

stands on the right side of the couch, grasps the patient's right heel with his right hand and steadies the knee with his left hand. The knee is flexed to the limit the patient will tolerate. While pressing on the outer side of the knee with the left hand the knee is extended while the tibia is alternately internally and externally rotated by the right hand (Fig. 109). If positive, a 'clunk' accompanied by some discomfort to the patient is felt over the displacing cartilage. If this does not produce the characteristic response, the manœuvre is repeated while the left hand presses on the inner side of the knee. The former technique is more likely to be positive where a medial cartilage is displaced, and the latter where the lateral cartilage is involved.

*Stability of the Patella.* With the knee extended, the patella is grasped and moved from side to side. An impression of excessive mobility may be gained when this is compared with the normal knee. Passive flexion of the knee while the patella is pressed laterally may reproduce the patient's symptoms or may even dislocate the patella.

**Tests for Degenerative Change in the Knee.** During active and passive movement of the knee palpation may detect crepitus or a grinding sensation, if osteoarthrosis is present. The character of the crepitus varies and the coarser it is the more extreme will be the degree of wear and tear in the articular cartilage.

Where the osteoarthrosis is localised to the patello-femoral compartment of the knee, moving the patella up and down against the femur (patellar grinding) will be painful and will be accompanied by crepitus. Similarly if the patient contracts his quadriceps muscle while the patella is pressed firmly against the femur, characteristic pain will be produced if the patella is the site of osteoarthrosis or of chondromalacia in the younger patient.

### The Leg, Ankle and Foot

The human foot has undergone great evolutionary changes. The tarsal bones have become massive and disposed in two layers. The metatarso-phalangeal segments now lie roughly parallel and instead of the central segment being the longest, the medial segment or hallux has become the longest and strongest component of the forefoot. Many feet fail to achieve this ideal and the first metatarsal remains relatively short and deviated medially in varus. The phalanges then deviate in the opposite direction and hallux valgus results. This is only one example of the many congenital defects found in the feet. In addition to this tendency to congenital abnormality, the feet have to bear the stress of the body weight on hard unyielding surfaces, often cramped and constricted by fashionable footwear. For these reasons many problems are encountered in the foot.

### ANATOMICAL FEATURES

The two feet placed side by side resemble an inverted soup-plate. Each foot corresponds with half a plate. The inner border of the foot is raised to form the longitudinal arch. The outer border, corresponding with the flange of the plate, lies on the ground. When the feet are placed together an arch, lying across the mid-tarsal region, is formed. When not bearing weight a further lesser transverse arch lies under the metatarsal heads. The arches of the foot act as shock absorbers when the foot takes the body weight and give spring to the gait. The flattened outer border gives stability when standing.

As an aid to the understanding of various deformities, the foot may be considered to have three main components—the talus, the calcaneus and the forefoot. The last includes the navicular, cuboid, cuneiforms, metatarsals and phalanges. When the patient is standing, the long axis of the talus, navicular, medial cuneiform and first metatarsal should lie in a straight line. This can be seen accurately only on radiological examination with the patient standing, but clinical examination will give some idea where this longitudinal axis is broken in foot deformity.

**Description of Foot Deformities.** *Talipes* is derived from the words talus and pes, inferring that there is a deformity involving the ankle and foot, and

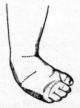
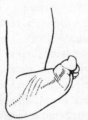

FIG.-110    Talipes Equino Varus.              FIG. 111    Talipes Calcaneus.

must be further qualified to have any meaning. *Talipes equinus* means that the foot and ankle are plantar flexed, like the foot of a horse which walks on the tip of one finger. *Talipes equino varus* means that in addition the hind foot is adducted and that the forefoot also is adducted or inverted at the midtarsal joint (Fig. 110). This is the typical clubfoot deformity. *Talipes calcaneus* indicates that the heel projects towards the sole of the foot (Fig. 111). When combined with valgus of the other parts of the foot, *talipes calcaneo valgus*, it is the other common congenital foot deformity.

Either of these deformities may be associated with deformity of the longitudinal arch. If flattened, the deformity is described as *planus*. If raised or increased, the deformity is described as *cavus*. It is possible, therefore, to have a talipes equino–cavovarus, etc.

*Pes* means foot and implies deformity involving the foot only and that the position of the ankle joint is normal. *Pes planus* means flat-foot. The axis of the longitudinal arch passing as a straight line through talus, navicular, medial cuneiform and first metatarsal may sag at either the talo-navicular joint or the naviculo-cuneiform joint. The most severe degrees of flat-foot are usually associated with the former. The normal heel is vertical when viewed from behind. In pes planus the heel is often abducted (valgus) and the whole foot pronated.

In *pes cavus* the longitudinal arch is raised and the heel seen from behind is often adducted (varus). In this position the foot is supinated and the toes are usually clawed. It is worth remarking at this point on the association of this deformity with abnormalities of the central nervous system, e.g. Friedreich's ataxia.

*Claw toes* are usually associated with a pes cavus deformity. The toes are extended at the metatarso-phalangeal joints and flexed at the interphalangeal joints. All the toes are commonly affected and eventually dorsal dislocation at the metatarso-phalangeal joints occurs.

*Hammer toe* often involves only the second toe and is not associated with other deformities of the foot. The metatarso-phalangeal joint is extended, the proximal interphalangeal joint is flexed and the distal interphalangeal joint is extended. A painful corn develops over the proximal interphalangeal joint.

*Hallux valgus* is probably the most common deformity in a shoe-wearing community. In addition to valgus deformity of the phalanges the metatarsal is often shorter than normal and deviated in the opposite direction—metatarsus primus varus et brevis (p. 363 ).

In *hallux rigidus* the hallux is often longer than the other toes and, perhaps because of this, develops degenerative change or osteoarthrosis in the meta-tarso-phalangeal joint. At first extension is diminished, but in the extreme instances the toe may become permanently flexed—*hallux flexus.*

### SPECIAL FEATURES IN THE HISTORY

In children pain in the feet directly related to the musculo-skeletal structures is not common. When not associated with obvious deformity or inflammatory changes the cause is usually osteochondritis involving the calcaneus, navicular or the metatarsal heads.

In the adult, pain localised to the foot usually has its origin there, but pain arising in the foot may be referred up the leg. The character and pattern of the pain will give some indication of the cause. Osteoarthrosis has the familiar pattern of pain and stiffness after rest, relieved temporarily by activity. Aching pain which gradually gets worse the longer the patient is on his feet suggests chronic ligamentous strain. Pain of a burning, tingling character radiating into the third and fourth toes and into the foot suggests a digital neuroma in the cleft between these toes. The patient notices that removing the shoe relieves this pain; on examination there is tenderness in the affected toe cleft, and sensation is depressed in the same toe cleft. Ischaemia of the feet in the elderly causes distressing pain, not always related to exercise, and often severe on first going to bed. Special enquiry should be directed at the condition of the feet in geriatric patients as severe but remediable disability can be caused by minor abnormalities such as callosities or overgrowth of a nail (onychogryphosis).

Perhaps the most common pain in the forefoot (metatarsalgia) is associated with claw or hammer toe deformity where the fibrofatty pad normally under the metatarsal head comes to lie under the toes, leaving the metatarsal heads exposed. The patient very appropriately describes pain as walking on the bones themselves, or likens it to walking on stones. This situation also develops in rheumatoid arthritis. Other causes of metatarsalgia are stress fractures of the metatarsal shafts usually the second or third, the so-called march fracture, and osteochondritis of the second metatarsal head in adolescence.

### EXAMINATION OF THE LEG, ANKLE AND FOOT

**Gait.** Stiffness without pain causes little alteration in the gait. Equinus deformity, as in the drop-foot gait, causes a high stepping gait in order to clear the ground, but differs from it in that the foot is fixed in the former but loose and flapping in the latter. The gait of calcaneus deformity lacks spring—the 'peg-leg' gait.

**Posture.** Apart from the effects of the congenital deformities already described, abnormal posture of the foot may result from a poor general posture. Surprising correction of flat-foot deformity is achieved by correcting the typical slouching, knee flexed, pronated feet stance of the disinterested adolescent.

**Palpation.** This is best performed with the patient sitting on the examination couch with the legs dangling over the edge. The calf is relaxed and foot movement is freer when the knee is flexed. The examiner sits on a low stool in front of the patient. The colour, texture and temperature of the skin give useful information concerning the circulation and nutrition of the foot. The condition of the nails is noted. The toes are separated and the area between them is inspected for evidence of fungal infection, in which condition the skin becomes thickened, whitish, sodden and fissured. Particular note is made of the site of any callosity or corn formation. Tenderness or other signs of inflammation are accurately localised. The pulses are palpated in the dorsalis pedis and posterior tibial arteries. If they are absent the perforating peroneal artery is sought in front of the inferior tibio-fibular joint.

**Movements.** While the patient is erect, the ability to stand on the toes, on the heels and on the inner and outer borders of the feet is tested. The active range of non-weight-bearing movement is then noted and finally the range of passive movement is reviewed.

FLEXION AND DORSIFLEXION OF THE ANKLE. The foot is in the neutral position when it is at right angles to the long axis of the tibia. The true position of the foot in relation to the leg is more easily appreciated when viewed from the outer side. In dorsiflexion the broader anterior surface of the talus is engaged in the ankle mortice and no other movement can take place in the ankle joint. In plantar flexion the narrower portion of the talus is engaged and some abduction and adduction can take place. In practice this cannot be differentiated from movement in the subtalar joint.

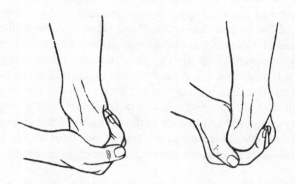

FIG. 112    Inversion and Eversion of the Hind Foot.

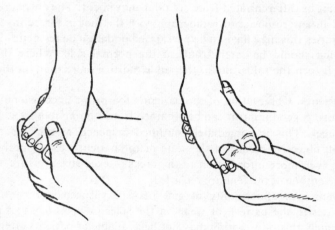

FIG. 113    Inversion and Eversion of the Forefoot.

INVERSION AND EVERSION OF THE HIND FOOT. The examiner holds the heel with the foot at right angles to the leg (Fig. 112). The heel is then adducted and abducted. These movements take place mainly in the subtalar joint.

INVERSION AND EVERSION OF THE FOREFOOT. The heel is held in one hand and the forefoot in the other and the forefoot is adducted and abducted in relation to the hind foot (Fig. 113). These movements take place in the mid-tarsal joint, between the talus and calcaneus posteriorly and the forefoot anteriorly.

TARSO-METATARSAL MOVEMENT. The range is so small that it cannot be assessed on clinical examination.

### Tests of Stability

1. TENDO ACHILLIS. The diagnosis of ruptured tendo achillis is often missed, perhaps because it is not realised that the foot can still be plantar flexed by the toe flexors. The classic signs are a palpable gap in the tendon, excessive active and passive dorsi-flexion of the foot, and inability to stand on tiptoe on the affected foot. However, these signs may be difficult to assess because of pain and swelling at the time of injury. The *squeeze test* does not suffer from this handicap. With the patient prone or kneeling, the calf is firmly but gently squeezed just distal to its maximal circumference. Where the tendon is intact the foot plantar flexes. Where the tendon is ruptured, no plantar flexion occurs. This test will also differentiate ruptured tendo achillis from the other common injury to the calf—alvusion of the medial head of the gastrocnemius muscle. Performing the test causes pain locally at the site of the avulsed medial head of gastrocnemius and none when the tendo achillis is ruptured.

2. LATERAL LIGAMENT OF ANKLE. It is impossible on clinical examination to know if this ligament is ruptured because abnormal movement at the ankle joint cannot be differentiated from subtalar movement. The only sure method is to take an antero-posterior radiograph with the foot in forced inversion. In recent injuries this may have to be performed under an anaesthetic. The same examination should be carried out on the normal side. Where the lateral ligament is torn the talus tilts in the ankle mortice more than on the normal side.

**Foot Prints.** Observation of the patient's footprints is occasionally useful in diagnosis. A good imprint can be obtained from a damp foot by standing on brown paper. This is immediately outlined in pencil or ink and affords a permanent objective record of the state of the patient's foot. Special rubber pads give even more information as the areas of excessive pressure as well as the simple outline of the foot are recorded.

**Footwear.** An abnormality of gait may be suspected or confirmed by irregularities in the pattern of wear on the soles or heels of shoes or boots. Unfortunately this information may not be available as patients often come to the clinic wearing their best and newest footwear.

## FURTHER INVESTIGATIONS

### Radiological Examination

Radiological examination plays a very prominent part in the further investigation of abnormalities involving the locomotor system. It is essential, for clinical and medico-legal reasons, if a fracture is suspected. At least two views must be taken, in planes at right angles to each other, to demonstrate properly the position of the bone fragments. If only one view is taken, the fragments may appear to be in good position when, in fact, they are overlapping and the bone ends are not in contact with each other. Two views may fail to show a crack fracture. When a fracture of the carpal scaphoid is suspected, at least four views are taken. If none is visible but the clinical findings suggest that a fracture is present, a plaster is applied and the radiological examination is repeated three weeks later. Any fracture will then be revealed by the reaction in the adjacent bone.

In children the epiphyses may be confused with a fracture, especially in the elbow. Comparable views of the normal joint will clarify the situation.

The extent of injury to the soft tissues can be demonstrated by special radiological techniques. Rupture of ligaments allows the related joint to dislocate to a lesser or greater degree and this abnormal position can be shown on a radiograph. For example, a sprained lateral ligament of the ankle cannot be differentiated from a rupture of that ligament on clinical examination. An antero-posterior view of the ankle is required with the foot held in forced inversion. If the lateral ligament is ruptured the talus will be seen to be tilted in the ankle mortice.

Abnormalities in the intra-articular structures can be revealed by arthrograms. Either air or a radio-opaque fluid is injected into the joint. In either case the soft tissues displace the contrast medium and their shape is outlined. This technique is occasionally helpful in injuries to the semilunar cartilages in the knee and in defining the position of the labrum of the acetabulum in congenital dislocation of the hip. Similar techniques are used to outline space occupying lesions in the spinal canal by injecting dye into the theca, myelography.

If loose bodies are present in a joint, more than the routine antero-posterior and lateral views will often be required. For example, in the knee additional intercondylar views are necessary. Special oblique views may be required for the adequate demonstration of certain joints particularly in the spine, for example the sacro-iliac joints which are involved in the early stages of ankylosing spondylitis and the facet joints when spondylolisthesis is suspected.

Where there is destruction of bone its extent may be demonstrated by tomography. To be visible by ordinary radiographic examination such a lesion must be at least one cm. in diameter. Bone scanning provides a more accurate and positive method of detecting destructive processes involving bone.

When examining the radiographs of the skeleton the opportunity should always be taken to look at the whole film for other abnormalities, as, for example, at the apices of the lungs in antero-posterior views of the cervical spine. Similarly, the examination of films of the lumbar spine should include a careful scrutiny of the soft tissue shadows of the psoas muscles, the abdominal viscera and the diaphragm.

# THE METHODS IN PRACTICE—AN EXAMPLE

## The Detection of the Malingerer

A malingerer is an individual who feigns disease or illness for personal gain or in order to avoid an adverse situation. Hysteria is induced by the same ultimate gains, but at a subconscious level. In clinical practice the clear distinction between malingering and hysteria is often blurred, but both conditions have one thing in common—apparent disability with no organic cause. In the locomotor system in general, and after industrial injuries in particular when claims for compensation are pending, these disorders of the mind are commonly encountered. Their recognition depends upon the observation of clinical features which do not conform to those expected from organic causes or from the injury in question. Without great experience this may be very difficult, or the complaints may be so bizarre as to be readily recognisable. The following comments are intended merely as a guide to the analysis of situations which may have an infinite number of variations.

**History.** The malingerer's symptoms do not form a consistent pattern as noted on page 331. When pain is the main complaint it is constant and not relieved by rest in contrast to most pains of organic origin except those due to advanced disease which is usually obvious. An absolutely symmetrical distribution of pain is rare in organic disease. When malingering or hysteria is suspected the patient should be asked to indicate the site of the pain on a rough diagram of the body. Absolute symmetry suggests a functional disorder.

**Demeanour.** The malingerer is on the defensive even though this may present as an aggressive attitude. The hysterical patient is often strangely indifferent to, or even cheerful about his disability.

**Gait.** When the complaint is of pain in the lower limbs the rhythm of the gait may be atypical in that the weight is not taken off the allegedly painful limb quickly. Rather the drama is heightened by standing on it for even longer than usual.

**Movements Inhibited by Pain.** The conscious or subconscious perpetuation or exaggeration of disability caused by pain is particularly common in cases where compensation is concerned. This is perhaps the most difficult problem to assess, but application of the principles mentioned in the section on interpretation of abnormal joint movement will reveal inconsistencies which will confirm the diagnosis. For example, a patient complaining of severe backache may, when standing, be unable to reach anywhere near his toes with his legs straight and, when lying, straight leg raising will be limited to a similar degree. If at the extreme of straight leg raising the knee is flexed, the genuine patient with sciatic root tension will allow further hip flexion to occur, but not so the malingerer. The posterior tibial nerve stretch (Fig. 96) may also help to differentiate the genuine sufferer from the false. Whatever the findings, the doctor should continue the examination and finally, with the patient still supine, examine the chest. The patient is then asked to sit up to permit of access to the back of the chest. Almost invariably the malingerer will do so with the legs straight out on the examination couch in a position which is equivalent either to touching his toes while standing or to normal straight leg raising while recumbent.

**Sensory and Motor Changes.** Apparent neurological defects are apt to be claimed by the malingerer or the hysteric, especially after trauma, and they are therefore mentioned briefly here. These commonly take the form of sensory loss or paralysis.

If anaesthesia is present, the distribution tends not to follow an anatomical pattern and is often of a glove or stocking configuration affecting a single limb. It must be borne in mind, however, that a symmetrical loss of sensation affecting all four limbs simultaneously and of a glove and stocking distribution is characteristic of polyneuritis.

Paralysis may be feigned but again can be detected through inconsistencies due to the patient's lack of knowledge of anatomy. The patient with a 'dropped wrist' will be unable to extend the fingers or wrist, but when asked to clench his fingers will, if malingering, produce a normal fist, unaware that the wrist extensors are playing a part in what he thinks is purely flexion of the fingers. Similarly, passive movement through the range of paralysis may be actively resisted by the patient.

Lower motor neurone paralysis or disuse of muscle leads to wasting which is best judged, in the early stages, by eye. Measurement is also of value in following progress and as objective evidence which can be recorded. Gross apparent weakness in the absence of wasting is always suspect.

The undiscerning patient, when asked how far he used to be able to lift an arm or leg, or what it is that he cannot do as a result of the accident, may actually perform the movement which he claims is impossible. It may be worth asking this question casually at the end of the examination.

**Attitude of the Examiner.** Throughout the proceedings the examiner must maintain an impersonal or friendly manner. Nothing is gained by browbeating the patient. Accurate records of the findings should be made at the time, especially if any legal issue is involved.

# CHAPTER 10
# The Infant and Child

'Children are not men nor women; they are almost as different creatures, in many respects, as if they never were to be the one or the other; they are as unlike as buds are unlike flowers, and almost as blossoms are unlike fruits.'

W. S. LANDOR

## GENERAL CONSIDERATIONS

In previous chapters the main emphasis has been on the adult, on the elucidation of symptoms and signs of disease as they present when physical and mental maturity are well advanced or have been achieved. In this chapter we are dealing with the infant and child, with the epoch in life preceding the development of adulthood but progressively leading towards it. Further, we are dealing here with all systems. Paediatrics is a speciality bound by age and not by system. It concerns itself with a whole individual undergoing rapid growth and change.

In turning at this stage to the clinical examination of the child we are following the practice which has long pertained in undergraduate clinical teaching—consideration of the adult first and of the infant and child subsequently. Although chronologically illogical this practice can be justified. The adult patient is in the main a more co-operative subject on whom the student may practise his clinical art, and does not exhibit the wide variations in physique, mentality and psychological status shown by the child. In adult life physiological normals are much more constant and are confined within a much narrower range than is the case in infancy and childhood. Weight is an obvious example of this. The variations within infancy and childhood may necessitate considerable adaptation of standard methods of approach, or new methods, and considerable modification or extension of the techniques of clinical examination. The student who does not appreciate this may come to have a seriously distorted approach to the clinical examination of children. He may feel that the child is merely an adult reduced in size, and, thinking in this purely quantitative way, may fail to appreciate the great qualitative differences which exist. He may not understand the need to orient his mind towards growth and development, which are such essential parts of paediatrics, and away from the established physical and mental status and degenerative processes which are inherent in adult medical practice. He may fail to interpret symptoms and signs and physical measurements in infancy and childhood against the wide range of physiological normals appropriate to the age of the patient. He may try to apply to the child clinical methods which are impracticable or will yield little information, and may fail to employ methods which may yield much. He may interpret as indicative of disease signs which, bearing pathological significance in the adult, are without significance in the child and he may ignore important signs peculiar to infancy and childhood.

While there is much that is common to the clinical examination of adults and children there is much that is different. A large proportion of what has already been said in preceding chapters is relevant to children in greater or lesser degree. This chapter would be inadequate, however, if it indicated merely those points where the clinical examination of the child differs from that of the adult. A disjointed collection of notes and comparisons would result and would give little guidance to the important considerations of emphasis and sequence. It would be difficult on this basis to present the methods of clinical examination of children in proper perspective. Accordingly, an attempt has been made to write the chapter as a whole with the emphasis on signs and symptoms peculiar to, or of special significance in, infancy and childhood.

A few examples may illustrate some of these points. A static weight in a child is abnormal and may be a sign of disease; in the adult it is normal; vomiting in a baby may have little significance or it may be of great import, whereas in the adult it is likely to have a much more constant pathological significance; a liver edge which is palpable one finger-breadth below the costal margin would probably indicate hepatomegaly in an adult while it would be normal in a child; the fontanelle is available for examination in infancy only; on the other hand, mapping of the visual fields in infants and toddlers may be impossible; head retraction is more likely to be associated with meningitis in the older child or adult than in the infant, in whom it tends to be a late sign of meningeal irritation but a common one in association with respiratory difficulty; slowly rising intracranial pressure in the infant is likely to reveal itself by increasing head size without papilloedema, and in the older child and adult by headache, vomiting and disturbance of gait with papilloedema; an extensor plantar response below one year of age has a different significance from such a response beyond this age; haemoptysis in a child is most commonly related to nasopharyngeal bleeding or to the traumatic effect of coughing, and hardly ever to pulmonary infarction which would be a likely possibility in the adult; the trachea is much more mobile in children than in adults and tracheal deviation does not have the same significance in younger patients; measurements of the position of the apex beat from the midline which are suitable for adults, are inapplicable to children; rigors are rare in childhood and febrile convulsions common, whereas the reverse is true in older patients.

## Age Periods

It is convenient to divide the period of infancy and childhood into certain age periods:

N

| Infancy | First year of life |
| Neonatal period | First month of life |
| Childhood | 1–15 years |
| Pre-school child | 1–5 years |
| School child | 5–15 years. |

## THE HISTORY

The history of disease in childhood is seldom obtained direct from the patient but usually through an intermediary, commonly the parent. This does not mean that the child should be ignored as a source of information. While infants and young children clearly can give little or no history, the older child may give a very accurate account of his symptoms and will usually answer simple questions accurately and without bias. Where appropriate, a supplementary history should be obtained from him. The examiner will also have to decide whether the history from the parents should be taken in the presence of the child or in his absence. The wishes of the parent, the age of the child and the nature of his complaint will determine this.

That so much of the history of childhood illness has to be obtained through a second party creates certain problems. The parent may seek to place his own interpretation on symptoms and signs rather than to describe these precisely as they occur. Further, the parent may fail to realise the misinterpretation which children may put on words. For example, a young child may generalise from past experience and use a phrase such as 'sore tummy' to describe any pain or discomfort anywhere, but the parents may not appreciate this. Only careful questioning on the part of the examiner, a shrewd appreciation on his part of the degree of insight which the parents have into their child's symptoms, and experience, will enable these difficult differentiations to be made. Further problems may be created by previous medical advice. The doctor who feels that he must suggest a specific diagnosis even when this is not possible may be storing up trouble for the future. If in the presence of a unexplained fever—a common situation in childhood—he frequently attaches the convenient but erroneous label 'tonsillitis', the parents may be inclined to attribute all other pyrexias to the tonsils and may recount a long list of attacks of 'tonsillitis' which on closer questioning and examination are unsupported by any real evidence of pain in the throat, tonsillar inflammation or tonsillar gland enlargement. Such parents, presenting with the confident assertion that, 'It is his tonsils, Doctor', may themselves be deceived and may mislead the examiner unless he is aware of such pitfalls.

### History of Present Illness

There are two main aspects of history-taking. In the first place the parent or parents should be encouraged to give a spontaneous account of the child's illness subject only to such curbs on irrelevancy or verbosity as the examiner deems expedient. Secondly, there are specific questions from the examiner designed to amplify and clarify the parents' description. These may include the following:

**Age and Sex.** Date of birth and sex should be ascertained.

**The Symptoms or Abnormalities complained of, and their Duration.** These may require clarification and more precise definition.

**The Precise Order of Symptoms.** This should include current symptoms and also the order of events in repeated episodes, as in asthma or epilepsy.

**Changes noted since the Onset of the Illness.** This question is designed to bring out the main presenting aspects of the child's illness by contrasting his present condition with that prior to the onset of symptoms.

**Activity or Apathy.** These may be gauged by the child's performance in normal household activities and in play, his willingness to walk to school or to the shops and his interest in people and things. Is he active in the house or does he tend to sit or lie about? Does he tire easily or not? Does he return early from play?

**Feeding and Appetite.** Determine whether the appetite is temporarily or persistently impaired, and if necessary calculate the caloric intake. With babies an accurate account of the total daily intake of milk (number of scoops of dried milk powder or volume of cow's milk or evaporated milk) can usually be obtained. With older children where there is a complaint of poor appetite enquiry should be made about the type and amount of food actually taken per day. Enquiries should of course include the amount of liquid food taken. A child, whose mother states that he eats nothing, may be drinking two pints of milk per day and almost completely satisfying his caloric needs from this source alone.

Food fads and dislikes on the part of the child or any unusual ideas regarding diet on the part of the parents should be enquired into, as should the intake of vitamin supplements such as cod liver oil, orange juice, rose hip syrup and proprietary preparations.

**Difficulty in Swallowing.** This is more likely to be functional than organic in children. The most common cause is over-persuasion of a child to eat against his will, resulting in choking and gagging. Organic dysphagia may occur rarely.

**Thirst.** Where there is any suggestion of thirst an attempt should be made to obtain a quantitative estimation of the total daily intake of fluid.

**Vomiting.** If vomiting has occurred, the amount, frequency and duration should be ascertained. Is it effortless, forceful or projectile? Is there any associated pain or screaming as in appendicitis or intussusception? Is the vomiting accompanied by diarrhoea as in gastro-enteritis, or by constipation as in intestinal obstruction or pyloric stenosis? What is the nature of the vomitus, and is it stained with bile or blood? If the patient is a baby, does he make any unusual movements with his mouth prior to vomiting (as with rumination)? Is there any abdominal distension? Has the child been fevered?

**Abdominal Pain.** What is the evidence that abdominal pain is or has been present? Enquire about the nature and timing of the pain. Does it interfere with ordinary activity? What is its duration? Is it constant or intermittent? Is is precisely located or is it of a general character? Does it radiate? Is the pain aggravated by breathing or by movement? Is there any relationship to bowel movement or to micturition? Is there any associated diarrhoea, melaena, constipation or vomiting? Sore throat may be associated with mesenteric adenitis, cough with pneumonia or purpura with the abdominal lesion of anaphylactoid purpura. Is appetite affected?

**Abdominal distension.** Grosser degrees of this will be evident to parents. Intermittent distension may be reported (e.g. due to congenital bands). The degree of distension and any associated symptoms should be enquired into.

**State of Bowels and Character of Stools.** The neonatal stool is semi-solid and mustard-coloured and several are passed per day. The frequency of bowel movement should be routinely ascertained in terms of number of stools per day and enquiry should be made into any involuntary faecal soiling (encopresis) or any unusual reactions to defaecation such as reluctance to allow the bowels to move or crying during the act (as in anal fissure). Questions should be asked about the character of the stools—are they hard or soft, watery, accompanied by mucus, blood-streaked or mixed with blood, bulky, normal in colour or dark or pale, floating on water or not, or malodorous?

**Loss or Gain in Weight.** Few mothers are aware of the exact weight changes of their children. They will be able to say whether a child has appeared fatter or thinner, whether his clothing has become too tight or too slack recently, whether his limbs have wasted or have become swollen, whether his eyes have become sunken or his face puffy, and whether these processes have been of sudden or gradual onset. Thus will genuine weight loss or obesity or oedema become evident.

**Discharge from Eyes, Ears, Nose or other Sites.** Enquire about the duration and note the character of the discharge, e.g. purulent, watery or blood-stained, profuse or scanty, continuous or intermittent.

**Sore Throat.** This is likely to be a symptom only in older children. Younger children may have obviously painful lesions in the throat and yet make little in the way of localising complaint.

**Cough.** This is one of the most common symptoms in childhood. For how long has the cough lasted? Is the cough 'dry' as in the early stage of pneumonia or bronchitis, or 'moist' as in the later stage of these diseases? Does it occur in paroxysms? Is it more severe by day or by night or is it continuous? Does it disturb sleep? Is there a whoop or accompanying vomiting? If there is sputum does the child swallow this or expectorate it and what is the character of the sputum—watery, mucoid, mucopurulent or blood-stained? Is there any pain on coughing as in pleurisy, or associated dyspnoea as in asthma or severe respiratory infection? Is there any associated nasal discharge or obstruction as in chronic sinus infection or gross adenoidal hypertrophy?

**Breathlesssness.** If present, does this occur on exertion only or also at rest? Is it persistent as in some types of congenital heart disease or intermittent as in asthma? If intermittent, do attacks come on gradually or suddenly? Is breathlessness worse at night? Is breathing noisy or not? Is there any breath-holding? Is there any associated cyanosis or cough? Ascertain degree of breathlessness and the amount of exertion of which the child is capable.

**Mouth Breathing and Stridor.** Does the child sleep with his mouth open or shut? Does he make a crowing noise when breathing, indicating stridor? What is the duration of the stridor? Is it associated with other symptoms such as dyspnoea or cough?

**Wheeze.** Does this occur or not? Is the onset sudden or gradual, at night or by day? Does any particular factor or group of circumstances precipitate attacks of wheezing? Does the child tend to put things in his mouth (and therefore run a greater risk of aspirating a foreign body into a bronchus)?

**Abnormalities of the Breath.** Has the breath been abnormal, e.g. due to acetone, or to foetor in certain mouth infections?

**Localised Swellings.** Site, size (including variations in size), shape and consistency as noted by the parents should be recorded, as should the presence of local pain or tenderness on palpation, mobility or adherence to underlying structures.

**Rashes or other Skin Lesions.** At what site did the rash occur? What was its appearance, e.g. colour, size of lesions, number of lesions, raised or not, vesicular, duration? Was the rash itchy? In the case of ulcers, site, size and duration should be known.

**Jaundice.** Note time of onset and whether intermittent, static, diminishing or increasing. Has any paleness of the stools or darkness of the urine been noted? Have there been any accompanying symptoms such as vomiting or hepatic tenderness?

**Cyanosis.** Blueness of the lips and shadows under the eyes are frequently described by mothers where no significant disease is present. Enquiry should be directed to determine the distribution of the blueness, e.g. extremities only or generalised, and the circumstances in which it occurs, e.g. in response to cold, exercise or respiratory infection.

**Pallor.** Many healthy children are pale, but pallor tends to cause anxiety in mothers. Is the pallor intermittent or permanent? Intermittent pallor, for instance that commonly seen in a sleeping infant or in a child exposed to cold, will be much less significant than persistent pallor.

**State of the Musculature.** In infancy this is most likely to be appreciated by the mother's experience on handling the child. Hypotonicity is likely to be revealed by the fact that he is 'floppy' and tends to slip through his mother's hands when lifting him or bathing him, hypertonicity by the fact that she feels that his limbs are rather stiff. With older children the development of muscle weakness will show itself by inability to perform activities which were previously possible, such as walking up stairs.

**Changes in Posture or in Walk.** Does the child hold his head or trunk in any unusual way (e.g. torticollis or scoliosis)? Has there been any change in the manner in which he walks or in the manner in which he rises from the sitting position (e.g. the broad based unsteady gait of cerebellar ataxia or the 'climbing up the legs' method of rising in muscular dystrophy)?

**Co-ordination of Movement.** Has he been dropping things or spilling fluid from cups? Can he perform fine movements such as writing and buttoning clothing? Has there been any change in his speech? These questions may be important, for instance in differentiating chorea from a tic.

**Involuntary Movements.** Obtain a full description of the nature of the movement. Is the same movement repeated or is there a series of movements? Has the child suffered any injury as a result of the movements? Does emotional stress aggravate them?

**Convulsions.** Obtain a full description, including the state of the child prior to the convulsion, and apparent precipitating factor (such as pyrexia), any premonitory symptoms, the types of movement observed and the duration of various stages. Was there any localised twitching? Was the child unconscious? Did he fall down? Was he incontinent? Did he bite his tongue or damage himself in any way? Was he pale or blue during the convulsive attack? Was there any associated pyrexia? Did he fall asleep? Was he disorientated afterwards or did he continue with his previous activities?

**Defects in Vision.** In a baby we are concerned with a gross assessment, (e.g. does he follow moving objects with his eyes?) and in older children with selective visual changes. Can he read print? Does he have any difficulty in reading the blackboard at school?

**Headache.** Young children seldom complain of headache. With older children the site of the headache, manner of onset, duration, severity (e.g. does he have to leave the school class or stop play) and accompanying symptoms such as vomiting, are relevant.

**Hearing.** With a baby, does he respond to various noises such as his mother's voice; with an older child is there any apparent inability to understand the spoken word, or to hear common noises such as the door bell?

**Dysuria.** Enquiries should be directed to ascertain whether any pain which might be dysuria is in fact related to micturition.

**Frequency of Micturition.** Enquire about frequency both by day and night.

**Bed Wetting and Incontinence.** Have these symptoms always been present or developed recently? How frequently does the bed wetting incontinence occur? Are the symptoms diurnal or nocturnal or both? Is he passing more urine than normal? Are there any circumstances which aggravate the symptoms or alleviate them? Is there an associated dysuria or frequency of micturition or thirst? What is the parent's reaction to the child's symptoms?

**Volume of Urine.** In the presence of frequency of micturition or incontinence the mother may have gained an exaggerated impression of the amount of urine passed per day but statements of an excessive or a diminished output of urine should be carefully assessed.

**Character of Urine.** What is the colour—amber, red, smoky, 'like tea', etc.? Bacterial decomposition of urine in napkins gives an ammoniacal odour.

**Behaviour and Mood.** It may be more appropriate to question a mother alone about her child's behaviour in the home, in school, or in play with other children. She may describe disobedience, negativeness, aggressiveness, reluctance to go to school, withdrawal from company and from social activities, inability to go to sleep, fear of the dark, nightmares and night terrors, abnormal jealousies, increased tendency to show emotional disturbance in the face of difficulty, nail biting and thumb sucking. The child's natural disposition should be ascertained, whether carefree or anxious, fastidious or careless, 'highly strung' or placid, volatile or stolid. An account of the child's relationship with his parents, with his siblings and with other children may be revealing as may his reaction to school and his relationship with his teachers.

**Treatment already given.** Any treatment already given to the child for his present illness should be noted even though the mother may not know its precise nature.

**Selectivity of Questioning.** Not all of the questions indicated above will be asked in every instance. Some are secondary and dependent on a positive answer to a primary question, while others will be irrelevant to the current symptoms. It is always better to ask too many rather than too few questions as a wide interrogation may uncover aspects of an illness which the parent may not have mentioned because they were considered irrelevant or had been forgotten.

### Previous History

**History of the Birth.** The manner of birth may have a profound effect on an infant's subsequent health and development. A history of the birth should thus be obtained for all infants and most children presenting for examination, and in certain types of disease such as cerebral palsy, mental retardation or epilepsy this will be of particular importance.

Enquiry should be directed to any illness or accident from which the mother suffered during pregnancy. She should be asked about drugs taken or exposure to radiation. Memory for events early in pregnancy is likely to be less accurate than that for later pregnancy, yet the profound effect which certain disorders such as rubella may have in early pregnancy makes enquiry into events at this time important.

Although the mother's knowledge of the duration of her labour, of the presentation of the foetus, of the type of delivery (e.g. forceps) and of any difficulties during delivery may be incomplete, an adequate account of these facts may be relevant and important. It may be necessary to obtain precise information from those who were responsible for the delivery.

Most mothers are aware of their children's birth weights—fathers can very seldom supply this information. The birth weight, the length of the period of gestation and the place of delivery should always be recorded.

Information should also be sought about the neonatal period. How long after birth was respiration established? Did the child suffer from convulsions, breathing difficulties, blueness, jaundice, vomiting or any other abnormality?

**Feeding.** A history of past feeding can be most conveniently combined with the present history as discussed above. In infancy we are concerned with such matters as difficulty in the establishment of feeding in the neonatal period, the duration of breast feeding, the type of artificial feeding, and the composition, volume and frequency of the feeds. With older children information on diet, on the past state of the appetite and on the amount of vitamin supplements taken should be recorded. Attention should be paid to any peculiar dietary habits.

**Previous Illnesses.** Previous illnesses and operations should be recorded together with their date of occurrence, duration and severity. The mother may require some time to recollect the necessary information.

**Contact with Infectious Illness.** Questions should be asked about infectious illness in other members of the family and in playmates. In such enquiries the symptoms of the more common infectious illnesses (e.g. rash, diarrhoea, spasmodic cough, jaundice) may have to be specified. Threadworms often have a familial distribution. A knowledge of contact with animals may be relevant, e.g. in the presence of lymphadenopathy due to toxoplasmosis.

**Age of Control of Bladder and Bowels.** At what age did the child become dry by day and at night? When did he gain control of his bowels? Does the mother have any strong views about 'pot training'?

**Residence Abroad.** A history of periods of residence abroad may indicate the need to consider the possibility of diseases which do not occur in this country.

**Immunisation.** Any prophylactic inoculations or vaccinations which the child has received should be recorded, including their approximate dates.

## Family History

The ages, present state of health, past health and possible consanguinity of the parents should be ascertained. The ages and sexes of other children in the family (and thus the position of the patient in the family), the occurrence of any stillbirths or miscarriages and past and present illnesses of siblings should also be noted. If any child in the family has died, the age at death and cause of death should be ascertained. Is there anything to suggest child abuse? Illnesses in the parents or in other relatives living with the family should be recorded. With certain disorders (e.g. allergic disorders, bleeding diseases or mental disorder) specific enquiries may require to be made about a much wider circle of relatives than the patient's immediate family. In the case of an adopted child, any available medical history about the natural parents should be noted.

### Social and Environmental History

The occupation of the father and of the mother if she works, the financial status of the family, the attitude of the parents to each other, divorce or separation of the parents, and the attitude of the parents to their children and to their parental responsibilities are all important.

Many disorders in childhood have a psychological basis. In understanding such disorders history is of paramount importance. For example, in tics, changes in behaviour and mood, enuresis, encopresis, cyclical vomiting, migraine and emotional disturbances the most rewarding investigation may well be the unravelling of the psychological interrelationships of the patient with the members of his family, his friends and his personal contacts in school and at play. An appreciation of the stresses which his environment, both at home and school, imposes on him, and of his intelligence, particularly as it affects his ability to meet the demands of education will also be relevant. A great variety of social and environmental factors may cause psychological disturbance in childhood but there are certain provoking situations which recur—a new baby in the home, the death of an immediate relative, absence of one or other parent from the home, first attendance at school, a change of school class or a new teacher, change of residence to another district with loss of playmates, bullying at school, scholastic difficulties, too rigid enforcement by parents or others of a desired pattern of behaviour.

Enquiries should also be made about the size and conditions of the home, including the number of occupants and about any special environmental circumstances of possible physical or psychological significance.

## PHYSICAL EXAMINATION

The examination of infants and children is an art demanding qualities of understanding, sympathy and patience, and at times finesse and subtlety. The paediatric patient who enters the consulting-room or who is ill in bed may be a bawling infant whom nothing will pacify, a toddler clinging to his mother and burying his tearful face in her lap at the slightest movement of the examiner towards him, a more robust young man of early school age who stoutly and persistently resists all attempts to remove his clothing particularly his trousers, a mentally retarded hyperactive child who moves rapidly round the room deploying his destructive interest against the inkwell, the torch or the examiner's glasses, or an apprehensive schoolgirl who just retains her self-control during questioning but recoils in terror at the production of a sphygmomanometer or an ophthalmoscope. In contrast there are many children who exhibit exemplary co-operation and self-control. Experience, practice and understanding of children enable much to be done to overcome difficulties. The examiner must not be too conscious of his own dignity; impatience or irascibility on his part is only likely to close the door to much of the information which might otherwise be available to him. As he outwardly manifests friendliness, sociability, tolerance and, if necessary, good-natured playfulness or great restraint, he must all the time be noting, observing, appreciating and taking advantage of every opportunity to obtain further information.

It would be impossible to describe an all-embracing technique to meet the manifold problems of approach which occur in the clinical examination of children; a few suggestions will suffice. During the history-taking the examiner should be able to gauge the type of child with whom he is dealing and to judge his approach accordingly. He may have to decide whether he should examine the child on the mother's knee or an examination couch. Although it is highly desirable to remove the child's clothing for an adequate physical examination, this may require to be done in a piecemeal or regional way in certain instances. The examiner must remain patient and confident, even if sorely provoked. He should allay the concern which mothers commonly experience that a fractious child's behaviour is annoying him or is in any way outside his normal experience. Loud noises tend to alarm children. A soft persuasive voice is much more likely to be effective than stentorian exhortations. With active noisy babies and toddlers, gentle stroking of the skin with one finger may result in a brief cessation of movement and of noise. The examiner should attune his attitude and conversation to the level of his patient's understanding. A great deal of examination and manipulation can be carried out without the child being very aware of it if his attention is held, and to achieve this the examiner may well have to appear to identify his interest with an appropriate current interest of the child—a rattle, a torch, a teddy bear, the recent exploits of a favourite space-man, or the current fashions in the dressing of dolls. With older children, simple explanations about the various aspects of an examination should be given. Although the examiner may have in his mind an established routine of examination, he must be prepared to depart from this as circumstances demand. Procedures which tend to frighten children, such as examining the throat or taking the blood pressure, can usually with advantage be carried out at the end of the examination.

## General Inspection

The examiner's assessment of a child from both physical and mental aspects begins from the moment of first meeting. Much may be learned from the child's appearance, his demeanour, his reaction to his environment and to the examiner, his relationship to his parents, any sounds he utters or even smells which may accompany him.

The general inspection will give information on his size relative to age, his state of nutrition including obesity or wasting, his state of activity whether increased or decreased, his posture and bodily habitus whether upright or recumbent or associated with torticollis, short neck, head retraction or scoliosis, and obvious deformities. Major external injuries and haemorrhage will be evident.

The facial expression may reveal pain or anxiety, the blankness of mental retardation or the spasmodic localised movement of the tic. It may show evidence of weight loss, dehydration or oedema or it may be characterised by the features of mongolism, cretinism or gargoylism. Enlarged adenoids and nasal obstruction may be deduced from mouth breathing. Pallor, cyanosis or jaundice may be observed.

Any rash should be observed and its character inspected. Light touch will determine whether the rash is raised or not. An erythematous rash, blanching on pressure, can be differentiated from a purpuric rash, recognised by its colour and by its failure to blanch. Petechiae can be differentiated from larger macules, macules from papules, papules from vesicles. The content of any vesicles, whether serum, pus or blood, should be observed. The distribution of a rash will be noted, for example flexural in eczema, centripetal in chicken-pox, at the periphery of the limbs, especially the lower, in anaphylactoid purpura and interdigital in scabies. Scratch marks will indicate whether the skin is itchy or not. A characteristic rash such as that of measles may provide an immediate clue to diagnosis. A rash such as that of erythema nodosum may suggest several diagnoses. There may be other abnormalities of the skin; ulceration; evidence of septic infection such as pustules, boils or impetigo; abnormal formation, as in the dry scaling of ichthyosis or the papery appearance of the neonatal placental insufficiency syndrome; angiomata; pigmentation. Sweating may be prominent. The dry skin and loose skin folds of dehydration may be evident, the skin remaining in folds when plucked up and not flattening immediately as it does in the normal elastic state of the skin in health. The shiny tenseness and pitting on pressure of oedema may be noted. There may be visible external swellings.

A first glance will reveal much of the patient's level of consciousness, whether he is fully conscious, semi-conscious or unconscious. A few moments' observation may tell much about a child's psychological make-up and intelligence—whether he is nervous, excitable, distractible, withdrawn, intelligent or stupid, and about difficult emotional relationships with his parents.

Disturbances of respiration rate and pattern and abnormal respiratory effort may be visible. Abnormal sounds such as a high-pitched cry, cough, wheeze, stridor or whoop may be heard. Body odours may reveal lack of cleanliness; the breath may smell of acetone; to those with an acute sense of smell a mousey odour may suggest phenylketonuria. In older children bodily form, character of the voice and manner may differentiate between states of pre-pubescence, pubescence and adolescence.

Much may be learned from an adequate general inspection. It is unwise to rush this or curtail it in the premature pursuit of more direct methods of examination, such as palpation, auscultation and instrumental examination. It is probably true to say that with children a much higher proportion show no abnormality on application of these procedures than with adults. The frequent paucity of specific localised physical signs in the child as compared with the adult results in a relatively greater contribution to diagnosis being made in the former by the history and general inspection.

PHYSICAL MEASUREMENTS

**Weight.** The most useful single measurements of physical development in infancy and childhood are weight and height. A comparison between actual and expected weight should be routine in any examination. Expected weight according to age can be calculated in a number of rough and ready ways or may be more accurately determined from tables. In the early weeks of life the average infant should gain approximately one ounce or 25 g per day after the tenth day, at which time the birth weight should have been regained. Thus at six weeks the expected gain in weight would be 2 lb or almost 1 kg. By five months of age the birth weight should have doubled and by a year should have trebled. For the next few years the expected weight can be calculated approximately from the formulae—age in years plus three, multiplied by five for pounds, and age in years plus four multiplied by two for kilogrammes. A table of average weights for infants and children from birth to 15 years (Table 4) is given in the Appendix (p. 459). In using it, it should be remembered that the average is not necessarily the normal for any individual. The normal weight for a child of small parents may be well below the average and an average weight for another child, with parents of large stature, may be below normal. Thus weight in the individual child must be interpreted against a number of background factors. Changes in weight of the individual child have a more specific significance.

**Length.** Length is the other valuable parameter of growth. It can be measured as standing height in toddlers and older children and as crown-heel length in infants who are recumbent. Table 4 (Appendix, p. 459) gives average heights from birth to 15 years. In regard to length the same considerations concerning 'normal' and 'average' apply as with weight.

Under certain circumstances a crown-rump length or sitting height (stem length) may be of value for comparison with crown-heel length or standing height, for example in achondroplasia where there is shortening of the limbs. In the recumbent position (e.g. in the infant) the crown-rump length is measured from the top of the head to a board placed against the extremity of the buttocks with the thighs at right angles to the trunk and the knees flexed. A table of crown-rump lengths (Table 5) will be found in the Appendix (p. 460). After the age of three years sitting height is usually measured.

A correlation normally exists between height and weight. A knowledge of the expected weight for any particular height and an appreciation of any dissociation between these measurements may be of value. In hypothyroidism, for instance, height may be reduced and weight normal, in Marfan's syndrome height increased and weight normal. In a wasting disorder height may be normal and weight reduced, in obesity height normal and weight increased. A correlation of these parameters can be made from tables or from charts such as those shown in the Appendix (pp. 462, 463), where the normal ranges for expected height and weight at different ages are charted. Such charts have as their primary function the recording of serial estimations of weight and height.

**Head Size.** Head size both above and below normal may have considerable significance in respect of childhood disease. Average occipito-frontal head circumferences for different ages with the measuring tape placed round the maximal occipito-frontal circumference are given on page 461.

**Temperature.** In the presence of any constitutional upset one of the most common instrumental observations made either in the home or in the hospitals is that of temperature. For most purposes skin temperature is adequate, but the site selected should not have been unnaturally cooled by exposure or heated by any artificial means. In infants the groin is probably the best site with the thigh held flexed on to the abdomen; in older children the axilla is more suitable. Some prefer the rectal temperature in infants. Where the temperature does not record on a standard clinical thermometer, as for instance in so-called neonatal cold injury, special low-reading thermometers covering the range from 30° to 43°C should be used routinely. The accepted dividing-line between normal and abnormal temperatures, namely 37°C, is appropriate for infants and children where a skin temperature is taken. The normal rectal temperature would be higher by about 0·25°C. Somewhat lower temperatures are normal in premature infants.

### Examination of Individual Regions and Systems

We can now turn to the examination of individual systems. It is easiest to consider these in sequence but it is not always possible to examine them in this way. Certain children, particularly younger ones, tire easily during an examination and it may be expedient for the examiner to begin in such cases with the system which is likely to yield the most valuable information. Thus it may be advisable to auscultate the heart before a child becomes fractious and cries. On the other hand it may be necessary with a child who cries initially to delay cardiac auscultation until he is quiet. The examiner must remain flexible in his approach and exploit any advantageous opportunities as they arise.

### HEAD AND NECK

**Cranium.** Observe the size and the shape, e.g. brachycephaly, scaphocephaly, plagiocephaly, oxycephaly, microcephaly or hydrocephalus (Fig.

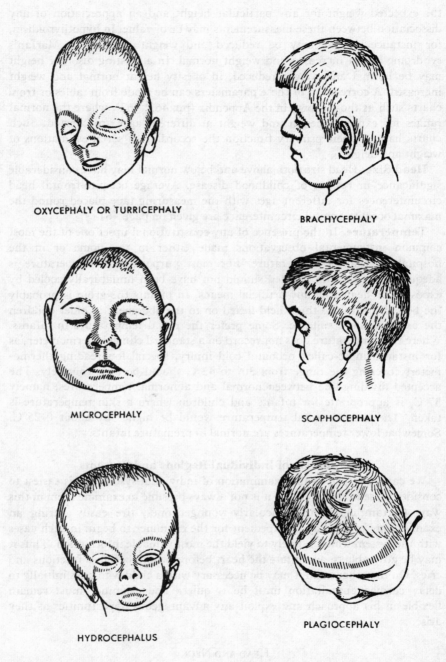

OXYCEPHALY OR TURRICEPHALY

BRACHYCEPHALY

MICROCEPHALY

SCAPHOCEPHALY

HYDROCEPHALUS

PLAGIOCEPHALY

FIG. 114   The Cranium as a Diagnostic Aid. (The disorders associated with these changes are discussed on p. 385.)

114). Head shape and size may have special associations with certain developmental disorders and disease processes, e.g. brachycephaly with Down's syndrome; plagiocephaly with prematurity; microcephaly with mental retardation; scaphocephaly and oxycephaly with craniostenosis; hydrocephalus with spina bifida. Measure the occipito-frontal head circumference. Note the amount, colour and consistency of the hair. A lowered hair line posteriorly may a feature of such diseases as the Klippel-Feil syndrome and Turner's syndrome. Fair hair, blue eyes and a 'mousy' odour may accompany phenylketonuria (p. 436).

The *fontanelles* are peculiar to the period of infancy and the anterior fontanelle in particular may provide information of the greatest value. The posterior fontanelle normally measures not more than 0·5 cm wide at birth. This fontanelle closes shortly after birth. Its persistence beyond this time or an increase in its size beyond normal may indicate increased intracranial tension or an abnormality of the cranial bones. The anterior fontanelle normally measures approximately 2·5 cm by 2·5 cm at birth and does not close until 18 months. Delay in closure beyond 18 months may be another pointer to diseases such as rickets, increased intracranial tension or abnormal development of cranial bones. Early closure may occur in premature synostosis. Fontanelle tension should be assessed at the same time as fontanelle size. Increased tension in the fontanelle can be detected chiefly by palpation, but also in some instances by the observation of bulging. Decreased tension with a sunken fontanelle—as in dehydration—is likely to be visible and palpable. An abnormally large fontanelle under increased tension and a large head may be associated with long-standing increased intracranial pressure and an enlarging head as in hydrocephalus. Increased fontanelle tension without significant increase in head size is likely to indicate an acute process such as meningitis or intracranial haemorrhage.

In conjunction with increased fontanelle tension the cranial *sutures* may be abnormally wide. At birth the main sutures such as the sagittal and coronal are easily palpable but the bone edges are not widely separated. In cranial synostosis the sutures may be prominent ridges prematurely fused.

Alteration in the consistence of the *cranial bones* is seen most commonly in infancy in, for instance, prematurity or rickets. The phenomenon of *craniotabes* is detected by placing the infant's head, face towards the examiner, between the examiner's hands and exerting pressure over the parieto-occipital region with the tips of the fingers. 'Give' in the bone, such as would be experienced on pressure on a table-tennis ball, indicates craniotabes. Palpation of the skull will also reveal other *structural defects* in cranial bones, bony swellings or local tenderness, e.g. over the mastoid process.

*Cranial bruits* may be audible on auscultation with a stethoscope over the vertex of the skull, the occiput or the temporal region in for instance arterio-venous malformations or the severe type of idiopathic hypercalcaemia.

**Ears.** The external auricle may be congenitally deformed as an isolated lesion or in conjunction with congenital abnormalities in other sites, such as the renal tract. Low-set ears, abnormal formation and size of the external auricle or deformity of the external meatus may be found (Plate V).

*Infection* in the ears is common in childhood and auriscopic examination is an important procedure. The speculum used should be appropriate to the size of the patient. Wax or purulent discharge in the external auditory canal should be noted and also any other obstruction such as a boil. Further inspection may not be possible until wax has been removed by a loop, or discharge by dry mopping with cotton-wool (e.g. on an orange stick). The drum should be examined for colour, bulging, retraction and perforation. It will appear dusky and injected in the presence of acute infection and there may be some distortion of the cone of light normally extending forward from the tip of the handle of the malleus. A bulging drum appears to be displaced towards the examiner and the light reflex is usually lost. With retraction the malleus is unduly prominent. Perforations may occur in any part of the drum but are most likely to be present in the upper part. They may be of pin-hole size or large, involving almost all of the drum.

**Face.** The face may reflect many aspects of disease. The expression may indicate the emotional state of the child and reveal something of his psychological make-up. Facial tics may be evident. A specific diagnosis such as cretinism, Down's syndrome (mongolism) or gargoylism may be obvious at once (Plate V). Many other features may be of diagnostic value—the shape of the forehead, whether prominent as in certain types of cranial dysostosis, narrowed and receding as in microcephaly, or bossed as in rickets; the position of the eyes, especially an increased distance between them (hypertelorism) as in some types of mental retardation; the shape and angle of the palpebral fissure and the presence of prominent epicanthic folds as in mongolism or the Treacher Collins syndrome. Any periorbital oedema or haemorrhage will be noted. The colouring of the conjunctival mucous membrane will give an approximate measure of the haemoglobin level. Examination of the eyeballs will reveal any undue prominence or depression; obvious squint; conjunctivitis; conjunctival icterus or conjunctival haemorrhage; congenital defects of the iris (colobomata); abnormal pigmentation or the presence of Brushfield's spots (small whitish inclusions scattered round the iris having the appearance of grains of salt—seen in mongolism); opacities in the cornea, lens, or intra-ocular chambers.

The use of the ophthalmoscope is dealt with elsewhere (p. 412). The difficulties of ophthalmoscopic examination in children are often considerable. To maintain the young child's gaze in a fixed direction it is usually necessary for a second person to arrange some diversion which for the child has an element of expectancy about it. The examiner, after positioning himself and the patient appropriately, may say, 'Tell me when the torch flashes', the torch being held in an appropriate position by a helper who may

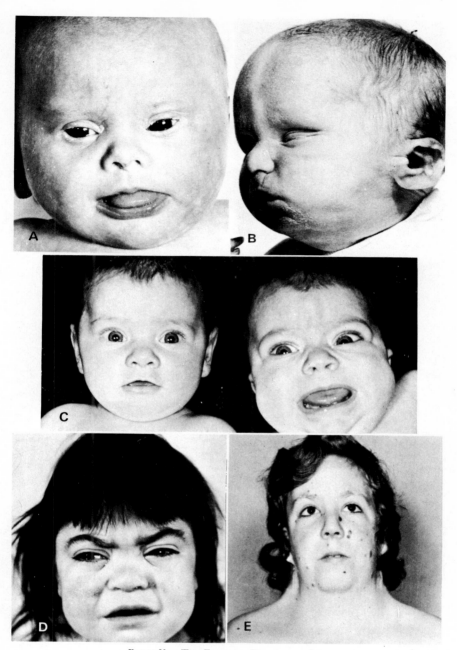

PLATE V. THE FACE AS A DIAGNOSTIC AID

A, Down's syndrome. Note palpebral fissures sloping laterally upwards and prominent protruding tongue associated with small oral cavity. B, Renal agenesis. Note small jaw, flattened nose, low set ears. C, Cretin with normal twin. Note large tongue, coarse features, bloated cheeks and double chin due to myxoedematous change. D, Gargoyle. Note wide nose with depressed bridge, prominent supraorbital ridges and eyebrows. E, Webbing of neck in Turner's syndrome. Pigmented naevi also present.

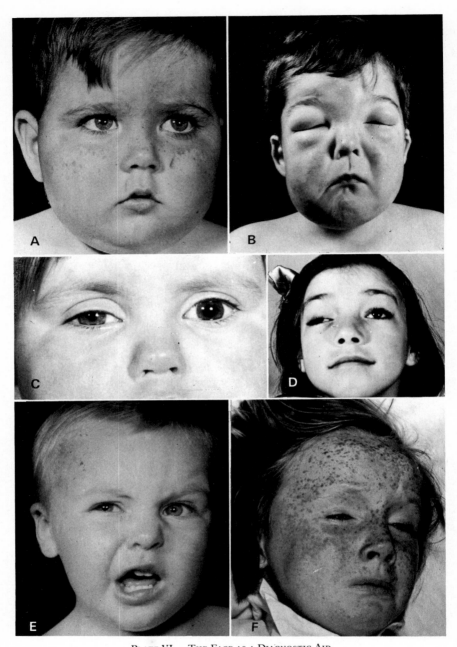

PLATE VI.   THE FACE AS A DIAGNOSTIC AID

A, Mooning of the face induced by corticosteroid therapy. B, Facial oedema in the nephrotic syndrome with peri-orbital involvement almost preventing opening of the eyes. (Photo by courtesy of Professor Gavin Arneil.) C, Right-sided Horner's syndrome – smallness of pupil (meiosis) enophthalmos and a narrow palpebral fissure. D, Ptosis (more marked on right side) in myasthenia gravis. E, Left-sided facial palsy. F, Risus sardonicus in tetanus; marked freckling of skin.

be mother or nurse, or 'Tell me how many fingers nurse has up—how many now?,' the nurse at the change of question changing the number of fingers and thus maintaining the child's attention while the examiner continues with his ophthalmoscopic examination. With younger children sedation (e.g. with quinal-barbitone) may be necessary and in certain circumstances even a general anaesthetic may be required. Dilatation of the pupil with Mydrilate (p. 413) may be necessary, for example with babies in whom the examiner has to carry out ophthalmoscopy without the co-operation of the patient and often while manually retracting the eyelids. To do this an assistant is usually necessary. Ophthalmoscopic examination will reveal opacities of the media and gross refractive errors. In the retina abnormal venous engorgement, haemorrhage, exudate, abnormal pigmentation, cherry-red spots (as in amaurotic family idiocy) and choroidal tubercles may be seen. The optic discs may show blurring of the margins, papilloedema or abnormal colouration.

The shape of the *nose* may be significant. It may for instance indicate racial origins or reveal the sunken bridge of gargoylism or the flattened tip of renal agenesis (Plate V). Movement of the alae nasi may provide supportive evidence of increased respiratory effort. In the child with a chronic cough, asthma or mouth breathing, the patency of each nasal passage should be tested in turn by blocking the other. Foreign bodies may block nasal passages. Any nasal discharge should be noted along with its amount and character (i.e. watery, mucoid, purulent, haemorrhagic). The state of the nasal mucosa should be observed, e.g. pale or congested, watery or dry.

Observe the formation of the *lips*, the presence of swelling, as in angioneurotic oedema, pallor or cyanosis, and cracking or ulceration. Check on their functional usage as in whistling or blowing.

**Mouth.** A child may open his mouth voluntarily. Refusal is likely to be encouraged where there is too much display of shiny instruments and too obvious an indication of intent to use them. Most children will react more willingly to the request to, 'Let me see your teeth', than to, 'Open your mouth', or, 'Show me your throat'. The demonstration of the teeth is more likely to be a matter of some childhood pride. Where reasonable persuasion has failed to make the child open his mouth, it may be necessary to use physical force. This should always be a last resort as it breaks the confidence which may have been built up between the examiner and his patient and may make all subsequent examination very difficult.

With a willing child, examination of the mouth will reveal possible abnormalities in the state of the mucosa—hydration, colour, ulceration, purpura; the white curd-like lesions of thrush which do not readily scrape off and leave bleeding points when they do; Koplik's spots (p. 82) disorders of the gums; etc.

The *teeth* should be observed for number, whether of the primary or secondary dentition, size and shape, discolouration (e.g. yellow colour of the primary dentition of prematurely born children who have suffered from severe neonatal jaundice, or children whose mothers have been given tetra-cycline during pregnancy), caries and enamel defects. The time of eruption of the teeth may be of some value as an index of normal development (p. 461).

Any defects in the *palate* will also be evident. *Tongue* size (large in cretins), shape (long and thin in mongols) and surface character will be noted. The ease with which the tongue can be examined does not justify the over-importance which in the past was attached to its appearance as an indicator of health.

The *tonsils* should be observed for size (varying with age and maximal in size at the age of 7–8 years) injection, presence of exudate or pitting, and the peritonsillar region for swelling and inflammation. The posterior pharyngeal wall should be observed for inflammation, swelling, postnasal discharge and the presence of lymphoid tissue.

At this point, if not earlier, the examiner will probably require to introduce a spatula into the child's mouth in order to see the *throat* clearly. A few children in saying ,'Aah', will depress the tongue sufficiently to avoid the need for assisted depression. In the majority a spatula will have to be used. As the child says, 'Aah', the spatula should be placed on the back of the tongue. If the child continues to co-operate depression of the tongue will reveal the oropharynx. If he is tense or actively resistant he will arch the tongue and defy depression of it. It is at this point that the examiner puts the gag reflex to use. By advancing the spatula to touch the posterior wall of the pharynx gagging will be induced, the posterior part of the tongue will be actively depressed and the throat exposed. The exposure is short lived and the examiner must take every advantage of it. One gag should usually be enough, as repetition will upset the child.

The non-cooperative infant or child should be either seated on the knee of the assistant or laid on a couch. Movement of the arms should be prevented by wrapping him in a blanket. If held on the knee, one of the assistant's arms should be placed round the child's body to prevent movement of his arms and trunk, the other should be placed round his head, holding his forehead. If lying on a couch, the assistant should hold the child's head between two hands and the examiner should restrain movement of the child's arms. The examiner should introduce a wooden spatula between the teeth at the side of the mouth and advance it slowly by gentle levering towards the posterior pharynx. It is possible to do this even although the child is clenching his teeth. When the tip of the spatula reaches the posterior pharyngeal wall the child will open his mouth and gag. In this brief moment, unless the performance is to be repeated, the examiner will have to observe all the features of the mouth which have been mentioned above.

**Neck.** Inspection from the front and from the back will detect any shortening (as in certain cervical vertebral anomalies), webbing (as in Turner's syndrome, Plate V), or positional deformity such as torticollis or head retraction. Limitation of movement may involve extension, flexion, rotation or lateral movement. Limitation of flexion (neck stiffness or rigidity) may be an important sign indicative of meningeal irritation due to infection or haemorrhage. It can be tested passively with the patient lying supine on a couch, the examiner placing his hand behind the occiput and gently raising the head. The infant or child may then resist flexion and cry, or his whole trunk may be raised. Alternatively, the child while in the sitting position with his knees drawn up, may be asked to put his nose on his knee. Abnormal swellings such as enlarged cervical lymph nodes should be sought for in the anterior and posterior cervical triangles and over the occipital region. Cystic hygromata are soft and transilluminable, while abnormal thyroid swellings are confirmed by palpation and by observing movement with swallowing. A sternomastoid tumour is a hard nodule or swelling in the sternomastoid muscle seen in infancy. Branchial cleft remnants may also be found.

## LYMPH NODES

Enlargement of certain groups of lymph nodes, particularly those in the neck and groin is a common occurrence in childhood. Submental lymph nodes and those in the anterior and posterior cervical triangles should also be examined. Involvement of the axillary lymph nodes is more significant of generalised lymphadenopathy. In the palpation of these the arm should first be moved out at right angles to the trunk to allow adequate access of the fingers to the axilla, and with the fingers in position the arm should be returned to a position beside the trunk. Palpability of epitrochlear lymph nodes at the elbow is another indication of lymphadenopathy. Examination of lymph nodes will be closely associated with examination of the liver and spleen.

## RESPIRATORY SYSTEM

**Inspection.** In the baby a cross-section of the thorax is roughly circular as opposed to the older child and adult where it is elliptical. The circular shape no doubt confers structural strength to withstand the stresses and strains of delivery, but as a circle cannot be so easily expanded as an ellipse it imposes certain functional limitations. The infant thus has a rounded chest normally and is a diaphragmatic breather.

Acute over-inflation of an infant's chest, such as may occur in bronchiolitis, results in expansion of the upper half of the chest anteriorly giving it a distended or 'blown' look. In the older child the antero-posterior diameter should be less than the lateral diameter. Increase in the former relative to the latter is likely to be due to a long-standing respiratory disorder such as asthma. This will also cause an increase in chest circumference.

In children, chest expansion is best determined with a measuring tape at the nipple line. The child is instructed to breathe out fully and then to take a deep breath. Less than 4 cm ($1\frac{1}{2}$ in) expansion probably indicates impairment. Asymmetry of movement on expansion is best detected by observing chest movement during a full inspiration. The method depicted in Figure 32 is of little value in young children due to the pliability of the chest wall. Other deformities of the chest, either as a result of previous disease or developmental anomalies, may be evident in childhood such as pigeon chest, pectus excavatum or Harrison's sulcus (p. 172). Praecordial bulging may be visible as a result of cardiac enlargement; spindle-shaped thickening at the costo-chondral junctions (the rickety rosary) may be present with rickets; the 'dinner fork' deformity of the costochondral junctions may occur with scurvy.

Observation of the *respiration rate* is of great value in respiratory infection because of the paucity of other signs which may exist in acute respiratory infections in infants and children. Crying or struggling will disturb the true rate and observation must therefore be made with the infant or child at peace, not crying, struggling or feeding. The upper limit of normal of the respiratory rate at various ages is as follows:

| 0–2 years | 2–6 years | 6–10 years | Over 10 years |
|-----------|-----------|------------|---------------|
| 40/min.   | 30/min.   | 25/min.    | 20/min.       |

In addition to the respiratory rate, the *respiratory rhythm* may be disturbed. In the premature newborn infant respiration may be irregular both in time and in amplitude. A similar pattern may occur with asphyxia in the newborn period. With older children the normal relationship between the phases of respiration may be disturbed with the occurrence of respiratory inversion. Thus normally the order of events in respiration is, inspiration—expiration—pause. In respiratory inversion the sequence is, expiration—inspiration—pause. The mother may describe this as a 'catch' in the infant's breathing. It is seen particularly in children with pneumonia. Normally the inspiratory phase of respiration is longer than the expiratory phase. In certain diseases, particularly asthma, expiration is longer than inspiration. In the infant or child suffering from respiratory failure, periodic breathing (Cheynes-Stokes respiration, p. 174) may occur. This is seen most commonly in the neonatal period when respiratory failure is relatively much more common.

The greater mobility and pliability of the infant's thoracic cage make certain signs related to chest movements much more common and more significant at this age period. Any increased respiratory effort or any obstruction to the free flow of air in and out of the lungs is likely to reveal itself by intercostal indrawing and costal margin recession. These signs are frequently found in common respiratory diseases such as bronchitis and pneumonia.

There may be abnormal sounds associated with disordered respiratory function. Stridor may be present, with laryngeal or tracheal obstruction. In lesser degrees this will be inspiratory only, but in more severe degrees both inspiratory and expiratory. With respiratory infection, respirations may be grunting in character and with certain metabolic disturbances, e.g. acidosis, hissing. Wheeze indicates the presence of airway obstruction of the smaller airways, such as occurs in asthma. It may give audible evidence of prolongation of the expiratory phase of respiration.

**Palpation.** Palpation of the chest with the flat of the hand may reveal palpable rhonchi or local tenderness or the crepitant sensation of subcutaneous emphysema. It will also reveal the position of the apex beat which is normally felt in the fourth or fifth intercostal space just within the mid-clavicular line. Due to its normal mobility and ready displacement with changes of body posture, deviation of the trachea is not of great value in the infant and toddler as an indication of mediastinal displacement.

**Percussion.** The thinner chest wall of the infant and child usually makes the percussion note in younger patients somewhat more resonant than in adults. Percussion should be lighter, particularly in infants. Alterations of percussion note may be absolute as in pleural effusion or extensive consolidation. Much more commonly, only a relative difference is detected by comparison with other areas of the lung. Fairly large areas of underlying consolidation or collapse can be present, as seen radiologically, without any impairment of percussion note, so that detectable impairment of percussion usually indicates an extensive lesion. In respiratory disease the significance of the area of cardiac dullness is usually in respect of reduction or loss of it as seen in emphysema or pneumothorax.

**Auscultation.** The fractious crying child as well as the co-operative one can be examined by auscultation. A child cannot cry during the inspiratory phase of respiration and the very act of crying makes him take a full inspiration. Auscultation is possible during this phase.

The *breath sounds* in infants and children are harsher (broncho-vesicular) than in adults. The auscultatory time relationships are: inspiration, expiration (following and approximately one-third of the duration of inspiration), then a silent period of the approximate duration of inspiration. In auscultatory examination the breath sounds themselves should first be assessed. Are they audible and if so are they of normal, diminished (as with a pleural effusion, pneumothorax or obstructive emphysema), or increased intensity (as with some types of consolidation and collapse)? Do they have the harsher quality which is commonly associated with bronchitis and bronchiolitis? Is the relationship of the various phases of the respiratory cycle normal, i.e. is there any prolongation of the expiratory phase of respiration (as with asthma) or is the abolition of the normal silent period, with inspiration and expiration of equal length and of an intense character (bronchial breathing)?

The significance of *added sounds*, i.e. rhonchi, crepitations and friction rubs, does not differ from that in the adult as described in Chapter 6.

Abnormal signs in the cardiovascular system are considered in the succeeding paragraphs. These can indicate respiratory as well as cardiac disease. Displacement of the apex beat, for instance, is as likely to be due to a pulmonary as a cardiac cause. As a corollary dyspnoea in infancy may well have a cardiac aetiology.

## CARDIOVASCULAR SYSTEM

**Inspection.** General inspection of the child may show signs which are due to a cardiovascular cause such as poor physical development, squatting, dyspnoea, tachypnoea, central cyanosis, oedema, clubbing of the fingers and toes and distension of superficial veins. Praecordial bulging associated with cardiac enlargement may be evident and there may be abnormal praecordial pulsations. In right ventricular hypertrophy there may be excessive pulsation of the central and superior parts of the praecordium leading towards the left sterno-clavicular joint, and in left ventricular hypertrophy an accentuated apical pulsation and visible lifting of the praecordium. The position of the apex beat, if visible, should also be noted. Assessment of the jugular venous pressure in the neck and of the venous pulse wave may be important (p. 120). In younger children inspection of the neck veins may not be easy because of the relative shortness of the neck and the mobility of the child.

**Palpation.** Palpation of the praecordium may reveal a right ventricular type of parasternal impulse or the heaving apex of left ventricular hypertrophy. It may also reveal the presence of a thrill. This is appreciated better with the palm than with the fingers. The site of maximal intensity of the thrill should be identified. A palpable second heart sound associated with pulmonary hypertension may be felt in the region of the second costal cartilage. The position of the apex beat (point of maximum impulse) should be identified, and normally in children should be within the mid-clavicular line in the fourth or fifth intercostal space.

The radial pulse can be used as an indication of heart rate, but in babies the difficulty of feeling it makes cardiac auscultation a much more reliable method. Pulse volume and the presence or absence of a collapsing pulse can, in older children at least, be assessed as in adults (p. 113). The pulse can also be used in the detection of arrhythmias. Sinus arrhythmia, i.e. an increase in heart rate on inspiration and decrease on expiration, is a common normal finding in most children. In any case of suspected congenital heart disease both radial pulses should be palpated to determine any difference between them, and the femoral pulses should also be felt. Absence or weakness of the femoral pulses or delay when they are palpated concurrently with the radial pulses is likely to be associated with coarctation of the aorta. In the same condition pulsation of collateral vessels may be detected by palpation in the scapular region.

**Percussion.** Percussion is not comparable with radiological examination in accuracy of assessment of cardiac size, but in the home, in the child welfare clinic and in the school, radiological facilities are seldom available. The thinner chest wall of the child makes him a more suitable subject for cardiac percussion than the adult, and the information which is obtainable by percussion of the upper (second intercostal space) and right (mid-clavicular line to right sternal edge) borders of the heart, used in conjunction with the position of the apex beat, is certainly of some value. An overall extension of the area of cardiac dullness is likely to indicate cardiac enlargement; displacement of the area may indicate mediastinal shift. Reduction of the area of cardiac dullness is likely to be due to emphysema.

**Auscultation.** The auscultatory signs of cardiac disease in infancy and childhood are basically the same as in adults, but as certain types of disease are more common in childhood there is a difference in incidence of the various signs. Congenital heart disease is much more common in infants and children while acquired heart disease is less frequently encountered.

Auscultation of the heart requires silence and a reasonably still patient. These may be difficult or at times impossible to obtain with infants and young children. There are occasions when cardiac auscultation may require to be abandoned till another day.

The heart sounds are usually more readily audible in normal infancy and childhood than in adulthood. Splitting of the pulmonary second sound on inspiration and a third heart sound are normal findings after the first year of life. The average heart rate varies with age and at each age there is a fairly wide spread. Ranges for the various ages (rate per min.) are as follows:

| Newborn | Infancy | Pre-School Child | School Child |
|---------|---------|------------------|--------------|
| 70–120  | 80–160  | 75–120           | 70–110       |

In auscultatory assessment we are concerned with the heart sounds themselves, cardiac rhythm, the presence of any murmurs—with their site, type, intensity, timing, propagation and variation with position, and the presence of any other adventitious sounds such as friction rubs. The scheme of auscultation set out in Chapter 4 can be applied to the child. As far as murmurs are concerned, those associated with congenital heart disease will preponderate. Thus a loud systolic murmur at the left sternal edge (e.g. ventricular septal defect), a systolic murmur in the pulmonary area (e.g. pulmonary stenosis or atrial septal defect), a systolic-diastolic murmur (machinery murmur or Gibson murmur) at the left sternoclavicular joint (e.g. patent ductus arteriosus), an aortic systolic murmur transmitted into the neck (e.g. aortic stenosis), pansystolic murmurs, and murmurs easily audible over the back (e.g. coarctation of the aorta) are more likely to be heard than the systolic or diastolic mitral murmurs or the aortic diastolic murmurs of established rheumatic heart disease. Mid-diastolic flow murmurs may be heard in congenital heart disease, e.g. at the apex with ventricular septal defect due to increased blood flow through the mitral valve and at the lower left sternal edge with atrial septal defect due to increased blood flow through the tricuspid valve. Presystolic mitral murmurs are relatively rare in childhood. A venous hum (p. 139) is common in childhood and must not be misinterpreted as signifying congenital heart disease.

**Blood Pressure Estimation.** The normal auscultatory method of blood pressure estimation can usually be carried out easily in children over the age of three years. It may be applied, but with more difficulty, to children younger

than this. For smaller children narrower cuffs are available of 5 cm (2 in) and
7·5 cm (3 in) widths. As the width of the cuff relative to the length of the
upper arm affects the pressure reading (the narrower the cuff relative to the
upper arm the higher the reading), a ratio of 2 : 3 (cuff width : upper arm
length) should be preserved. The determination of blood pressure in the legs
(e.g. in suspected coarctation of the aorta) by the auscultatory method may
be very difficult. The palpatory method of blood pressure determination can
be extended down to toddlers and babies, but with babies even this may be
difficult. In such circumstances the flush method may be employed. Two
operators are required. A suitably sized cuff is applied loosely round the upper
arm or thigh. The limb below the elbow or knee is blanched either by
wrapping an elastic bandage around it or by one of the operators compressing
it with two hands. The cuff is then inflated by the second operator following
which the compression of the limb is released. The limb remains blanched due
to the sphygmomanometer cuff preventing entry of blood into it. The
sphygmomanometer pressure is allowed to drop quite rapidly. The point at
which the blanched lower limb flushes is indicated verbally by the first
operator to the second who is watching the sphygmomanometer scale and who
notes the pressure. The flush pressure represents a pressure approximately
midway between the systolic and diastolic levels. Average blood pressure
readings (mm Hg) in infancy and childhood are as follows:

| | | |
|---|---|---|
| Newborn | 35–85 | (flush method) |
| Infancy | 80/55 | (auscultation) |
| Preschool child | 85/60 | (auscultation) |
| School child | 90/60 | (auscultation) |

The normal range of the auscultatory readings would be these means plus
or minus approximately 20 per cent.

**Examination of the Liver.** This is described below, but hepatic enlargement is such an important sign of cardiac failure in infancy that it is
mentioned here as part of the examination of the cardiovascular system.

### ABDOMEN

**Inspection.** Inspection of the abdomen will reveal whether it is distended
or not. The more it is distended the more shiny and tense will the skin appear.
A child who has lost weight may show a retracted (scaphoid) abdomen with
the skin of the abdominal wall lax and even wrinkled.

In view of the essentially diaphragmatic type of breathing in normal
infants, movement of the abdominal wall is very obvious with respiration.
Loss of this movement in infants and also in older children may therefore be
an important sign of intra-abdominal disease, such as peritonitis.

Visible peristalsis may be evident through the abdominal wall in a number
of obstructive conditions in the alimentary tract. It is seen most frequently
and most significantly during the first three to four months of life in

congenital hypertrophic pyloris stenosis—a common disease of male infants. It should be sought while the infant is feeding and when he is placed in such a position that a cross light is shining over his abdomen from his right side. The examiner, seated on the infant's left side and with his eyes just above the level of the abdominal wall, watches for gastric peristalsis moving from left to right across the epigastrium.

In obstruction lower down in the bowel there may be abdominal distension, visible peristalsis and a ladder pattern created by loops of gut.

A distended bladder may reveal itself by a uniform rounded central swelling in the suprapubic region.

Inspection of the abdominal wall will also reveal any abnormality of the umbilicus such as an umbilical hernia or umbilical infection, and any distension of veins of the abdominal wall as in portal obstruction.

**Palpation.** Abdominal palpation should normally be carried out with the patient supine and relaxed. The examiner is probably best seated beside the examination couch and his hands should be warm. Relaxation may be assisted by getting the child to draw the knees up and by diverting the child's attention by conversation or by some visual distraction (e.g. asking him to observe a fly crawling on the ceiling). With infants and children who cry on being laid flat it may be advisable to conduct the abdominal examination with the child sitting on the mother's knee if co-operation can better be obtained in this way. The abdomen cannot be adequately palpated when a child is crying. If all attempts at pacification fail a limited palpation can be carried out during the few seconds when the child stops crying to inspire. Momentarily during this period the child relaxes his abdominal muscles.

Loss of weight may be indicated by the ability to pick up loose folds of skin and subcutaneous tissue.

*Tenderness* should be sought by gentle palpation covering the whole area of the abdominal wall, progressing gradually to deep palpation. Throughout, the patient's face should be observed for expressions of pain. The extent of the area of tenderness and its site of maximum intensity should be determined. After deep palpation, rebound pain (p. 212) can be sought particularly where any doubtful area of tenderness is discovered. During light palpation any *guarding* (e.g. in early appendicitis) or *boarding* (e.g. in peritonitis or tetanus) of the abdominal wall will become evident.

Palpation for a *pyloric tumour* is an essential part of the diagnosis of congenital hypertrophic pyloric stenosis (Fig. 115). Under the same examination conditions and position as for the observation of visible epigastric peristalsis, the examiner palpates with the flat of his left hand on the abdomen, the fingers being directed towards the right hypochondrium with their tips lying below the hepatic edge just lateral to the rectus muscle. Gentle depression of the tips of the fingers, using particularly the middle finger, is employed seeking a walnut or hazelnut sized tumour which tends to harden intermittently. It is likely to be impalpable during relaxation and may harden

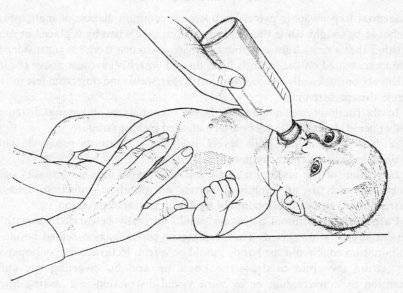

FIG. 115   Palpation for a Pyloric Tumour.

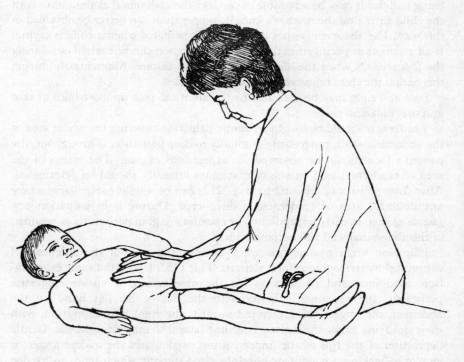

FIG. 116   Palpation of the Liver in the Child.

only once in 10 to 15 minutes. The examination must therefore be conducted for this length of time.

The lower border of the *liver* can normally be felt in infants; to palpate the edge the examiner should place one or both hands flat on the abdomen with their axes directed towards the costal margin and at right angles to it (Fig. 116). Palpation is conducted by gentle intermittent depression of the tips of the fingers. The increased resistance to palpation created by the liver can usually be felt just below the costal margin in the normal infant or extending further away from it in the presence of hepatomegaly. As palpation is continued at a progressively increasing distance from the costal margin, the edge of the liver will be felt. Its presence can be confirmed by approaching the liver from below using moderately deep palpation so that the tips of the fingers are deeper than the liver edge and rolling the tips of the fingers upwards over the edge. In a child who will co-operate, deep breathing assists the examination. On inspiration the liver edge descends and becomes more superficial and the fingers can be rolled more easily over the edge to identify its position. In a crying child the periods of abdominal relaxation between cries will have to be used for these manoeuvres.

The *spleen* may be just palpable in about one in ten healthy children. The technique of palpation does not differ from that in the adult described on page 216 (Fig. 43). The spleen is a superficial organ. If the fingers are dug into the abdominal wall they may go below the spleen. With minimal enlargement the tip of the spleen will be felt descending below the costal margin on deep breathing. Greater degrees of enlargement will be evident without deep breathing. In these cases the tips of the fingers should be placed far enough away from the costal margin to define the splenic edge. In infancy the spleen enlarges towards the left iliac fossa while in older children, as in the adult, it enlarges towards the right iliac fossa.

The *kidneys* can often be felt in normal children and especially in the newborn infant. Sitting beside the patient, the examiner should place one hand behind on the renal angle and the other in front and conduct bimanual palpation (p.217 ). The hands are approximated during expiration and the shape and size of the kidney defined. A rounded pyriform swelling is palpable in the suprapubic region when the *bladder* is abnormally distended. Other masses of varying size, site and consistency may also be felt. *Faeces* may be palpable along the line of the descending colon. In other cases more extensive scybala may give rise to widespread hard lumps throughout the abdomen. *Mesenteric nodes*, may be palpable as somewhat rubbery masses. Other swellings such as those due to neuroblastomas and Wilms' *tumour* are likely to be easily felt if present. The soft sausage-shaped tumour of an *intussusception* in the upper right quadrant of the abdomen may be much more difficult to feel. It may be associated with a detectable emptiness in the right iliac fossa. *Hernias* may be present—e.g. a soft swelling seen to develop in the inguinal region on crying and reducible by palpation. When strangulated there is likely to be evident discomfort and a tender, harder, irreducible swelling.

**Percussion.** The chief value of abdominal percussion lies in the detection of free fluid in the abdomen and in the differentiation of gaseous distension from distension due to solid or liquid containing masses. The technique for percussion in the flanks for shifting dullness is as valid in the child as in the adult (p. 218 ); so too is the elicitation of a fluid thrill (p. 219). A distended bladder will result in impairment of the percussion note in the suprapubic area.

**Auscultation.** Bowel sounds, tinkling and crackling in character, are normally intermittently audible on auscultation of the abdomen with a stethoscope. These will be accentuated where there is increased peristalsis, as in obstruction. They will not be heard in the absence of peristalsis, e.g. in ileus, associated with infection as in peritonitis, occurring post-operatively or associated with a condition such as neonatal cold injury.

## PERINEUM AND GENITALIA

The *anus* should be examined; anterior positioning may occur or there may be an abnormal opening into the vagina. The formation of the anus should be observed. In ano-rectal atresia it may be noted to be imperforate; in myelomeningocele it may be abnormally open and patulous. The presence of prolapse of the rectum will be very obvious. Introduction of the finger may reveal diminished tone, increased tone or stenosis.

*Rectal examination* is carried out as with adults except that with babies and toddlers the smallest finger should be used to avoid undue stretching of the anus. Gripping of the finger by the narrow rectal segment of Hirschsprung's disease is more likely to be encountered in infants and children than in adults.

In the female, inspection of *the genitalia* should detect the presence of labial adhesions, enlargement of the clitoris (e.g. in the adreno-genital syndrome), abnormal vaginal discharge or abnormal positioning of the vaginal introitus or urethra.

In the male the size and shape of the penis should be noted, and also any abnormal development (such as hypospadias) or infection (such as balanitis). The position of the testes should be checked (i.e. in the scrotum, palpable in the inguinal canal or not palpable in either of these locations). Any testicular swelling or tenderness or an inguinal hernia or hydrocele will be noted.

## NERVOUS SYSTEM

Examination of the nervous system in the older child can be conducted with the same exactitude as in the adult. With the younger child, and particularly with the infant, the central nervous system has not reached a stage of development at which it is capable of the functional precision with which it operates later and, integrally with this, mental development has not reached a stage at which the co-operation which is an essential part of so much neurological examination can be achieved. With younger children and infants neurological examination is thus much more objective in its approach and less precise in its application. Chapter 8 covers the neurological examination as applied to the older child. Here we shall concentrate on the younger child and infant.

**Inspection.** In the developing child neurological disorder is often linked with disorders of intellect and behaviour. Thus an assessment of these characteristics in a child is important in the neurological examination. After the age of five it usually becomes fairly easy to test *intelligence* separately from motor function. The younger the child the more difficult is this as many of the tests by which intelligence is assessed in infancy and early childhood depend on motor functional ability. This is one of the major difficulties of intelligence testing in children who have suffered neurological damage. The child may appear to be less intelligent than he is or, alternatively, the presence of a nervous disorder may wrongly be assumed to explain a poor performance in tests of development when impaired intelligence is the real cause. Bearing these pitfalls in mind, we should as part of the neurological examination attempt to assess the intelligence which a child possesses and likewise observe his behaviour and his reactions to his environment.

*Level of consciousness* may be closely related to neurological disease. Hyperexcitability, unresponsiveness, drowsiness, semi-consciousness and unconsciousness may accompany such disorders as meningitis, encephalitis, the post-epileptic state, cerebral injury and others. A somewhat finer appraisal will assess the child's degree of alertness, interest and memory for events in relationship to his age.

*Disorders of posture and movement* may be gross or may be minimal. What position does the child adopt voluntarily—standing, sitting, recumbent, attitude of flexion or attitude of extension? Can he at the appropriate age adopt the sitting or the standing positions or does his illness prevent him from doing so? Is there an obvious limitation of his ability to carry our certain movements of trunk, head or limbs (e.g. neck stiffness in meningitis, loss of power in poliomyelitis or in nerve injury)? Are there any abnormal movements such as the writhing movements of choreo-athetosis (e.g. following kernicterus), intention tremor on reaching for objects, tics (repetitive involuntary movements) or rolling movements of the eyes (e.g. in blindness)? Are there any convulsive movements associated with impaired consciousness such as generalised convulsions, or localised twitchings, e.g. of the limbs or face? The so-called salaam attacks (myoclonic spasms) are epileptic in nature; the sitting infant suddenly and momentarily falls forward or drops his head abruptly. Does the child in making spontaneous movements exhibit any evidence of inco-ordination or clumsiness (e.g. in certain types of cerebral palsy and cerebral tumour)? If he is walking, does his gait reveal any abnormality such as the broad-based groping walk of ataxia; or the rather stiff legged movements of spasticity, associated possibly with inability to put the heels to the ground and excessive wear of the toes of the shoes; or the scissors gait of cerebral diplegia; or the slight outward fling and stiffness of the leg seen in hemiplegia with failure to swing the arm on that side; or the staggering gait of cerebellar disturbance? Has any change been noted in the child's normal hand or foot dominance? Inspection may also reveal some obvious peripheral nerve damage such as facial palsy, wrist drop or Erb's palsy.

*Cry and speech* may be affected in other than neurological disease (e.g. the hoarse voice of laryngitis, the gruff one of cretinism and the nasal speech of cleft palate), but they are probably disturbed in a wider range of disorders of the nervous system than of any other system. The infant may have a high pitched cerebral cry (e.g. in cerebral birth injury or meningitis), the child's sppech may lack intelligibility in varying degree (e.g. in cerebral palsy), speech may disappear (e.g. aphonic chorea), or there may be well marked stammer (e.g. in psychological disturbance) or monotony and lack of expression (e.g. certain post-traumatic states following head injury or with impaired hearing). Delay in the onset of speech may also be noted, as in mental retardation or deafness or infantile autism. The range of vocabulary and language may also give some indication of mental and cerebral functional status.

**Cranial Nerves.** Specific methods for examining the cranial nerves have been described in Chapter 8. In older children these will be applicable in their entirety; the younger the child the greater will be the limitations imposed by age. Specific appreciation of *smell* does not develop until later childhood. *Vision,* to the extent of appreciation of light and darkness, is probably present at birth. At approximately four weeks the child will watch his mother as she speaks to him. By six weeks he will be beginning to watch moving objects, but the arc of visual movement will not be more than 90°; by eight weeks he will be fixing, converging and focusing, and by 12 weeks his arc of visual movement will be approximating to 180°. Thus by six to eight weeks defects in visual perception, and from 12 weeks disordered eye movements, begin to be evident. The accurate testing of visual fields is hardly possible until the child reaches the age of 5 years.

*Strabismus.* This is common in children. A certain amount of transitory squinting occurs in the early weeks of life. Thereafter a squint becomes significant and we must determine whether the squint is paralytic or non-paralytic (concomitant) in type. In the former the paralysed eye will constantly fail to move in one or more directions, e.g. when a slowly moving light is being followed. Thus the angle between the axes of the eyeballs will vary according to the direction in which the child is looking, e.g. in paralysis of the right sixth nerve the squint will be evident on looking to the right and on this movement the eyeball axes will converge due to movement of the left eye; they will remain parallel when the eyeballs look straight ahead or to the left. With a concomitant squint the two eyes maintain the same relative position in whatever direction the child looks. This type of squint is not necessarily persistent. It may be much more evident at the end of the day when the child is tired or when he is unwell. The squinting eye can be determined by getting the child to look at an object and covering alternately one and then the other eye. When the dominant eye is covered the squinting eye will look at the object but its gaze will move away from the object when the dominant eye is uncovered. The dominant eye will look at the object both when the squinting eye is covered and uncovered.

The testing of *hearing* is discussed on page 405.

Although testing of *other cranial nerves* is normally carried out with the voluntary co-operation of the patient, some testing can be carried out in younger children incapable of co-operating by observing spontaneous movement. Thus a facial palsy, even of the upper motor neurone type, can be readily diagnosed in the new-born when the infant cries. The normal depression of the corner of the mouth and screwing up of the face with crying does not take place on the affected side. Likewise palatal and tongue movements can be observed.

**Muscle Tone.** Handling of the child and passive movements of his limbs will give a general idea of muscle tone. Hypotonia will be indicated by softness of the muscles, floppiness on handling and excessive laxity of the joints due to poor muscle support; hypertonia by excessive firmness of the muscles and stiffness on movement of the limbs. Commonly, hypertonicity in children is 'clasp knife' in type, movement of the muscle beyond a certain range resulting in sudden relaxation of tone. Hypotonicity is usually generalised as in mental retardation, but it may have a local distribution (e.g. in certain types of cerebral palsy). Hypertonicity may be generalised but is much more likely to show a specific regional distribution (e.g. unilateral with predominant lower limb involvement in hemiplegia). Certain groups of muscles especially the adductors of the thigh and plantar flexors of the foot are more prone than others to be affected by hypertonicity (spasticity).

**Motor Power.** In the infant, loss of motor power may be deduced from lack of activity or limited movement without obvious cause. In an older child, active tests of motor power can be used. An assessment can be made of the presence or absence of weakness of the grip, flexion or extension at the elbow against resistance, pronation and supination of the forearm, abduction and adduction at the shoulder, raising the knee against pressure while in the recumbent posture, dorsiflexion and plantar flexion of the foot against resistance and abduction and adduction of the hip joint.

**Co-ordination.** This can be actively tested by asking the child to carry out specific movements requiring co-ordination, e.g. picking up pins, or in younger children by giving them the opportunity to perform similar movements for their own interest. A certain amount of ingenuity will enlarge the range of testing.

**Sensation.** In the infant the crying response or the withdrawal response can be used to test pin-prick sensation and muscle tenderness. It may not be possible to test light touch and position sense until the child reaches an age at which co-operation is possible.

**Reflexes.** In infancy a number of reflexes peculiar to that period of life are recognised and the absence or impairment of these or their persistence beyond the normal time of disappearance may have diagnostic and predictive value. The *sucking* and *swallowing reflexes* are present in all normal newborn infants and persist until voluntary control of these activities is achieved. The *Moro reflex* may be elicited by a a sudden noise or vibration but is probably best stimulated by holding the baby in the supine position with his shoulders, back and buttocks supported on one hand and arm of the examiner, and the head (occiput) in the other hand. If the head is allowed to fall back about an inch while the body remains supported, the arms rapidly abduct then come together again with an embracing movement. This reflex normally disappears at two or three months. The *grasp reflex* is also present in normal newborn babies. It is elicited by placing the examiner's forefingers in the palms of the infant's hand. The baby's hand closes on the examiner's finger. This reflex also disappears at two to three months. The *rooting reflex* is present in normal infants and helps them to find the mother's nipple. When light contact is made with the infant's cheek, the infant turns towards the point of contact. The *tonic neck reflex* is elicited with the baby in the supine position. Rotation of the head to one side produces increased tone in the arm on the same side with partial extension of it and there may be flexion of the knee on the contralateral side. This reflex normally disappears at two to three months. The Moro reflex, grasp reflex, rooting reflex and tonic neck reflex may be absent in a baby suffering from cerebral birth injury or certain types of cerebral dysgenesis. In cerebral palsy or mental retardation they may persist beyond the time at which they normally disappear. The *light reflex* is present almost from birth. The *knee and ankle jerks* are of limited value in the neonate but develop in intensity after a few weeks. The *abdominal reflexes* are present from birth but great patience may be required to elicit them in the newborn. They show the adult pattern of response. The normal adult type *plantar reflex* (p. 305) is seen in children over one year of age. Under one year, an equivocal response is normally obtained. In certain disorders (e.g. meningocele) loss of the *anal reflex* (constriction on stroking the perianal skin) may be of some value.

**Tests of Meningeal Irritation, etc.** One or two other neurological tests are commonly employed in children. Kernig's sign is valuable and should be carried out as in the adult (p. 309). It may be associated with Brudzinski's sign which is positive (e.g. in meningitis) when on flexing the head the thighs and knees also flex, or with inability of the child, in the sitting position with the knees drawn up, to touch the knees with the nose. The straight leg raising sign—limitation of the angle to which the leg can be lifted due to the development of sciatic pain—may be of use where the lower spinal nerve roots are subject to pressure as, for example, by a spinal tumour.

**Hearing.** Defective hearing in a child may go unsuspected for years and have a serious effect on the development of speech and education. Ability to hear certain sounds may give the impression of normal hearing whereas partial deafness may be present.

The possibility of deafness may well not have occurred to parents when they describe delayed or abnormal speech, inattentiveness, apparent backwardness or tantrums in their child. The examiner should bear this possibility in mind in the presence of such symptoms. The testing of hearing in infancy and childhood is difficult. If a doctor has reason to suspect impairment of hearing he may make observations on the child which will help him to confirm or refute his suspicions and he may apply a few simple tests involving a range of common sounds, but he is unlikely to be able to rely entirely on his results and should usually refer the child for more expert examination.

With an infant or child suspected of deafness, a fairly prolonged period of observation in a peaceful environment in the presence of his mother is likely to be required. Impairment of hearing and of comprehension of speech may reveal themselves by general indifference to sound, lack of response to the spoken word and response to noises rather than voice Vocalisation and sound production may be defective. From about four months onwards babies laugh aloud and vocalise freely with such sounds as 'ba', 'ka', 'goo', etc. At 7 months a tuneful repetitive babble of the 'dad-dad', 'bab-bab', 'mam-mam' variety is to be expected, followed at 10 to 12 months by a few words understandable to the mother only and at 14 months by a few recognisable words. Any delay in reaching these stages of vocalisation should arouse the suspicion of deafness. Sound production may also be abnormal in character, monotonous in quality and indistinct. Laughter may be lessened and pleasure, annoyance and need may be expressed by yelling and screeching.

Loss of hearing may increase visual attention and alertness to gesture and movement. Gestures may be markedly imitative and vehement.

Social rapport and adaptation may be affected. This may be evident in vocal nursery games. His facial expression may be unexpectedly enquiring, surprised or thwarted.

Disturbances of emotion may be evident. He may indulge in tantrums to draw attention to himself or to his needs. Obstinacy, irritability at not making himself understood and outbursts of self-vexation may occur.

*Objective tests of hearing in young children* have been developed but require to be carried out exactly as specified to give accurate results and require practice and experience. There is a series of more simple tests for infants and children from six months to seven years. These utilise sounds made by familiar objects. For infants of 6 to 14 months a soft-pitched rattle, the crinkling of tissue paper, a small handbell, the stroking of a spoon round the rim of a cup and the spoken voice are used. The sounds are made at 18 in from the infant at a level with his ear and with the examiner outside his range of vision. The child should react by turning his head in the direction of the sound. For children from 15 months to 2 years similar sounds and a series of verbal tests are used. In the latter a number of common objects such as a cup, ball, toy motor-car and doll are displayed and verbally identified. The child is then asked to pick out individual articles when they are named. For two-year-olds further objects are added such as spoon, fork, knife and cubes, and thus the conversation related to the larger group of objects is extended to include a wider range of sounds. The child's own speech and his phonetic usage will at this stage further indicate his ability to appreciate sound.

At 3 to 4 years and at 5 to 7 years the general principle is followed of widening the range of sounds addressed to the child via the examiner's voice. By the latter age the child should be capable of co-operating in more formal testing to the extent of covering one ear and repeating a list of words spoken at 10 ft into the uncovered ear, identifying a watch tick, etc. By this age, too, the spoken language of the normal child is usually fluent and correct.

## LOCOMOTOR SYSTEM

Examination of the nervous system will inevitably involve some examination of the locomotor system. The more specific examination of this system may reveal other defects.

**Fractures.** These may be suspected because of bony deformity, crepitus (should not be actively elicited), local pain and tenderness on attempted movement. Bony tenderness and swelling may also be present in other conditions, such as osteomyelitis.

**Deformities of the Trunk and Neck.** These may take the form of scoliosis, kyphosis or lordosis. They should be sought with the child unclothed and standing in the erect position or lying free. Scoliosis may be suspected if the skin creases in the flanks are asymmetrical and if they fail to disappear when the spine is passively flexed to the opposite side. In association with scoliosis, kyphosis and lordosis absence of ribs may be detected. Anterior positioning of the shoulders may be found to be associated with absence of the clavicles. Torticollis is excluded by a full range of passive rotation of the head. If a tuft of hair is visible over the lumbo-sacral region, spina bifida occulta may be present and may be palpable.

**Deformities of the Limbs.** In the upper limbs a number of deformities may be evident. There may be an increased carrying angle at the elbow in Turner's syndrome or, in the absence of the radius, severe flexion and lateral twisting of the hand at the wrist. There may be other flexion deformities or absence of part of the arms or fingers, extra digits, or incurving of the little finger (as in Down's syndrome), or a variety of other abnormalities. Functional deformities such as the dinner fork deformity of the wrist with the hands outstretched (as in chorea) may be evident.

In the lower limbs examples of deformity would be genu valgum, talipes equino varus (club foot), absence of part of the limbs, and shortening or unequal development, e.g. hemi-atrophy or hemi-hypertrophy. Pes planus is best observed with the child standing, when eversion of the foot and deficiency of the normal plantar arch will be evident.

**Muscles.** The muscles should be examined for evidence of general or local wasting or absence of individual muscles. Hypertrophy may also be noted, as in the calves in pseudo-hypertrophic muscular dystrophy. Assessment of muscle tone has been described on page 403.

**Joints.** Examination of a joint will assess its range of movement, the presence or absence of swelling, tenderness, pain on active and passive movement and any local rise of temperature. Swelling of a large joint may be seen in conditions such as rheumatic fever, haemophilia, and of small joints in rheumatoid arthritis. Congenital dislocation of the hip must be diagnosed as soon as possible after birth, on the basis of routine screening using the Ortolani test (pp. 355, 356).

## DEVELOPMENTAL DIAGNOSIS

The progressive acquisition of the various body movements and motor skills which characterises normal development is closely related to the maturation of all systems but especially to that of the nervous system. The dates of passing so-called milestones of development may be of great predictive value both in the assessment of intellect and in the diagnosis of physical disease. Some of the milestones of normal development from 4 weeks to 5 years of age are given on page 458.

## EXAMINATION OF THE NEWBORN INFANT

The majority of infants born in Britain are now medically examined at birth. If any abnormality is present this may be obvious on casual inspection, as with a gross congenital disorder such as spina bifida, or may only be uncovered after a careful and thorough clinical examination. While the principles and practices described throughout this chapter apply in the main to the newborn infant, there has to be some selectivity in the methods of approach on the grounds of practicability, and the limitations of clinical examination at this age period have to be recognized. Underlying disease may be present, but the signs by which it can be recognized may not yet have developed. A gross congenital cardiac defect such as transposition of the great vessels may be present without murmurs, without clinical evidence of cardiac enlargement or cardiac failure and without cyanosis (which will develop later); severe infection may occur with little temperature response; gross mental defect may be present yet its recognition may be impossible; vision has not yet developed; the range of facial expression is limited; hypothyroidism may be present without any of the signs of cretinism. While the difficulties have to be recognized, they should not discourage the routine clinical examination of the newborn infant. This may reveal much and the information obtained and recorded at this time may be of great value in the future should the infant later develop any abnormality. As the methods have largely been described already this section will indicate chiefly the breadth and scope of the neonatal examination rather than the technique.

The *medical history of the parents and other relatives* is relevant, as for example in disorders which have a strong hereditary tendency such as haemophilia, haemorrhagic telangiectasia or the Treacher-Collins syndrome, and these with a weaker but definite hereditary tendency such as cleft lip and spina bifida. The history of the mother's pregnancies may indicate factors such as recurrent prematurity or postmaturity. Her age may be important (e.g. Down's syndrome). Disease such as rubella, syphilis or toxoplasmosis may have affected the mother during pregnancy and may have had a profound influence on the foetus. Enquiry about siblings may reveal familial disease such as cystic fibrosis, the adrenogenital syndrome, mental retardation of albinism.

In the newborn infant the history of previous illness consists largely of the *birth history* (p. 379 ). This will include information on foetal distress, e.g. slowing of the foetal heart rate or meconium staining of the liquor; early rupture of the membranes; induction of labour; prolonged or rapid labour; difficulties of delivery—forceps delivery or caesarean section; maturity; birth rank; birth weight; asphyxia, such as that associated with delayed onset of respiration or irregular or periodic breathing; respiratory distress with increased respiratory effort and costal margin recession; twitchings and convulsions or disturbances of consciousness; jaundice, pallor or cyanosis.

Weight, length (crown-heel or crown-rump) and head circumference are *standard measurements*. If available, the weight charted from the time of birth is valuable.

The following are a few examples of *deformities* which, when present, will be obvious in most cases:

Spina bifida or webbing of the neck.
Deformities of the limbs such as achondroplasia or hemimelia.
Abnormalities in cranial shape and size such as hydrocephalus, excessive moulding or cephalhaematoma.
Abnormalities such as the characteristic facies of Down's syndrome or the flattened nose and low set ears of renal agenesis (Plate V).
Absence of, for instance, digits or ribs.
Tumour masses such as sacro-coccygeal teratoma.

Areas of local swelling such as an umbilical hernia or a cystic hygroma should also be obvious.

The character of *the skin* may be revealing; it may be elastic and pink as in the healthy infant, cracked and parchment-like as in placental insufficiency, abnormally pallid as a result of foetal exsanguination, cyanosed as a result of asphyxia or severe congenital heart disease, jaundiced to varying degrees, loose and inelastic in association with a deficiency of subcutaneous fat as in prematurity, dry and turgorless as in dehydration, blemished as with superficial angiomata or milia (pinpoint-sized white spots due to retention of sebaceous material within sebaceous glands) or infected as with pustules. The character of the umbilical cord or the presence of umbilical bleeding or infection will be noted. Skin temperature may be roughly assessed by palpation with the dorsum of the middle phalanges (e.g. hypothermia in neonatal cold injury). If necessary more accurate assessment can be made rectally with a thermometer. This would certainly be done in the presence of any unexplained loss of weight, anorexia or vomiting.

The *state of consciousness* of the child, for example the unresponsiveness of severe apnoea or the open eyes and hyperactivity of cerebral irritation, will be evident and the response to stimuli such as pinching of the skin noted. The amount of spontaneous movement may be significant. Convulsive movements if present may be localised, as with twitching of the face or a limb, or generalised.

The *mouth* will be examined for deformities such as cleft palate, drying of the mucous membranes, ulceration, or infection. The size, shape and tension of the *anterior fontanelle* and the degree of closure of the *posterior fontanelle* may be important.

The shape of the *chest,* the pattern of respiration (e.g. regular in time and force, or periodic and of varying depth), the respiration rate, the presence of respiratory distress, respiratory depression as in the failure of establishment of adequate respiration, moisture in the chest (the 'mucousy' baby), abnormalities in the breath sounds such as diminished air entry or adventitious sounds like crepitations, may all be important observations.

The *heart* will be examined for position, for the presence of any abnormal praecordial pulsation and for murmurs. The radial and femoral pulses may be palpated and if indicated the blood pressure will be estimated in the arms and legs (probably by the flush method).

In the abdomen any impairment of the normal movement with respiration will be observed and also the shape of the abdomen—scaphoid in certain types of oesophageal atresia or distended or exhibiting peristaltic waves as in intestinal obstruction. The abdomen should be palpated for masses.

The infant may with advantage be watched while *feeding,* for vigour and co-ordination of sucking, character of swallowing, vomiting and evidence of visible abdominal peristalsis.

The *genitalia* will be examined for conditions such as hydrocele or undescended testes in the male or for clitoral enlargement (as in adrenogenital syndrome) in the female. Any imperforation of the anus or malposition of the urethral orifice as occurs in hypospadias will be noted.

In the *locomotor system* any limitation of joint movement such as occurs in arthrogryposis, the click of congenital dislocation of the hip on Ortolani's manoeuvre, any reduction in muscle tone as may occur with cerebral damage or specific muscle disease or increase in tone which again may occur with cerebral damage, will be appreciated by handling the infant.

In the *nervous system* local pareses, for instance of one side of the face in facial palsy or of the lower limbs in spina bifida, will be looked for. The Moro reflex and the grasp reflex may be absent in the presence of cerebral injury. The character of the cry may be revealing such as the high-pitched cry of cerebral irritation or the 'cri-du-chat' syndrome.

The performance of certain basic activities in the newborn infant such as sucking, swallowing and crying and a normal sleep pattern (about 20 hours asleep and 4 awake) are dependent on the integrity of the nervous system. Any deficiencies in these abilities or disturbances of pattern raise the question of neurological damage. Examination should include observation of the infant's ability to suck and swallow and an appreciation of his pattern of sleep and wakefulness.

Enquiries can be made about the passage of meconium and the frequency and character of the *stools*. The stools may be examined. Likewise there may be indications for examining the *urine* visually, chemically, bacteriologically and for measuring daily volume. Further biochemical or bacteriological or radiological examination may be indicated.

## FURTHER INVESTIGATIONS

### Collection of Specimens

**Urine.** This should be examined routinely in any clinical examination of an infant or child. At the uncooperative ages specimens may not be easily obtained when required. Infants tend to pass urine after feeding so that the chances of success in obtaining specimens are higher at this time. Polythene bags for urine collection are available with an opening surrounded by adhesive material which sticks to the skin round the pubis, groin and perineal areas. These can also be used for the collection of 24-hour specimens. The average daily output of urine at different ages is as follows:

| | |
|---|---|
| First and second days | 30–60 ml |
| Third to tenth day | 100–300 ml |
| Tenth day to two months | 250–450 ml |
| Two months to one year | 400–500 ml |
| 1–5 years | 500–700 ml |

For bacteriological purposes a mid-stream specimen must be obtained. The younger the child, the more are patience, luck and a steady hand on the receptacle required.

**Faeces.** Specimens of faeces should be collected in sterile containers using a spoon or spatula to transfer the specimen from the pot or the napkin. Where a specimen of faeces for bacteriological examination is unobtainable a rectal swab may be taken but is less satisfactory. An ordinary throat swab is introduced into the anus for an inch or so for this purpose.

**Sputum.** In younger children sputum, if present, is difficult to obtain. A cough swab may be taken in an attempt to obtain a sample for bacteriological examination. A throat swab is introduced as far back as possible and the child is encouraged to cough. Gastric aspiration may occasionally enable swallowed sputum to be obtained.

**Throat Swab.** The procedure already described for visualising the nasopharynx is employed (p. 390) and the tonsils and pharynx are swabbed.

**Gastric and Duodenal Juice.** In babies the passage of a fine polythene tube into the stomach through the mouth or nose is easy, as active swallowing is not necessary. In older children, in using a Ryle's tube, persuasion, encouragement and even demonstration may be required. Intubation of the duodenum is not usually easy in young children, but by leaving the tube down for some hours and by placing the child on the right side its passage through the pylorus will be encouraged.

**Blood.** Venepuncture is much more difficult in infants than in older children and adults due to the smaller size of the veins, their greater mobility and the plumpness of the limbs which is usually present. The external jugular vein, the veins in the antecubital fossa, the femoral veins and scalp veins may be used. The femoral vein lies medial to the femoral artery which can be identified by palpation.

For many purposes an adequate quantity of blood can be obtained by heel puncture.

**Sweat.** In the diagnosis of cystic fibrosis (mucoviscidosis) it may be necessary to collect sweat. The skin is first cleaned with distilled water then dried with a gauze swab. A piece of sodium and chloride free filter paper is applied to the skin (usually of the back) and is covered with a piece of polythene which has been washed in distilled water and dried. The polythene is sealed down with adhesive. After some hours the filter paper is removed with forceps and placed in a chemically clean container which is then sealed and despatched to the biochemistry laboratory. Alternatively iontophoresis using pilocarpine can be used.

**Cerebrospinal Fluid.** The technique of lumbar puncture is essentially the same in the infant and child as in the adult. Some prefer the child to be in the upright position, others in the lateral position. Smaller lumbar puncture needles are available for infants and toddlers.

# CHAPTER 11
# The Use of the Ophthalmoscope

'The first model was constructed of pasteboard, eye lenses, and cover glasses used in microscopic work. It was at first so difficult to use that I doubt if I should have persevered unless I had felt that it must succeed; but in eight days I had the great joy of being the first who saw before him the human living retina.'

HERMANN VON HELMHOLTZ, 1821–1894

The tradition dies hard that the ophthalmoscope is difficult to use and that its subtleties can be mastered only during the long training of the eye specialist, the neurologist or the consultant physician. In fact, modern ophthalmoscopes are so constructed that Helmholtz's initial difficulties have long since been overcome and attention to a few simple details of technique will suffice to enable the student to see the fundus without difficulty. In different subjects, the colour and the form of the visible structures will be seen to vary like complexion and facies; familiarity with the range of normal appearances is therefore essential. The ophthalmoscope, like the stethoscope, should be accepted as a necessity at the start of the student's career. Indeed, at least during the undergraduate years, inspection of the fundus should be included as part of the routine clinical examination. The very life of the patient may depend upon the discovery by ophthalmoscopic examination of abnormalities such as those indicative of malignant hypertension, miliary tuberculosis or raised intracranial pressure.

## The Ophthalmoscope

Direct ophthalmoscopy is nothing more or less than looking at the fundus with a suitable light. If batteries are used it is advisable to buy the leakproof type in order to avoid corrosion of the instrument's casing. The light is focused on to a mirror set at the top of the instrument so that the beam is deflected through a right angle. The observer looks through a small hole or slit in the mirror and shines the light into the patient's eye (Fig. 117). At the head of the ophthalmoscope there is also a wheel carrying up to 30 lenses in a regular order according to their focal length and they may be placed in turn behind the hole in the mirror. Those marked with a red number or '+' are convex, while the white numbered or '−' lenses are concave. In American instruments these colours are reversed. The number of each lens corresponds with its focal length expressed in dioptres. (One dioptre is the strength of a lens whose focal length is 1 metre, 2 dioptres correspond to a focal length of $\frac{1}{2}$ metre, 20 dioptres to $\frac{1}{20}$ metre and so on.) There are variations of detail among different makes of ophthalmoscope, but these should not cause confusion if the principle is understood. Some of the more expensive models incorporate a

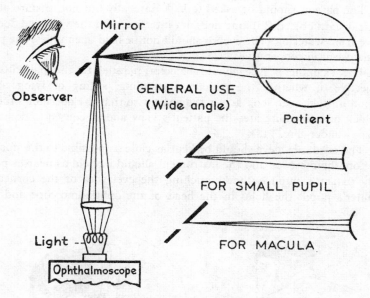

FIG. 117   OPHTHALMOSCOPY.   Basic Principles.

wheel bearing a series of black circles ranging from 1 to 10 mm in diameter to match with the pupil and thus measure its size. Before buying an ophthalmo- scope it is advisable to learn to use those that are available in hospital wards or from friends, and then to select the type which suits best. If a model which has an interchangeable auriscope headpiece proves to be satisfactory, so much the better.

## Technique in the Use of the Ophthalmoscope

For routine work, the optic disc and sufficient of the surrounding areas to include most of the common lesions can be seen through the untreated pupil in the majority of cases. For thorough examination of the fundus the patient's pupil should be dilated by dropping a mydriatic solution into the conjuctival sac. Mydrilate (cyclopentolate hydrochloride in 0·5 to 1 per cent solution), is to be preferred to homatropine as it acts more rapidly and for a shorter period. After the examination it is essential to constrict the pupil by means of 1 per cent pilocarpine or 2 per cent eserine sulphate drops. This will avert the danger of precipitating acute glaucoma.

If detailed attention is paid to each of the following points, there should seldom be any difficulty in examining the fundus.

1. The environment should be darkened whenever possible.

2. The instrument should be held in the right hand with the forefinger on the lens adjustment wheel and the right eye used to look at the patient's right eye, and vice versa for the left eye.

3. The patient should be asked to look naturally but not to stare at some specific distant object. Blinking does not interfere with the view and does save the eye from watering. The eyelids should not be held open unless the patient is comatose or uncooperative.

4. The examiner's face should be kept parallel to the patient's face, irrespective of whether the patient is standing, sitting or lying. A very common mistake is to look across the patient so that the operator's forehead or a lock of hair obliterates the patient's view and in consequence his gaze tends to wander (Fig. 118).

5. The examiner's eye should be kept as close as possible to the small hole in the ophthalmoscope and the instrument should be held as near as possible to the patient's pupil without touching the eyelashes or the cornea. The examiner's pupil, the holes in the head of the ophthalmoscope and in the

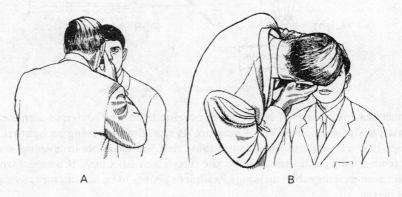

A                                        B

FIG. 118A  OPHTHALMOSCOPY.                FIG. 118B  OPHTHALMOSCOPY.
The Correct Method. The patient's gaze can be   The Wrong Method. The patient's view is
fixed on a distant point.                  obstructed and he is unable to fix his gaze on a
                                           distant point.

mirror, and the patient's pupil make five small holes in a row; the closer they are the better the view.

6. It is important to look past the light reflected from the cornea at the fundus beyond. This will eliminate the beginner's difficulty from this reflected light.

7. Breathing is apt to create problems. Considerate beginners and patients tend to hold their breath; this is not only undesirable but unnecessary if the position described above is adopted.

8. To follow the blood vessels and to examine the peripheral parts of the fundus, rotate the ophthalmoscope, and your head with it, so that the light is always on the pupil. Beginners tend to move the instrument up and down or from side to side; the light immediately leaves the pupil and they are left wondering why their glimpse of the fundus was so fleeting.

9. Inspection of the macular region or more detailed examination of small lesions of the fundus may be facilitated by narrowing the beam of light. This may be achieved in some types of ophthalmoscope by sliding the outer casing of the head up on the stem and in others by placing a small aperture in front of the mirror (Fig. 117). Some models have no such adjustments.

10. The examination of detail is possible only if the instrument is steady. This is best achieved by resting the middle and ring fingers of the holding hand against the cheek of the patient. If in addition the ulnar border of the other hand rests on the patient's forehead, the thumb can be used to steady the upper end of the ophthalmoscope, while the fingers form a useful shield to shade the eye.

### Difficulties from Opacities and Errors of Refraction

A clear view of the fundus will be obtained only if it is in focus and if all the intervening structures are transparent.

A useful routine is to examine the cornea first and then work back through the aqueous, iris, lens and vitreous to the fundus. The iris and lens can be examined with a +20 or +15 lens. If the blurred red reflex of the retina is all that is seen, the wheel is turned in an anticlockwise direction, one lens after another, until the retinal vessels come sharply into focus. Any opacity in the vitreous will become evident during this manœuvre. Occasionally crystals in the vitreous may reflect light and show as moving, glistening particles. A short-cut for discovering opacities or verifying the clarity of the media is to look at the red reflex at a distance of about 15–25 cm using no lens ('0') in the ophthalmoscope. Dense opacities reflect the light and the red reflex cannot be seen. Lesser opacities cast black shadows by obstructing the light reflected off the retina. If there are no opacities, close in to the normal position and adjust the lenses if necessary until the retinal vessels are in sharp focus. If the observer's and the patient's eyes are both normal then no lens ('0') is required; the fundus although only about 3 cm from the examiner's eye, is in perfect focus owing to the refractive power of the cornea, lens and vitreous body amounting in all to about 60 dioptres (Fig. 119). The necessity for a plus lens indicates hypermetropia, while a minus lens is required for a myopic eye

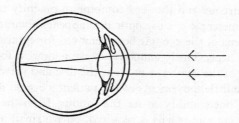

FIG. 119. THE EMMETROPIC (NORMAL) EYE.
The retina is in focus without a lens.

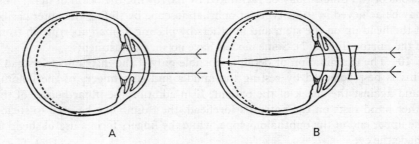

FIG. 120   THE MYOPIC (SHORT-SIGHTED) EYE.

(A) The eye is too long and the retina is not in focus when no lens is used.
(B) The use of a concave (minus) lens brings the retina into focus.

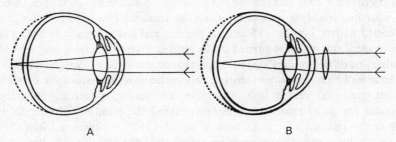

FIG. 121   THE HYPERMETROPIC (LONG-SIGHTED) EYE.

(A) The eye is too short and the retina is not in focus when no lens is used.
(B) The use of a convex (plus) lens brings the retina into focus.

(Figs 120, 121). Myopia is common, and in very short-sighted persons it may be necessary to use a −20 lens before a clear view is obtained. Many ophthalmoscopes have no more than a −20 lens so that exact focus may not be possible. If the examiner, for a reason other than astigmatism, wears spectacles, these should be removed and an appropriate allowance made for the correction.

The cornea, vitreous and the lens combine to magnify the features of the fundus. In an emmetropic eye the optic disc appears about four times its true diameter. If the lens of the eye has been removed for cataract it will be noted that the retina of a previously emmetropic eye is now in focus at about +10 lens, a large area of the fundus is in view, the disc and vessels look very small and the inevitable little movements of the patient's eye do not have the usual adverse effect on one's ability to see the fundus. If on the other hand, in a myopic eye, a strong minus lens is required, only a small area of the fundus may be in view, the disc and the vessels appear very large, and any little movement is magnified. A very myopic patient can be asked to wear his

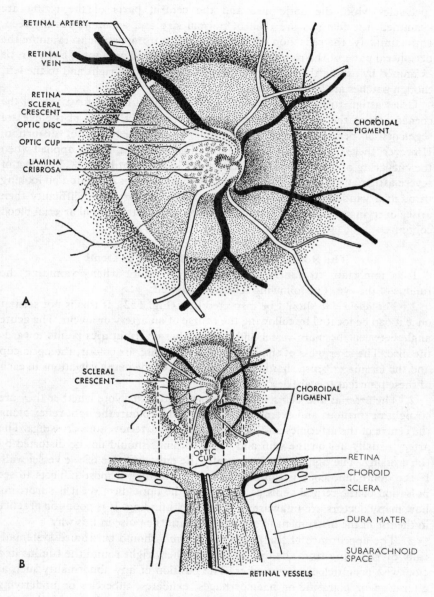

RETINAL ARTERY

RETINAL VEIN

RETINA

SCLERAL CRESCENT

OPTIC DISC

OPTIC CUP

LAMINA CRIBROSA

CHOROIDAL PIGMENT

A

SCLERAL CRESCENT

CHOROIDAL PIGMENT

OPTIC CUP

RETINA

CHOROID

SCLERA

DURA MATER

SUBARACHNOID SPACE

RETINAL VESSELS

B

FIG. 122   The Normal Right Optic Disc.

spectacles while the optic disc and the central parts of the retina are examined; the features are then of normal size and are more readily seen. Unfortunately, the reflection off the glass makes it impossible to examine the peripheral parts of the retina in the usual way. A good area may, however, be examined by asking the patient to look up, down, to the right and to the left, though patches are liable to be missed.

Gross astigmatism may also cause some difficulty. If the curvatures of the cornea and of the anterior and posterior surfaces of the lens of the eye are segments of perfect spheres, the fundus is magnified without distortion. However, there is commonly some degree of astigmatism, a term applied when the curvature of any of these surfaces varies in different planes. The effect of severe astigmatism is to distort the image just as one sees distortion on looking through a window pane that is slightly defective. Particular difficulty then arises in trying to recognise segmental narrowings of the retinal arterial blood columns.

### The Routine Inspection of the Fundus Oculi

It is important to adhere to a routine procedure when examining the fundus of the eye. The following scheme is advised.

1. The *optic disc* should be inspected first (Fig. 122). If this is not seen at once it can be located by following the course of an artery or a vein. The acute angle between the main vessel and its branches or tributaries points towards the disc. The sharpness of the edge of the optic disc, its colour, the optic cup and the lamina cribrosa should be noted. Some of the many variations in each of these four features are described on page 419.

2. The *arteries and veins* should be inspected next. Note whether they are straight or tortuous and examine their width and colour, the light reflex along the centre of the arterioles and the appearance at arteriovenous crossings. The artery usually lies on the vein and blood columns should not be distorted by the crossing. The light reflex is normally the only evidence of the vessel wall. If the ophthalmoscope is quite steady, it is possible in most subjects to see pulsation of the retinal veins as they lie on the optic disc, yet it is surprising how many doctors are unaware of this normal finding. It is good for practice in the use of the instrument to attempt to count the pulse in this way.

3. The appearance of the *fundus as a whole* should be studied systematically by radiating from the disc to the periphery right round the fundus in a clockwise or anticlockwise manner. The position of any abnormality such as alteration of pigment, or haemorrhages, exudates, tubercles or underlying choroidal changes should be noted as if the fundus was a clock with the optic disc as its centre.

4. Finally the *macula and its surroundings* should be examined. Unless the pupil is dilated, it is probable that a narrow beam will be required for inspection of the macular area. It can be seen at once if the patient looks directly into your light. The macula is situated about two discs'

width to the temporal side of the lower pole of the optic disc. It appears as a small dull red patch, darker than the remainder of the retina. In the centre there is often a little glistening white dot which is due to reflection of light from the fovea. Lesions in this area tend to cause serious loss of vision.

## Common Ophthalmoscopic Appearances

**Cornea.** Light shone on the cornea obliquely will show up a scar as a whitish opacity—just enough to have made the optic disc look rather hazy had the scar not been observed. The lesion may follow corneal ulcer or injury. Bilateral corneal scarring is more commonly due to a systemic condition such as measles in childhood.

**Lens.** While examining the cornea of elderly patients by oblique light the lens is often seen to be opaque, yet it is clear by transmitted light. Cataract seen by transmitted light is also extremely common in elderly patients. Other lens opacities may be congenital, traumatic or inflammatory in origin or may form as a complication of systemic disorders such as diabetes mellitus or hypoparathyroidism.

**Vitreous.** In myopic eyes especially, irregular, drifting, black masses of various sizes, known as vitreous floaters, may be seen. The vitreous sometimes contains fixed or mobile shiny crystals which reflect the light. Occasionally the fetal hyaloid vessels, or more commonly vestiges of them, may be seen between the optic disc and the posterior pole of the lens. None of these appearances is of diagnostic value, but, like anterior opacities, they may obscure the fundus.

**Optic disc and its immediate surroundings.** Before describing abnormal appearances of the optic disc, it is necessary to give some account of normal variations. The edge of the disc is usually sharply defined on the temporal side, but it is often indistinct on the upper, nasal or inferior margins. It is common to see a line of pigment at some part of the edge of the optic disc. This is due to redundant choroidal pigment heaping up at the edge of the optic nerve. A deficiency in the choroidal pigment and vessels near the disc is also common and gives rise to a white crescent adjacent to the disc due to the sclera seen through the transparent retina (Fig. 122). Crescents and the myopic changes described below are also liable, like large optic cups, to be mistaken by the beginner for optic atrophy. It is usually possible to differentiate between the edge of the disc and the crescent by careful inspection. As an occasional congenital abnormality of no significance, some of the nerve fibres may be opaque due to myelination. They may be recognised as broad white brush-like streaks radiating for a short distance from the edge of the disc, and commonly obscuring the vessels at this site. They may rarely occur elsewhere in the retina.

In colour the disc is paler than the fundus. Pallor or redness beyond the normal range occurs in certain pathological states (p. 420). Normally the optic cup varies from not being visible at all to being so large as to occupy the greater part of the optic disc. It is whiter and deeper than the rest of the disc. In order to focus on the base of the cup, as much as two dioptres may be required, though the depth is variable. At the base will be seen a fine white network of sclera with darker pits in the mesh where the nerve fibres make their exit; this is the lamina cribrosa (Fig. 122). Glaucoma may lead to deepening and enlargement of the cup right up to the edge of the disc and the vessels crowd towards the nasal side. Sometimes glial fibres like a spider's web of variable density lie on the disc, which are persistent remnants of the hyaloid artery of the foetus.

*Hypermetropia* is associated, for the optical reason already mentioned, with a small disc and vessels. In addition, the colour of the disc may be unusually pink, there may be no optic cup and the vessels may bulge forward giving a false impression of papilloedema.

*Myopia* on the other hand causes the disc to appear large, and stretching of the inner coats of the eye frequently causes degenerative changes, especially in the adjacent choroid. The disc may become surrounded by white crescents or large irregular white patches due to a shift or disappearance of pigment and to atrophy of the choroidal vessels, so that the sclera is visible. Pigment masses may be seen in or around these white areas.

*Papilloedema* must be suspected by noting details which appear during the course of its development. The veins are engorged and cease to pulsate, the disc looks pinker than normal, the optic cup becomes obliterated, the edges of the disc blurred and the disc swollen so that the vessels come into focus in front of the rest of the retina (Plate VII). In advanced cases the vessels around the disc may be obscured by oedema and there may be radially arranged haemorrhages. While the choked disc of advanced papilloedema is unmistakable, the recognition of the condition in its early stages may be impossible, and suspicion may require confirmation by fluorescein angiography. In addition the appearances of papillitis secondary to optic neuritis are similar to those of papilloedema and the differentiation depends on features other than the ophthalmoscopic findings (p. 247).

*Optic atrophy* shows as a peculiar whiteness and flatness of the disc due to gliosis and loss of capillaries (Plate VII). The causes are discussed on page 247.

**Blood Vessels.** In the retinal arteries and veins only the blood is visible. Light is reflected off the vessel wall and is seen as a thin bright white line running along the centre of the arteries in particular. *Thickening of vessel walls* is mainly recognised by narrowing of the blood column. The arterioles may show pallor and diffuse or segmental narrowing, widening of the light reflex and sometimes sheathing due to hypertensive sclerosis. Sometimes a vessel may be white. This is due to extreme thickening so that the blood column can no longer be seen, or to total occlusion. Atheroma is rare; it shows as a dense yellowish-white opacity obscuring part or the whole of the blood

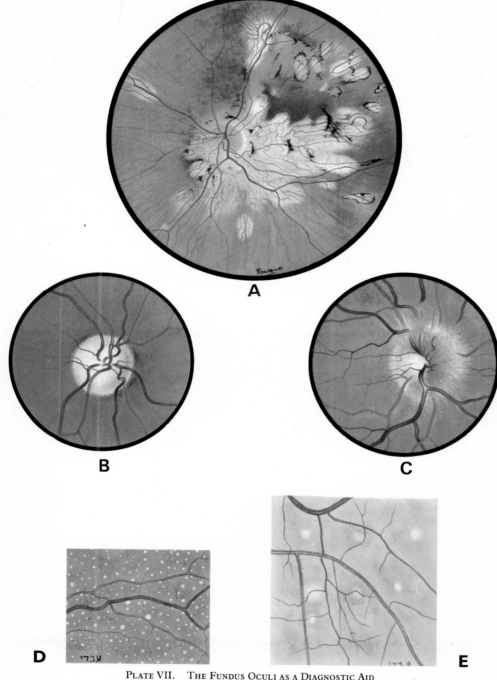

PLATE VII.  The Fundus Oculi as a Diagnostic Aid

A, Healed choroiditis. As a result of inflammation there has been a shift of pigment exposing the sclera and overlying choroidal vessels. The cause in this case was syphilis. B, Optic atrophy. Note the pallor and structureless appearance of the disc. C, Papilloedema. The veins are congested; the optic cup is still visible but the lamina cribrosa is not seen; the edge of the disc is blurred, particularly on the nasal side where the vessels are obscured by the oedema. The cause in this case was papillitis. D, Colloid bodies. Note the round yellowish-white discrete spots. They occur in older persons and are of no pathological significance. E, Miliary tuberculosis. Note the foci of varying size beneath the retinal vessels. This condition is now rarely seen in Britain.

From Ballantyne, A. J. & Michaelson, I. C. (1970). *Textbook of the Fundus of the Eye.* Edinburgh and London: Churchill Livingstone.

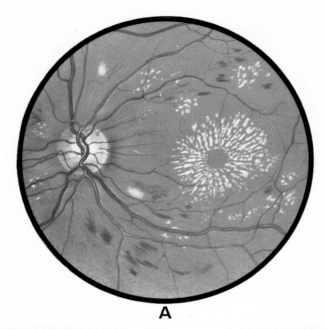

**A**

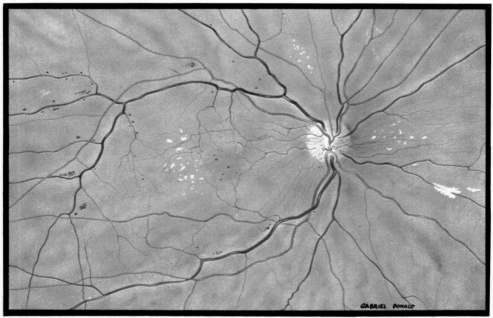

GABRIEL DONALD

**B**

PLATE VIII.    THE FUNDUS AS A DIAGNOSTIC AID
A, Hypertensive retinopathy. Note haemorrhages, two soft exudates, numerous hard exudates including a macular star and irregularity of the calibre of the arterioles. B, Diabetic retinopathy. Note microaneurysms and a few hard exudates.
From Ballantyne, A. J. & Michaelson, I. C. (1970). *Textbook of the Fundus of the Eye*. Edinburgh and London: Churchill Livingstone.

column and sometimes projecting beyond it. The appearance is comparable to the plaques of atheroma which can be seen through the walls of the arteries of the Circle of Willis at post mortem examination of most elderly subjects. *Dilatation of the veins* appears especially in conjunction with chronic respiratory failure, papilloedema, diabetes and polycythaemia. A ratio of 2 : 3 between the normal artery and vein is approximately valid but only when branching of the vessels is comparable as in the superior temporal quadrant of Figure 122. Changes in the ratio may be due to narrowing of the arteries or dilatation of the veins.

*Arteriovenous crossings.* The artery and vein share their media and adventitia at these crossings. Hypertensive sclerosis therefore commonly distorts or obscures the venous blood column. Senile arteriosclerosis with thickening of the adventitia may cause similar appearances so that the arteriolar changes described on page 420 provide the more direct evidence of hypertension. However, distension of the vein distal to the crossing usually indicates arteriolosclerosis; it is apt to be complicated by venous thrombosis.

**The Background.** The normal cornea, aqueous, lens, vitreous and retina are transparent. The red background of the fundus is due largely to blood in the massive meshwork of choroidal vessels whose detail is fogged by the retino-choroidal pigment layer on which the rods and cones lie. If the pigment layer is missing, as in the albino, or is thin, as in some fair haired people, then the choroidal vessels will be clearly seen lying on a white background of sclera. In contrast, dense pigment, commonly present in dark skinned or black haired people, is often arranged in streaks between the main choroidal vessels and gives a tigroid appearance to the fundus. The pigment also tends to become finely granular with advancing years, and the retina loses the shiny appearance seen in the child and young adult.

Nerve fibres, interspersed by their cell nuclei, run vertically from the light receptors in the deepest layers of the retina until they reach the internal limiting (hyaloid) membrane where they turn horizontally and converge upon the optic disc. The retinal vessels lie in this anterior horizontal layer of nerve fibres and nourish the inner third of the retina while the choroidal vessels supply the outer two-thirds. The hyaloid membrane separates the horizontal layer from the vitreous. Consideration of these facts explains the shapes of haemorrhages according to their depth and other background appearances now described under the broad headings of red, white and black lesions.

RED LESIONS. These are due to haemorrhages, microaneurysms or new vessel formation. The causes of haemorrhages include arterial hypertension, diabetes mellitus, retinal vascular occlusion, severe anaemia, papilloedema, microvascular diseases such as systemic lupus erythematosus, bleeding disorders, infective endocarditis and any toxic state such as that associated with advanced malignant disease.

In the nerve fibre layer, haemorrhages are linear, or fan or flame shaped as seen in arterial hypertension (Fig. 123 and Plate VIII). In contrast, in diabetes

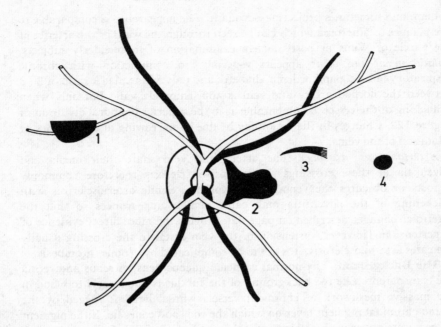

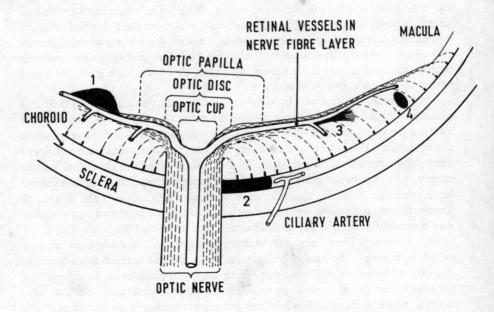

RETINAL VESSELS IN NERVE FIBRE LAYER

MACULA

OPTIC PAPILLA

OPTIC DISC

OPTIC CUP

CHOROID

SCLERA

CILIARY ARTERY

OPTIC NERVE

FIG. 123   SITES OF RETINAL HAEMORRHAGES
1: Subhyaloid Haemorrhage.  2: Choroidal Haemorrhage.  3: Haemorrhage in nerve fibre layer.
4: Deep Haemorrhage in diabetes.

mellitus most haemorrhages are in the deeper layers and they are therefore roundish—the blots of the so-called 'dot and blot haemorrhages'. The dots are, in fact, the small, dense, persistent, well circumscribed microaneurysms which may rupture to form blot haemorrhages (Fig. 123 and Plate VIII). Diabetes mellitus may also cause primary neovascularisation or new vessels may form secondarily to the organisation of pre-retinal and vitreous haemorrhages.

Occlusion of a retinal vessel, especially a vein, is accompanied by haemorrhages and patches of oedema in the segment affected and may be followed by the development of collateral vessels and microaneurysms.

A choroidal haemorrhage is less common; it is often large with a wavy, map-like margin, and dark owing to the fact that it lies beneath pigment of variable density (Fig. 123). It may be mistaken for a melanotic tumour but, like all other haemorrhages in the fundus, it tends to disappear without trace in a few weeks. Microaneurysms on the other hand, in spite of their small size, can be identified by the fact that they remain unchanged for many months.

A subhyaloid (preretinal) haemorrhage bulges forward and lies between the retina and the vitreous. A light reflex may be seen somewhere near its centre. Roundish at first, it usually sediments to give a flat topped lesion (fig. 123). The blood may burst into and mix with the vitreous, and obscure the fundus by total darkness. Alternatively it may cause streaky pools in the vitreous which are seen to lie in front of the retinal vessels. Vitreous haemorrhages may become organised by fibrous tissue. A subhyaloid haemorrhage is most often seen in company with subarachnoid haemorrhage, but may also be observed in almost any other condition in which retinal haemorrhages occur.

WHITE OR WHITISH LESIONS. Sclera is exposed in albinos, in congenital and myopic crescents around the disc, and in choroidal lesions such as congenital gaps (colobomata) or post-inflammatory or degenerative changes (Plate VII). Soft exudates (Plate VIII) are fluffy and ill-defined. They are infarcts caused by arteriolar occlusion: they often displace or obscure retinal vessels, indicating that they lie superficially. Their causes include arterial hypertension, diabetes mellitus and other microvascular diseases such as systemic lupus erythematosus and they also occur in severe anaemia. In the context of arterial hypertension they indicate a bad prognosis unless effective treatment is instituted. If soft exudates are inspected at intervals, it will be seen that, like haemorrhages, they disappear in a few weeks, leaving no trace. Hard exudates (Plate VIII) are small, dense, white spots which, when numerous, may merge into dense white patches. They lie deeply and consist of lipid deposits. They disappear in time on treatment with clofibrate.

The arrangement of nerve fibres has a bearing on the distribution of lesions. In the peripheral retina a single nerve fibre is distributed to about 80 light receptors. In the macular region each cone has its own nerve fibre; the number is so great that the fibres have to radiate outwards from the macula before turning towards the optic disc. This accounts for the star-like pattern of lesions in this area (Plate VIII).

Colloid bodies (Plate VII) are hyaline deposits in the pigment layer which appear with advancing years and are nearly always present in elderly subjects. Miliary tubercles (Plate VII) which commonly lie in the choroid, are rare in Britain but are important because they may be visible sometimes when a radiograph of the chest is negative.

Fibrous (glial) tissue occurs, especially in diabetic retinopathy, in association with neovascularisation, and the prognosis for vision is poor. In contrast a patch of myelinated nerve fibres is a harmless congenital anomaly (p. 419). Thick or occluded blood vessels show as white streaks (p. 420), and there are also a few other whitish lesions of too great a rarity to merit description here.

BLACK LESIONS. The tigroid fundus and the deposits of pigment at the disc edge have already been mentioned (p. 421). Occasional black spots of congenital origin occur which are comparable with benign melanomas of the skin. Other pigment disturbances indicate choroidal or deep retinal lesions. Choroidal degeneration in myopia or in healed choroiditis causes irregular clumps of pigment on or around a white background of sclera (Plate VII). In the hereditary disorder, retinitis pigmentosa, characteristic pigment patches giving the appearance of bird's footmarks occur in the midzone, while visual acuity relentlessly deteriorates. Lastly, but not least, is the rare but very fatal malignant melanoma which is also sometimes determined by a dominant inheritance.

CONCLUSION

It would be a fruitless task to attempt to portray adequately in words the manifold appearances of the fundus oculi in health and disease. Although there is no real substitute for direct experience, modern colour photography has much to offer and the students is advised to study an atlas of ophthalmoscopy as an introduction to the clinical appreciation of this field. A few examples have been reproduced in Plates VII and VIII to illustrate the wide range of information which may be made available by the use of the ophthalmoscope.

# CHAPTER 12
# The Examination of Urine, Blood, Vomit, Faeces and Cerebrospinal Fluid

'First we must consider the nature of man in general and of each individual and the characteristics of each disease. Then we must consider the patient—his mode of life, his mannerisms, his silences, his thoughts, his habits of sleep or wakefulness and his dreams. Next we must note whether he plucks his hair, scratches or weeps. We must observe his paroxysms, his stools, urine, sputum and vomit. We must determine the significance of all these signs.'

HIPPOCRATES, 5th Century B.C.

This comprehensive view of the scope of clinical examination emphasises the fact that the physical examination is not complete until several simple observations have been made on the patient's urine and, in appropriate circumstances, on his blood, vomit, faeces, sputum and cerebrospinal fluid. The methods employed must be used with reasonable precision and attention to detail. Nevertheless, they ought to be within the capacity of every hospital doctor and, in most instances, of the medical practitioner in his consulting-room. Procedures of a more elaborate nature, which generally constitute part of the subsequent investigation of the patient, are not described.

## EXAMINATION OF URINE

The urine should be tested in every case and this is usually most conveniently carried out immediately before or after the physical examination. Some diagnoses may become apparent only after this is done; for example glycosuria may be the sole manifestation of diabetes mellitus. Many renal disorders are unattended by any obvious physical abnormality and the patient's complaints may be non-specific. Significant renal disease is almost invariably accompanied by urinary abnormalities and their detection may be the only means of establishing the correct diagnosis. The development of simple and reliable methods of analyses has also resulted in urine testing becoming an important way in which early diagnosis of some diseases may be achieved by screening large groups of the population.

Although in special circumstances, the urine can be submitted to a large number of biochemical and biological investigations of varying degrees of complexity a few simple observations and tests suffice for routine purposes. These concern the volume, colour, opacity and smell, the measurement of specific gravity and pH, and tests for blood, protein and glucose. If protein is present or if there are clinical indications of renal disease or disorder of the urinary tract, the centrifuged deposit of a specimen should be examined microscopically. If glucose is present, a test for ketone bodies should be made. When the clinical features point to disease of the liver or biliary tract, tests for bilirubin and urobilinogen are indicated. All tests should be carried out on fresh specimens.

### Volume of Urine

The volume of urine excreted in 24 hours is determined by the fluid intake, the amount of solute to be excreted, and the capacity of the kidneys to form a concentrated or a dilute urine. In health and in temperate climates this volume varies within the range of 800 to 2500 ml. Measuring the volume of urine is important in many clinical circumstances both as a guide to the state of hydration and as a means by which oliguria or polyuria may be recognised. When the urine is being collected over a period of 24 hours the bladder should be emptied at a convenient hour immediately before the start of the 24-hour period, e.g. 8 a.m. All the urine passed in the next 24 hours up to and including the same hour next day is collected in a clean polythene or glass bottle.

Without special attention to detail it is often more difficult in hospital than in the home to collect the total output of urine over a period of 24 hours. A succession of nurses may empty the bedpan, domestics may remove the urinal, and through failure of communication or human memory, specimens are lost. Whenever possible the close co-operation of the patient should be enlisted; even when this can be obtained, a proportion of the urine may be lost unwittingly, especially during defaecation.

Formerly tests for most abnormal chemical constituents of urine were relatively complicated and involved the use of reagents, test tubes and heating. Now simple and convenient methods using commercially prepared tablets or strips containing the necessary reagents have become established as reliable alternatives to many of the classical methods. For satisfactory results these tests must be performed under clean working conditions and the tablets or sensitive ends of the reagent strips should not be touched.

### Appearance of Urine

Normal urine is clear, but its colour varies greatly from one individual to another and from day to day. Little significance should be attached to colour changes unless they are marked, and no estimate of urinary concentration should be based upon them. Certain definite colour changes should be confirmed by appropriate qualitative tests. These include:

| | |
|---|---|
| Bile | Brownish with yellow froth 'like beer'. |
| Blood, haemoglobin or methaemoglobin | Red, brown or 'smoky'. |

| Porphobilinogen | Red on standing if the urine is acid. |
| Melanogen | Urine darkens on standing. |
| Homogentisic acid | Urine darkens on standing. |
| Dyes, e.g. from methylene blue or sweets | Green. |
| Beetroot | Pink. |

The colour of urine may occasionally be altered by the presence of certain drugs or their derivatives as follows:

| Tetracyclines | Yellow. |
| Phenindione | Orange. |
| Phenolphthalein purgatives | Reddish orange, colour disappears on acidification. |
| Methyldopa | Dark grey. |
| Jectofer (intramuscular iron) | Grey or black. |

The urine may be cloudy and a sediment may be present because of the presence of mucus, pus or blood, or because of precipitation of some of its constituents on standing, e.g. phosphates or urates. The nature of such deposits can best be determined by microscopic examination.

## Smell of Urine

Most people are aware of the peculiar odour of concentrated urine. An ammoniacal smell is the result of bacterial decomposition and is commonly present on babies' napkins or in urine which has been standing for many hours. Food and drugs may cause distinctive smells. For instance, asparagus causes an unpleasant smell due to methyl mercaptan, while turpentine was taken by Cleopatra to give her urine the scent of violets. A smell of fish is caused by infection with *Esch. coli*. In patients with ketosis it may be possible to smell acetone in the urine.

## Specific Gravity of the Urine

For most clinical purposes and in the absence of glycosuria, determination of specific gravity affords a sufficiently close approximation to the osmolal concentration of urine. Its determination in a random sample of urine is of limited value. It is most useful as a measure of the extent to which the renal tubules are capable of establishing an osmotic gradient between the blood and the urine in the collecting ducts under conditions of hydropenia or hydration.

**Maximal Concentration of Urine.** The maximal capacity of the kidneys to concentrate urine may be determined either after depriving the patient of fluid for a standard time or by the injection of pitressin. In health, fluid deprivation results in a rise in serum osmolality which acts as a stimulus for release of vasopressin from the posterior pituitary. The urine becomes progressively more concentrated as fluid deprivation is continued, and in experimental subjects increasing values for urine osmolality are found up to three days. This is far too long a period for clinical application and it is customary to determine the degree of urinary concentration after 18 to 24 hours. With this procedure urinary concentrations corresponding to specific gravity of from 1·022 to 1·040 are obtained in healthy individuals. Restriction of fluid to this extent is nearly always unpleasant and may on rare occasions be dangerous. The test should be discontinued if more than 5 per cent of body weight is lost during the period of restriction. As an alternative to fluid restriction the patient may be given 10 units of pitressin tannate in oil by intramuscular injection, the specific gravity of all specimens of urine passed in the next 24 hours being measured. During this time eating and drinking need not be restricted. The results obtained with this method are slightly lower than those found after fluid restriction, but, in health, values of 1.020 or above are found. If a random specimen of urine is found to have a specific gravity of 1·020 or more there is clearly no need to carry out the formal tests.

**Minimal Concentration of Urine.** The minimal concentration of urine that can be attained is determined after the ingestion of one litre of water or the intravenous infusion of one litre of 5 per cent dextrose in water to the fasting subject. No longer than 20 minutes should be taken to give the fluid and the urine should be collected hourly thereafter for four hours. During this time the normal subject excretes at least 80 per cent. of the water load and the concentration of at least one specimen should be below 1·004.

THE USE OF THE CLINICAL HYDROMETER. The specific gravity of the urine specimens is normally determined using a clinical hydrometer which is a relatively inaccurate instrument. In order to minimise errors of technique it is important to adhere to the following instructions: (1) The hydrometer should be tested in distilled water before use and care should be taken to see that the calibration is accurate at this point (1·000 at 15°C.). (2) The urine to be tested should be allowed to cool to room temperature as hydrometers are calibrated to read at 15°C. (3) The hydrometer should be pushed deeply into the urine and gently rotated, care being taken to see that it floats freely without contact with the walls of the vessel.

### ABNORMALITIES IN THE CONCENTRATION OF URINE

Diminution in the power to concentrate the urine may be due to (1) an inability to produce vasopressin in response to fluid deprivation such as occurs in diabetes insipidus; (2) failure of the renal concentrating mechanism to respond to vasopressin or administered pitressin; this category includes patients with a wide variety of acute and chronic primary renal diseases (e.g. pyelonephritis, glomerulonephritis) and extrarenal conditions such as hyperparathyroidism and other causes of hypercalcaemia, potassium depletion and adrenocortical insufficiency; or (3) the existence of an osmotic diuresis which occurs for example in the course of diabetes mellitus.

Although defects in urinary concentration are usually accompanied by restriction in renal diluting power, this is not invariable and the latter may persist long after concentrating power is lost. This is especially liable to happen in the presence of uraemia.

## Reaction of the Urine

In health and on a normal diet, 40 to 80 mEq of acid is excreted daily in the urine. The greater part of this acid is excreted buffered partly in the form of dihydrogen phosphate, which constitutes the bulk of the titratable acidity of the urine, and partly as ammonium ions. A very small amount of free hydrogen ion is also excreted and it is this which is measured when the pH is determined. Little information is gained from the routine determination of urinary pH in random samples. The urine is normally more acid than pH 6·0. Occasionally the finding of a urine with a pH of 7·0 or above is due to the consumption of alkali or a vegetarian diet, or to infection in the urinary tract by organisms other than *Esch. coli*. In certain circumstances, however, the ability of the renal tubules to excrete hydrogen ions is depressed and the accurate demonstration of this is of clinical significance.

**The Tubular Capacity to Secrete Acid.** The administration of ammonium chloride by mouth to the normal subject rapidly leads to a fall in the urinary pH and to a progressive rise in titratable acidity and in the amount or urinary ammonia. This is due to the conversion of the $NH_3$ in the ingested salt to urea, leaving HCl to be buffered in the body and subsequently excreted in the urine.

For most clinical purposes this function is tested by the oral administration of 0·1 g/kg body weight of $NH_4Cl$ in gelatin-covered capsules taken over a period of 60 minutes in the fasting state with one litre of water. Urine is collected without catheterisation at one- to two-hourly intervals for seven hours and the pH of each specimen is determined. This may be done approximately by the use of narrow range indicator paper (B.D.H.) or Johnson Comparator papers. More precise information regarding the power of the kidneys to secrete acid may be obtained by sending the urine specimens to the laboratory for the determination of titratable acidity and ammonia. The pH can also be determined there more accurately using a glass electrode.

Normally the pH of the urine falls to 5 or below and this value is also reached in most patients with chronic acquired renal disease. Failure to acidify the urine following ammonium chloride is characteristic of distal renal tubular acidosis occurring either as an inherited or acquired defect, and may also occur in potassium deficiency and in some patients with hypercalciuria and nephrocalcinosis.

## Proteinuria

The detection of protein in the urine by either of the two methods described below is always of clinical significance. Proteinuria does not usually occur with disease of the lower urinary tract, though a trace of protein may occur in the presence of severe inflammatory or haemorrhagic processes. Proteinuria almost invariably indicates the presence of parenchymal disease of the kidneys but its magnitude bears no relation to the degree of renal failure.

**Salicylsulphonic Acid Test.** 0·5 ml of 25 per cent salicylsulphonic acid are added to between 5 and 10 ml urine in a test-tube. In the presence of protein, mucoprotein and Bence Jones proteins, a cloudy precipitate forms. The test is sensitive and detects as little as 10 mg per 100 ml. Positive results are also found in patients taking tolbutamide, sulphonamides, penicillin or para-amino salicylic acid or who have been given radio-opaque substances such as biligrafin.

**Albustix.** The use of Albustix is the most convenient method available for the detection of protein in the urine and is almost as sensitive as salicyl-sulphonic acid. The test strips are impregnated at one end with buffered tetrabromphenol blue and are dipped momentarily into the urine. The yellow test end of the strip should not be touched nor should the strip be left in the urine or passed through a urine stream. Protein, if present, is absorbed on to the strip and produces a greenish-blue colour, which should be compared immediately with the appropriate colour chart. The amount of colour change varies roughly with the concentration of protein in the urine, the + colour block corresponding to about 30 mg albumin per 100 ml urine. It is best to read the strip in bright white light. Albustix is combined with other tests in Bili-Labstix (p. 431).

Positive results are occasionally seen in patients receiving large doses of phenothiazine drugs. Urine which has been acidified for purposes of preservation may give a negative reaction although protein is present, and protein-free urine which has become very alkaline through bacterial activity may give a positive reaction. Contamination of the urine with detergents or antiseptics, particularly those containing quaternary ammonium compounds, may give falsely positive reactions.

When Bence Jones proteins are present in concentrations above 150 mg per cent the test is positive. The technique, however, may fail to detect this protein if the concentration is less than this.

**Bence Jones Proteins.** These are rarely found in urine but they are important because their presence is practically diagnostic of myelomatosis though they are detected in less than 50 per cent of cases. Five-parts of urine are mixed with one-part of 50 per cent acetic acid and three-parts of saturated sodium chloride solution. Bence Jones proteins are precipitated at once at room temperature, dissolve on boiling and reappear on cooling. Other urinary proteins are precipitated by these reagents but do not disappear on boiling.

**Semi-quantitative Estimate of Urinary Protein.** For clinical purposes the total 24-hour excretion of protein may be determined using Esbach's method. Esbach's tube consists of a cylinder bearing two marks 'U' and 'R' and is calibrated to read directly in grams of protein per litre. An aliquot is taken from a 24-hour collection of urine and is made acid by the addition of a few drops of 20 per cent acetic acid. The urine is quantitatively diluted to a specific gravity of 1·010 or below, and is added to the tube up to the mark 'U'. Esbach's reagent (1 per cent picric acid and 2 per cent citric acid) is added to the mark 'R' and the two solutions are mixed by inversion. The tube is then left in the vertical position undisturbed for 24 hours, and the level of precipitate is then read. The appropriate corrections are made for any dilution of the urine and the total 24-hour excretion of protein is calculated as follows:

$$\frac{\text{Reading of Precipitate (Corrected)}}{1000} \times \frac{\text{24-hour}}{\text{volume in ml.}} = \frac{\text{g/24}}{\text{hours}}$$

## Glycosuria

**Qualitative Test for Glycosuria.** The presence of glucose in the urine is best detected using a test paper impregnated with glucose oxidase, o-tolidine, a peroxidase and a red dye which plays no part in the reaction (*Clinistix*). When dipped into urine containing glucose and withdrawn, the glucose is oxidised by atmospheric oxygen in the presence of glucose oxidase to form gluconic acid and hydrogen peroxide. The latter reacts with o-tolidine in the presence of the peroxidase to produce a blue compound which mixes with the red dye to give a purple colour. The colour change is observed in exactly 10 seconds. For all practical purposes the reaction in the test paper is specific for glucose, and is sensitive to quantities greater than 10 mg per cent. Lactose, which may be present in the urine during the latter part of pregnancy and during lactation, and other reducing substances do not give a positive reaction.

Although specific to glucose, the reaction is affected by such factors as temperature, pH and the amount of ascorbic acid present and, for this reason, the test is not quantitative. Ascorbic acid in the urine of patients receiving this vitamin for therapeutic purposes may be present in sufficiently high concentrations to reduce the sensitivity of the test. False positive reactions can occur if the urine container has been contaminated with hydrogen peroxide, hypochlorite (e.g. household bleach) or detergents containing sodium perchlorate.

Used as a routine screening procedure in infancy and childhood, this enzyme test might lead to failure to recognise the rare condition of congenital galactosaemia, for the adequate treatment of which early diagnosis is essential. For this reason the less specific quantitative test for glucose described below is recommended for infants as a screening procedure. In older children and in adults the simple specific enzyme test is adequate since failure to detect rare abnormalities such as pentosuria or fructosuria is not likely to have serious consequences.

COMBINED REAGENT STRIPS. *Bili-Labstix* combine six standardised colour tests for pH, glucose, protein, ketones (p. 433), bilirubin (p. 434), and blood

(p. 436) in urine and can be read in 30 seconds. The specificity, sensitivity and limitations are as for the individual reagent strips.

**Quantitative Test for Glycosuria.** Benedict's test has been used for many years to detect the presence of glucose in the urine and as a semi-quantitative method. The test, which depends on a reduction of a cupric to a cuprous ion, has now been modified and is available as a self heating tablet. The test is carried out as follows: with the special dropper provided, 5 drops of urine are placed in a clean dry test-tube. The dropper is rinsed and 10 drops of water are added. One Clinitest tablet is then dropped into the test-tube and the reaction mixture effervesces. The tube should not be shaken during this period and the effervescence should be allowed to settle. Fifteen seconds after the effervescence has subsided the tube should be shaken gently and the colour produced compared with the colour scale provided, which ranges from blue (no glucose) to orange (2 per cent glucose).

If, while the reaction is taking place, an orange colour appears, even for a moment, and then changes to greenish brown, more than 2 per cent of sugar should be recorded. Failure to watch the reaction and to note the 'orange flash' may mean the final colour is compared with other colours on the scale, with misleading results. When used in this way Clinitest tablets possess the same sensitivity and fallacies as the original Benedict's reaction.

Apart from glucose, other reducing substances include fructose, lactose, galactose, glucuronides and phenolic drugs such as salicylates. In very concentrated specimens reduction may occur with creatinine or uric acid. Ascorbic acid in high concentrations may also give the reaction and the urine of patients with alkaptonuria has reducing properties. The different sensitivities of Clinistix and Clinitest occasionally result in a urine being found to be positive for Clinistix and negative for Clinitest. This result means that glucose is present in the urine in concentrations of between 0·01 per cent and 0·25 per cent. Tablets which have become discoloured should be discarded.

### The Determination of Blood Glucose

This can appropriately be discussed here. Dextrostix reagent strips are specific for the presence of glucose in the blood. Read visually they provide an approximate assessment of the level of blood glucose and may be used to distinguish between hypoglycaemia, normal or near normal concentrations of blood glucose and high blood glucose. The method is particularly helpful in an emergency or at night in detecting values outside the lower and upper ranges of normal, or in suggesting that the blood glucose may be sufficiently abnormal to account for the occurrence, for example, of coma. Until further experience is acquired, confirmation of an abnormal result observed with Dextrostix should be obtained as soon as possible by more accurate biochemical methods. An instrument is now available which measures the reflected light from the surface of the reacted Dextrostix and converts the measurement to a direct reading of the blood glucose which is claimed to be accurate and available within two minutes.

Capillary or venous blood may be used, but blood samples to which sodium fluoride has been added should be avoided as the enzyme in the test strip may be inactivated. A large drop of blood is spread over the printed side of the test area of the reagent strip; smears of blood must not be used. After exactly one minute the blood is washed off the strip with a fine jet of cold water conveniently kept in a plastic wash bottle and the colour of the strip is then compared at once with the colour chart provided.

Dextrostix reagent strips should be kept in their original container and protected from exposure to heat, light and moisture. They should be stored in a cool place (not in a refrigerator). The bottle should be recapped immediately and tightly after use. Any strips with a brown discoloration should not be used.

## Ketonuria

The detection and semi-quantitative assessment of ketonuria is of importance in patients with diabetes mellitus and in those suffering from starvation or persistent vomiting. In those conditions acetoacetic acid, acetone and $\beta$-hydroxybutyric acid appear in the urine as a result of their increased production in the body and concentration in the blood. There is no satisfactory method for the urinary detection of $\beta$-hydroxybutyric acid and in ketosis acetoacetic acid is present in concentrations about ten times more than that of acetone. The available tests for acetoacetic acid and acetone vary in their convenience and sensitivity, and their usefulness depends to some extent upon the circumstances in which they are employed.

**1. Rothera's Nitroprusside Test.** About 5 ml of urine are shaken with solid ammonium sulphate until saturation is achieved and a few drops of freshly prepared 5 per cent sodium nitroprusside solution (w v) are added. The solution is mixed and 5 ml of concentrated ammonia are then layered on to the surface of the urine. A purple colour due to the presence of acetoacetic acid or acetone develops at the junction of the two layers and its intensity should be assessed in 10 minutes. The presence of ammonium sulphate reduces interference by non-ketone substances and the final interpretation of the result in 10 minutes allows time for the red colour produced by sulphydril compounds within the first few minutes to fade.

Rothera's test has been modified and incorporated into a standardised tablet test (Acetest tablets) and a reagent strip test (Ketostix, Bili-Labstix). These are carried out as follows:

NITROPRUSSIDE TABLET TEST (Acetest tablets). The tablet contains sodium nitroprusside, glycine, disodium phosphate and lactose. One drop of urine is added to one tablet placed on a clean white surface. In the absence of ketone bodies the tablet becomes cream in colour. A lavender or purple colour develops in the presence of acetoacetic acid or acetone and the intensity of this should be read after 30 seconds and compared with the three shades of colour provided by the manufacturer.

KETOSTIX REAGENT STRIPS. These are an adaptation of the sodium nitro-prusside test in strip form. The Ketostix is dipped into a fresh specimen of urine and removed immediately. Excess liquid is removed from the strip by briefly touching the lip of the urine container; after 15 seconds the colour is compared with that on the chart. A lavender or purple colour indicates the presence of acetoacetic acid or acetone. This test is also incorporated in Bili-Labstix.

**2. Ferric Chloride Test.** A 10 per cent solution of ferric chloride (w/v) in 2 N HCl is added drop by drop to about 5 ml. of fresh urine. A precipitate due to phosphate frequently forms but redissolves on further addition of ferric chloride.

If acetoacetic acid is present a reddish brown colour develops rapidly. If this occurs another sample of urine should be boiled for about 10 minutes in an open beaker. If the boiled urine when cooled fails to give a positive result the presence of acetoacetic acid is confirmed. Persistence of the colour development after boiling indicates the presence of interfering non-volatile compounds of which salicylates and phenothiazine drugs and their meta-bolites are the most commonly encountered.

**Choice of Test.** For practical purposes all these tests may be regarded as detecting the presence of acetoacetic acid only. The ferric chloride test is negative with acetone and although Rothera's test, Acetest tablets and Ketostix theoretically detect the presence of this substance it contributes a very small part of the total colour. Of all the tests Rothera's method is by far the most sensitive. It is therefore the best qualitative test but should not be used semi-quantitatively. The ferric chloride test, on the other hand, is considerably less sensitive than is Rothera's method and covers a wider range of ketone levels. Used semi-quantitatively the depth of colour can be conveniently and easily assessed as varying from a trace to 4+. The ferric chloride test is therefore the most reliable of the three tests in judging the response to treatment in diabetic ketosis and in assessing its severity. The tablet test and Ketostix are intermediate in their sensitivity to the above two methods. They are both satisfactory routine qualititative tests but are unsatisfactory when used semi-quantitatively because most observers find difficulty in recognising the different degrees of colour induced by ketosis of varying severity. Acetoacetic acid is liable to decomposition to acetone which is volatile. Heat or the presence of bacteria or yeast rapidly cause the removal of acetoacetic acid from the urine. Refrigeration is the best way of preserving the specimens if analysis is delayed.

## Bilirubin in the Urine

Conjugated bilirubin is water soluble, and appears in the urine whenever there is interference with the excretion of bilirubin glucuronide in the bile, i.e.

in extrahepatic obstructive jaundice and some cases of hepatocellular jaundice. Bile pigment in the urine renders it greenish-brown in colour and a stable yellow froth is easily produced on shaking.

The presence of bilirubin is best detected by its reaction with a diazo compound, an analogue of the Van den Bergh reagent. This test is most conveniently carried out using reagent strips containing this compound, salicylsulphonic acid and sodium bicarbonate (Ictostix and Bili-Labstix). The reagent area of the strip is completely immersed in freshly passed urine and removed immediately, tapping the strip against the edge of the container to remove excess urine. The colour change should be read at 20 seconds; positive tests give a brown or purple colour recorded in three degrees of severity. In health the test is negative.

Protein in the urine gives a slight pink colour but this does not interfere with the sensitivity of the method. The test may be positive before jaundice can be detected clinically in the early stages of biliary obstruction or hepatocellular disease.

## Urobilinogen and Porphobilinogen in the Urine

These compounds appear in the urine in two entirely different disorders (see below); they are described together because they both give a colour reaction with Ehrlich's aldehyde reagent. This test is performed as follows:

Two ml of the reagent (2 per cent dimethylaminobenzaldehyde in HCl 7 mol/l) is added to 5 ml of fresh urine. Urobilinogen and porphobilinogen both give a pink colour within five minutes. To distinguish between these substances add 1 ml saturated sodium acetate solution and 2 ml chloroform. Stopper the tube and shake for one minute. Allow the chloroform and aqueous layers to settle. If the pink colour is due to urobilinogen it will be extracted into the chloroform (lower) layer, but if it is due to porphobilinogen it remains in the aqueous (upper) layer. In health the amount of urobilinogen in the urine is usually insufficient to be detected by this method unless the urine is highly concentrated, when a faint pink colour may develop.

Urinary urobilinogen can also be detected with *Urobilistix* which are dipped into fresh urine for 5 seconds. Remove excess urine by tapping edge of strip against container and read in exactly one minute. Results are expressed in Ehrlich units, one unit being equivalent to 1 mg urobilinogen/100 ml. Commonly a trace (1 mg/100 ml) is present and the scale rises to 12 units.

Urobilinogen is present in excess in haemolytic disease and in the early and recovery stages of hepatocellular disease. Porphobilinogen can be detected in acute intermittent porphyria, in variegate porphyria, and in certain drug induced porphyrinurias. Several substances interfere with the detection of urobilinogen and porphobilinogen. Positives occur with patients receiving sulphonamides and in the presence of acetone or during treatment with para-aminosalicylic acid.

## Blood and Haemoglobin in the Urine

Red blood cells may be detected in urine by microscopic examination as described on page 437. Chemical methods of detection, however, are equally sensitive and are capable in addition of demonstrating the presence of haemoglobin which may have been released from cells when the urine is hypotonic or has been standing for some time or in true haemoglobinuria. Chemical determination depends upon the peroxidase-like action of haemo-globin. In the presence of a peroxide, haemoglobin and its derivatives bring about the oxidation of a variety of substances including o-tolidine. The method is conveniently carried out using *Haemostix reagent strips,* the test end of which is dipped into urine and removed immediately. The colour of the strip is then compared with the appropriate chart after 30 seconds. A positive test goes blue within this period of time. This test is also incorporated in Bili-Labstix.

In health, urine will give a negative result with this method which is capable of detecting as little as 50 cells per $mm^3$ or 150 $\mu$g haemoglobin/100 ml urine. Significant degrees of haematuria below this level are extremely rare. Falsely positive results may be obtained if the urine contains iodide in high concentrations as may occur if, for example, the patient is being given potassium iodide.

## Phenylketonuria

Phenylketonuria is a rare genetically determined defect in the metabolism of phenylalanine which may lead to mental deficiency. Hence its early detection in infants is extremely important if the severity of the mental defect is to be minimised. In classical phenylketonuria phenylpyruvic acid and its derivatives are excreted in urine and can be detected by using *Phenistix.* Unfortunately in many cases screening of infants using Phenistix is unreliable and microbiological assay on blood obtained by heel prick is usually now employed, e.g. the *Guthrie test,* between the sixth and fourteenth days after birth.

## Salicylates in the Urine

Phenistix gives a reddish brown colour if salicylates are present in the urine. This reaction may be used as an aid to diagnosis in cases of coma or to ascertain whether patients advised to take paraminosalicylic acid are really doing so. A similar colour change can also be caused by phenothiazine drugs.

## MICROSCOPIC EXAMINATION OF THE URINE

Microscopic examination of the centrifuged deposit of a fresh specimen is the only reliable method of detecting the presence of red blood cells, pus and casts. These structures rapidly disintegrate if the urine is allowed to stand and the microscopic appearances become further confused by the appearance of various crystals which deposit as the pH alters and as the urine cools. The undergraduate should take every opportunity of becoming familiar with the technique and with the common normal and abnormal features.

Microscopy is indicated when certain conditions are under consideration, such as renal colic, urinary tract infections, infective endocarditis, glomerulonephritis or significant proteinuria. Examination of the deposit microscopically is also occasionally of value in recognising when opacity is due to bacteria. In appropriate geographical areas, microscopic examination of the last few drops of urine passed is the standard method for the discovery of the ova of *Schistosoma haematobium* (bilharzia, Fig. 124).

About 15 ml of urine should be centrifuged in a clean tube for two minutes at 3000 r.p.m. The supernatant urine is then removed by decanting, leaving about 0·5 ml in the centrifuge tube. Any sediment is then mixed by gentle shaking and a drop of this is placed on a clean microscope slide and a cover slip added. The specimen is examined at first under low-power magnification ($\frac{2}{3}$ inch objective lens). It is common in health to detect in each low power field one or two red cells and hyaline casts, an occasional epithelial cell and a few white blood cells. In many pathological states these cellular constituents are present in larger numbers and their nature should be confirmed by examination under higher magnification ($\frac{1}{6}$ inch objective lens).

**Cells.** Cells seen in the urinary deposit are illustrated in Figure 124. *Red blood cells* are recognised as round, refractile, non-nucleated discs. Shrunken crenated cells occur in concentrated urine. Enlarged cell 'ghosts' may be seen in hypotonic urine. *Epithelial cells* are two to four times larger than red cells, nucleated and cuboid in shape; *pus cells* are easily distinguished by their roundness, the refractile granularity of their cytoplasm and by the presence of lobed nuclei. These features may be rendered more prominent if a 10 per cent solution of acetic acid is run under the cover slip. These cells very often appear in clumps or groups and are slightly larger than red cells.

**Urinary casts.** Casts are cylindrical bodies of coagulated protein, so called because their shape represents a cast of the renal tubular lumen. Their presence in the urine therefore indicates that the proteinuria has its origin in the kidney. Hyaline casts are transparent, homogeneous structures best seen in subdued light with the microscope condenser at its lowest adjustment. Epithelial and granular casts are formed initially in the same way as hyaline casts. Tubular epithelial cells in varying stages of degeneration subsequently adhere to their surface. Red blood cell casts are composed of masses of conglutinated red cells which give them an orange or brown colour. Leucocyte casts are formed in a similar way. The various casts are illustrated in Figure 124.

Hyaline casts may be found in any urine containing protein of renal origin. Epithelial and granular casts indicate the presence of tubular damage and desquamation such as occurs for example in pyelonephritis. Red blood cell casts always reflect glomerular disease, of which the most common example is

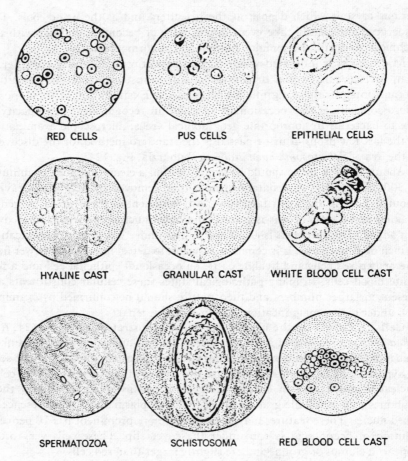

RED CELLS            PUS CELLS            EPITHELIAL CELLS

HYALINE CAST         GRANULAR CAST        WHITE BLOOD CELL CAST

SPERMATOZOA          SCHISTOSOMA          RED BLOOD CELL CAST

FIG. 124   THE URINARY DEPOSIT (x 375).

acute glomerulonephritis, and their presence is of great value in making this diagnosis.

**Crystals.** A wide variety of different crystals is often visible on microscopic examination of the urine but individual identification is seldom of value. A possible exception to this is the rare condition of *cystinuria*, in which hexagonal crystals of cystine are found. While the diagnosis may be suspected on the basis of the microscopic appearance of the crystals, it should always be confirmed by chemical analysis.

## Collection of Urine for Bacteriological Examination

For the detection of tubercle bacilli, three or more 24-hour specimens should be sent to the laboratory. For all other bacterial infections a fresh midstream specimen of urine is required, and detailed attention must be paid to the technique of collection. The patient is provided with a sterile collection bottle. He then urinates, and the specimen is collected by switching the container into the stream. For the ambulant patient the collection is conveniently made at a urinal or while sitting front to back on a lavatory seat. Women should sit astride the lavatory seat or squat over a bedpan or basin. While the labia are separated by the index and middle fingers of one hand, urine is passed and a wide-mouthed container is then switched into the stream with the other hand. For ill patients of either sex, some assistance and common-sense modifications of these techniques may be required. The collection of urine from infants and children is described on page 410.

The specimens of urine should be conveyed to the laboratory at once. Some bacterial contamination is almost unavoidable, and as each organism may divide into two every 15 to 20 minutes, a false result may be obtained if the urine is not fresh. Furthermore, a large population of contaminant may sometimes suppress the growth of pathogens. If immediate delivery is not possible, the specimen should be quickly cooled, preserved in an insulated container at 0 to 4°C and sent to the laboratory within 15 hours.

An alternative method is to use *dip innoculation culture (e.g. Uricult)*. A slide with nutrient agar on one side and MacConkey's agar on the other is dipped momentarily into a freshly voided specimen. Organisms are caught on the agar surfaces in numbers proportional to their concentration in the urine and the slide is returned to a securely closed sterile vial. Although claims have been made that, after 16–24 hours incubation at 37°C, direct reading of the bacterial growth can be made by comparing the appearance of the slide with colony density models, considerable experience is required if accurate results are to be obtained. Another disadvantage is that no information of antibiotic sensitivity is forthcoming. In spite of these shortcomings the technique offers the considerable advantage that if delay in sending specimens to a laboratory is unavoidable, reliable results are obtained by subculture of the slides after several days. Thus the technique is of particular value in screening tests for urinary tract infection.

## EXAMINATION OF THE BLOOD

The measurement of the haemoglobin concentration, the erythrocyte sedimentation rate and the study of a blood film are simple methods of examination of the blood which readily provide important information in a wide range of clinical circumstances and which are useful screening tests. The total and differential counts of the white blood cells are particularly helpful when determining the cause of pyrexia. The reticulocyte count assists in the differentiation of anaemias due to failure of production of red cells from those in which production does not compensate for loss of cells from haemorrhage or haemolysis. The platelet count and bleeding time are used when haemorrhagic disorders are suspected. The mean cell volume and the mean cell haemoglobin, which are often directly proportional to each other, are now accurately measured by electronic counters. Low values are found even in early iron deficiency anaemia and in other states where haemoglobin synthesis is impaired; high values are found in vitamin B12 and folic acid deficiency.

## Methods of Obtaining Blood

When only a few drops are required (e.g. for Hb determination, cell counts and blood films) sufficient blood may be obtained from capillary puncture. The pulp of a finger or the side of a finger nail base or the lobe of the ear in the adult and the heel in the young child are the recommended sites. The skin should be cleaned by the application of 70 per cent spirit which is allowed to dry. The part should be warm so that the blood flows freely. Squeezing of the area to obtain blood may not only close the wound but may also dilute the blood with tissue fluid. Because of the danger of transmitting hepatitis, a sterile skin-cutting needle, individually wrapped should be used for each patient. It is also possible to acquire serum hepatitis by accidentally swallowing blood being sucked into a pipette by mouth. Whenever possible automatic pipettes or a syringe should be used. This may be impossible in the case of the determination of haemoglobin and the white blood cell count which employ special pipettes. In these instances the pipette should be fitted with a long extension tube and trap and great care exercised to avoid aspiration.

When more than a few drops of blood are required, venepuncture is necessary. A tourniquet will usually be needed, but this should be applied for as short a time as possible to reduce, to the minimum, haemoconcentration distal to the site of the tourniquet. Blood withdrawn in this way is transferred to a small tube containing sequestrene and immediately mixed.

Changes in blood cell morphology occur quickly *in vitro*, but these are slowed if the blood is kept in a refrigerator until it can be examined. It is best to make films from sequestrene-treated blood within one hour after withdrawal and to do cell counts and ESR determination within eight hours. Platelet counting can be done accurately up to 24 hours after anticoagulation of blood with sequestrene (K2 EDTA).

## Haemoglobin Determination

The many methods which have been devised for the determination of haemoglobin reflect the difficulties involved in this estimation. The most accurate techniques are suitable only for laboratory use but a simplified version of the Gray Wedge photometer is available for use outside the laboratory. The Sahli method provides a useful approximation and is simple to perform.

**Sahli Acid Haematin Method.** This estimates oxy- and reduced haemoglobin by their conversion into acid haematin, the brown colour of which can be compared with that of a standard acid haematin solution or a non-fading coloured glass.

The test is carried out in a tube calibrated to give a percentage reading, 100 per cent representing 14·6g Hb decilitre of blood. 0·02 ml of blood is drawn up in a special 'haemoglobin' pipette and mixed with N/10 HCl which has previously been added to the tube to the level of the '20' mark. One of the difficulties of the method is that although the colour develops rapidly in the first few minutes it is not fully developed for 40 minutes in the adult and longer in the infant. Each Sahli comparator is therefore calibrated to be read at a certain minimum time, which is stated on the instrument, usually five minutes, after acidification of the blood. This time must be adhered to. Distilled water should then be added gradually to the tube until the colour is matched with that of the standard, the accuracy of which must be checked in a haematological laboratory every six months. Bilirubinaemia, meth-, sulph- and carboxyhaemoglobin influence the final colour and there may be as much as 10 per cent variation between the observations of different individuals.

## Erythrocyte Sedimentation Rate (ESR)

The mechanism of production of changes in the ESR is not completely understood. The concentration of protein in the plasma, the red cell mass and the specific gravity of the cells all seem to be implicated. The Hb level may certainly affect the ESR. Since it is only one of the many factors involved and since the effect on the ESR tends to be much higher in macrocytic anaemias than in anaemia due to iron deficiency, the elaborate corrections of the ESR for anaemia which are sometimes recommended are unnecessary.

The ESR is abnormal in many diseases and particularly when an inflammatory process or a disorder of globulin formation is present. An ESR in excess of 100 mm occurs in acute viral infections and myelomatosis. The normal upper limit of the ESR rises quite sharply in the elderly. The ESR may be low in cardiac failure or polycythaemia but in general a normal ESR is a reassuring finding.

The ESR is expressed as millimetres of fall of the level of the red cell column in the one hour after setting up the test and may be read directly from the graduations on the tube. By the methods described the normal upper limit for the ESR is 15 mm in the first hour.

Blood anticoagulated with sequestrene is used. Of this blood 2 ml is added to 0·5 ml of 3·8 per cent sodium citrate (w/v) and thoroughly mixed. The suspension is then drawn up to the mark on a Westergren tube (i.e. a long tube of 1 to 2 mm internal bore and graduated to 200 mm) using a syringe, and a short rubber extension; it is then set up in an appropriate ESR tube stand. In view of the length and narrow bore of the tube care must be taken to see that the tube is vertical otherwise there will be great variation in the ESR value. It should be pointed out that considerable inaccuracies may arise if the blood is not diluted as described. The test should be set up within eight hours of collection of the blood.

Sucking by mouth or a syringe into the Westergren tube and exposure to blood at all stages may be avoided by using suitably designed polythene containers which can be air sealed and into which a disposable Westergren-type pipette may be inserted, e.g. the Sedimat system. The pipette is filled by pressure exerted on the container and its tip remains under the blood on the bottom of the container during the test period.

## Blood Films

The preparation and staining of smears of peripheral blood on glass slides is essential for the study of the morphology of the red cells and white cells and for the determination of the relative proportions of the different cell types. Blood smears are also necessary for the recognition of certain human parasites such as those of malaria and trypanosomiasis.

**Preparation of the Blood Film.** A chemically clean slide free from dust must be used. A quick polish with a grease-free cloth can make all the difference between a good and an indifferent result. A small drop of the patient's blood is placed towards the end of the slide. The unbroken smooth edge of the end of another slide may be used for spreading the film. The spreading slide is placed at an angle of 45° to the slide bearing the patient's blood. The edge is then brought back into contact with the drop of blood which spreads out along the edge quickly. As soon as this takes place the spreader is advanced in a quick, even movement over the surface of the slide for a distance of 3 to 4 cm. Practice is required to produce a good film with some overlap of the red cells throughout most of the film's length, but with separation and lack of distortion of the cells towards the 'tail' of the film. Film thickness may be varied as desired by varying the angle of the spreader and the speed of spreading, e.g. thin films are preferred for the study of the red cells, thicker films for differential white cell counts and very thick films if search is being made for malarial parasites.

**Staining the Film.** Blood films should be dried rapidly by waving the slides in the air. They are then fixed and stained as quickly as possible after being spread, certainly within a few hours. The plasma adherent to the slide takes on a bluish tinge if staining is long delayed.

One or more of a group of similar Romanowsky stains are almost universally employed for the purpose of studying the morphology of the red and white blood cells and for the staining of marrow smears. These stains depend for their effects on the properties of the compounds which result from the inter-action of the basic dye methylene blue and the acidic dye eosin; they produce a wide range of shades between blue and red and are particularly helpful in distinguishing the cytoplasmic granules of different types of polymorph.

Most Romanowsky stains are dissolved in absolute methyl alcohol. When the quality of staining is consistently bad, enquiry should be made regarding the pH of the distilled water used in the preparation of stains and in the treatment of films. It is imperative to buffer the distilled water to pH 6·8 for consistently good results. Convenient buffer tablets, one of which when added to 1 litre of water corrects the pH to 6·8, may be obtained commercially. Leishman, Wright, May-Grünwald and Giemsa are all Romanowsky stains which may be employed. The combined use of the last two is recommended as they provide by far the most consistent results.

PROCEDURE. The slide is placed on a level staining rack (e.g. appropriately spaced parallel rods preferably of glass) which rests over a sink. The film is covered by 20 drops of May-Grünwald stain using a pipette. The methyl alcohol in the stain fixes the film. After two minutes 20 drops of buffered distilled water are added (i.e. the stain is now in 50 per cent dilution). After 12 to 15 minutes the slide is washed with buffered distilled water and is then shaken free of excess water. Then 20 to 30 drops of Giemsa stain freshly diluted to 5 per cent with buffered distilled water are added and allowed to act for a further 12 to 15 minutes before being washed off with a flow of tap water. The slide is dried at room temperature but the drying may be hastened by resting the slide against the warm box of a microscope lamp.

If Leishman stain is used the same technique as for May-Grünwald should be employed but the volume of the buffered distilled water added to the stain should be double the volume of the stain put on the slide.

While the times recommended will usually be found to be suitable, some adjustment by trial and error may be desirable to establish what is optimal for new batches of stains.

## Appearance of the Blood Film

In the well-made film there is some overlap of the red cells at one end with good separation at the other. The white cells are always irregularly distributed, the lymphocytes tending to predominate in the centre, polymorphs and monocytes at the edges and in the tail. In bad films there is often striking aggregation, clumping and distortion of the leucocytes at the edges.

**The Red Blood Cells.** In health the average cell is circular. Because of its biconcavity on cross section there is pallor of staining at the centre. It is described as being normochromic and normocytic. It is normal to find a small proportion of oval cells and otherwise misshapen cells and there may also be slight variation in size from the mean diameter of 7·2 μm. Cells which have a faintly bluish tinge (i.e. slight basophilia) and which are slightly larger than average are usually reticulocytes (p. 448).

Recognition of morphological abnormalities of the red cell has considerable diagnostic value. Iron deficiency leads first to reduction in the size of the cells *(microcytosis)* and when more severe, to thinner red cells which may have a reduced concentration of haemoglobin and appear pale in the centre *(hypochromia)*. There is variation in size *(anisocytosis)*.

Deficiency of vitamin $B_{12}$ and/or folic acid, on the other hand, leads to increase in the average cell size (*macrocytosis*) and to anisocytosis and usually to considerable variation in shape (*poikilocytosis*). The oval macrocyte is the most useful and important cell in recognising a megaloblastic change. This is often the only significant abnormality, appearing before other forms of poikilocytosis. Unless there is coexistent deficiency of iron (leading to a 'dimorphic' picture) the cells contain a normal concentration of haemoglobin and are normally stained. It should be pointed out that macrocytosis is not always the sequel of megaloblastic blood formation in the marrow and occasionally arises if there is brisk marrow activity, hypothyroidism, liver disease, or invasive disease of the marrow, in association with cytotoxic chemotherapy, and sometimes for reasons not understood.

In hereditary spherocytosis the typical cell is small, round and densely stained (*microspherocyte*); this cell may also be found in acquired haemolytic anaemias. Fragments of red cells (*schistocytes*) are seen from trauma to the red cells as occurs with a prosthetic heart valve or in disseminated intravascular coagulation. *Target cells* (red cells with a central dot of staining) suggest liver disease or haemoglobinopathies and when associated with a microcytic hypochromic picture, thalassaemia, if iron deficiency is excluded. The combined presence of target cells and red cells containing nuclear fragments known as *Howell-Jolly bodies* suggest previous splenectomy or splenic hypoplasia.

**The White Blood Cells.** The *polymorphs,* so named because of their multilobed nuclei, are readily distinguished from one another by the staining reaction of their cytoplasmic granules. The neutrophil granules are small, numerous and faintly acidophilic while those of the eosinophil and basophil are larger, fewer in number and distinctly orange or blue/black respectively. Frequently the eosinophil nucleus has only two large lobes and has the appearance of spectacles.

The *lymphocytes* contain a round well-defined nucleus composed of heavy clumps of chromatin. Most of the lymphocytes are 'small' (about 7 $\mu$m diameter) having only a narrow rim of pale blue cytoplasm. 'Large' lymphocytes (10 to 15 $\mu$m) differ only in respect of their more abundant cytoplasm which stains clear pale blue. In a well-stained film a few large cytoplasmic granules may be seen but this is an unimportant feature of lymphocyte morphology.

The *monocyte* is the largest white cell. The nucleus tends to be eccentric and usually indented if not actually kidney-shaped or lobulated. The cytoplasm which has a grey, frosted appearance, often contains many fine azurophilic granules and may be vacuolated.

A *differential white cell count* entails counting at least 100 white cells. Owing to the irregular distribution of the different types of leucocyte the count should be made by scanning longitudinal strips in the centre of the film head to tail.

### The Normal Differential Count

| | |
|---|---|
| Neutrophil granulocytes | 40–75 per cent $(2.0 - 7.5 \times 10^9$ 1$)$ |
| Eosinophil granulocytes | 1–6 per cent $(0.04 - 0.4 \times 10^9/l)$ |
| Basophil granulocytes | Less than 1 per cent $(0.01 - 0.1 \times 10^9/l)$ |
| Lymphocytes | 20–45 per cent $(1.5 - 4.0 \times 10^9/l)$ |
| Monocytes | 2–10 per cent $(0.2 - 0.8 \times 10^9/l)$ |

The numbers in brackets are the absolute figures for white cell counts within the normal range of $4.0 - 11.0 \times 10^9/l$.

In neonates and infants up to 1–2 years, the number of lymphocytes is relatively increased and may be up to 70 per cent of the total white cell count. At all ages the number of neutrophils rises in the presence of pyogenic infections but tends to be unaffected in viral infections. Eosinophils are increased in many hypersensitivity reactions.

**The Platelets.** Platelets appear as blue or purple non-nucleated granular bodies which are about a quarter to one-third of the diameter of a normal red cell. Giant platelets, up to the size of the red cell, may constitute 10 per cent of the platelets in normal blood. If platelets can be easily seen it can be assumed that the patient does not suffer from significant thrombocytopenia. This simple test is of considerable value in the rapid 'side-room' evaluation of an acute haemorrhagic illness.

**Abnormal Nucleated Cells.** *Normoblasts,* the nucleated marrow precursors of normal red cells, may be found in the peripheral blood whenever there is a brisk generative reaction in the marrow (e.g. after haemorrhage or in haemolytic disease), whenever the marrow is infiltrated by myelomatosis, leukaemia, carcinomatosis or fibrous tissue (myelofibrosis). These conditions may also cause the appearance of primitive white cells in the blood; the blood is then said to show a 'leuco-erythroblastic picture'.

*Megaloblasts,* the red cell precursors which appear in the marrow when anaemia is due to deficiency of folic acid or vitamin $B_{12}$, may appear in the blood particularly in severe cases. Experience is required in order to recognise these cells; they tend to be larger than normoblasts and the nucleus has a distinctive spotted appearance.

*Primitive white cells* of all types and stages of maturation are seen in the leukaemias. In chronic leukaemia the total white count tends to be higher than in acute leukaemia; it usually exceeds $50 - 10^9$ 1 in the untreated patient and may reach several hundred thousand. The type of leukaemia (myeloid, lymphatic or monocytic) is recognised by the predominant cell. The stage of maturation of the cells that are seen depends on the activity of the condition; the more chronic the disease, the higher the proportion of mature cells. When 'blast' cells are numerous (i.e. the nucleolated precursor cells) it may be assumed that the leukemia is of the acute type. In acute leukaemia the cells in the peripheral blood may be so immature that it is impossible to determine the cell series to which they belong. The platelet count (p. 449) is often helpful in differentiating between acute and chronic leukaemias, being usually profoundly depressed in the former and normally only slightly lowered in the latter.

On rare occasions *plasma cells, reticulum cells* and *cancer cells* may be seen in the blood. When the presence of such cells or of megaloblasts is suspected it is helpful to make smears of the top layer of cells from a centrifuged specimen of blood (i.e. the 'buffy coat'). In this way a high concentration of nucleated cells (and therefore also of the abnormal cells) is obtained.

A characteristic mononuclear cell is found in the blood of patients with *infectious mononucleosis*. Typically it is larger than a lymphocyte and shows considerable variation in the staining of the cytoplasm, there being areas of intense blue at the periphery changing to very pale areas elsewhere. The cell outline is irregular and pseudopodia are often seen.

**Miscellaneous Findings in Blood Films.** In a well-made film of blood from a healthy individual *rouleaux formation* of the red cells occurs only when the film is thick. Pronounced rouleaux formation in all areas of the film is abnormal. It occurs when there is a high level of globulin and perhaps also of fibrinogen in the plasma. It is usually associated with a rapid erythrocyte sedimentation rate and is most frequently encountered in myelomatosis and septicaemia. Rouleaux formation may also occur, for a time, after the intravenous infusion of dextran; this observation explains why the giving of dextran may temporarily interfere with blood grouping and cross matching.

The *spirochaete* of relapsing fever and the *parasites* of malaria, filariasis, trypanosomiasis, kala azar and other forms of leishmaniasis are stained by the Romanowsky dyes. A textbook of tropical diseases should be consulted for the recognition of these organisms in the peripheral blood.

### Tests for Sickle Cell Haemoglobin

Haemolytic anaemia is recognised by a persistent reticulocytosis (p. 448) and excess urobilinogen in the urine (p. 435). It is often overlooked. Yet the World Health Organization has estimated that over 100 million people suffer from glucose-6-phosphate dehydrogenase deficiency and probably an ever greater number carry the gene for sickle cell haemoglobin. As a result of immigration there are now areas in Britain where sickle cell anaemia is the commonest anaemia in childhood.

**Sickling Test.** Sickling of red cells containing haemoglobin S may be demonstrated by depriving them of oxygen. This may be done most simply by sealing a wet film of the patient's blood under a coverslip with petroleum jelly or wax and incubating at 37°C. A normal control should always be set up. Distortion of the red cells into filamentous shapes is seen after two hours, especially in sickle cell disease. Sickling may be induced more rapidly by suspending the patient's red cells in a *freshly* made 2 per cent solution of sodium metabisulphite. The test technique is otherwise the same as for the sickling test except that sealing of the coverslip is not necessary as long as the slide is incubated in a moist chamber. The test can be read in half an hour. A positive sickling test may reflect sickle cell anaemia, haemoglobin SC disease or sickle cell trait. These can be differentiated by a stained blood film which in sickle cell anaemia is so characteristic with the presence of sickled cells that it will confirm the diagnosis in most cases. Target cells in the absence of sickled cells would be strongly suggestive of haemoglobin SC disease while in sickle cell trait the appearances are usually normal.

## Blood Cell Counts

It is now recognised that cell counts using conventional counting chambers are subject to considerable error. In unskilled hands this may be as much as 20 per cent and in the case of red blood cell counts such errors may render the results valueless. It is for this reason that red cells counts should normally be carried out only by laboratories equipped with electronic counting apparatus.

**The White Blood Cell Count.** The white cell count is subject to the same errors as the red cell count. However, an error of 20 per cent (i.e. the difference between $5 \times 10^9$ and $6 \times 10^9$ cells/l) has much less clinical significance than with the red cell count. A 1 in 20 dilution of blood is obtained by using either a white cell bulb pipette or the much less expensive haemoglobin pipette. The cell suspension is then thoroughly mixed and added to the counting chamber (improved Neubauer) under the special glass cover slip. When applying the cover-slip to the counting chamber the observer should look for the appearance of Newton's rings on the glass supports; these indicate that the cover-slip is properly and firmly in position. Ordinary thin glass cover-slips must not be used; they bend and thereby alter the volume of fluid in the chamber. Fluid must not be spilled into the moat around the edges of the counting area. After allowing three minutes for the cells to settle, the count should be undertaken at once.

The counting area is best located with a × 10 objective lens. The ruled area of the improved Neubauer counting chamber is illustrated in Figure

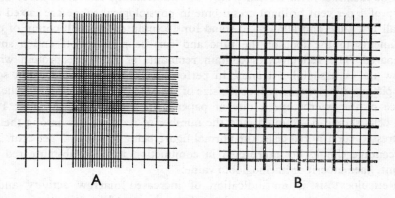

FIG. 125 Counting chambers.    A, Improved Neubauer.    B, Fuchs-Rosenthal.

125A. It will be seen that there are nine large squares each $1 \times 1$ mm and that the central area is subdivided into 25 squares each of which is further divided into 16 small squares. If the ruled area of the counting chamber is faint, better definition of the lines may be achieved by reducing the light intensity by lowering the condenser of the microscope.

Before proceeding it must be ascertained that the cells have settled, that they are evenly distributed over the counting area and that there are no debris or air bubbles in view. The cells are seen as small dots, and practice is required to distinguish the white cells from dots due to dirt and clumps of red cell stroma. It is important to realise that white cells cannot be differentiated from nucleated red cell precursors in this preparation.

The cells are counted in the $1 \times 1$ mm large squares preferably in all nine large squares in the ruled area.

*Calculation.* (Improved Neubauer counting chamber.)

> Each large square$=1 \times 1$ mm
> Depth of counting chamber$=0 \cdot 1$ mm
> Let W$=$total number of cells counted.
> Let Y$=$number of large squares counted.
> $Y \times 1 \times 0 \cdot 1$ mm³ of *suspension* contains W cells
> $0 \cdot 1$ Y mm³ of blood contain 20 W cells
> (original dilution)

$$1 \text{ mm}^3 \text{ of blood contains } \frac{20 \text{ W}}{10^{-1}\text{Y}} = \frac{200 \text{ W}}{\text{Y}}$$

The normal total white cell count in adults is from $4 \cdot 0 - 11 \cdot 0 \times 10^9/\text{l}$. It tends to be higher in infants where values of $15 \cdot 0 \times 10^9/\text{l}$ are found.

**The Reticulocyte Count.** Stippled or diffusely basophilic erythrocytes are reticulocytes, but in normal blood such cells are seldom seen, and reticulocytes can be identified with certainty only by vital staining. A drop of blood and a drop of 1 per cent brilliant cresyl blue in physiological saline are mixed in a small test tube and allowed to stand for 15 minutes. A small clump of cells sediments to the foot of the tube and can be pipetted off and a smear prepared. The reticulocytes contain remnants of ribonucleoprotein which show up as basophilic strands. In performing the reticulocyte count some people find it helpful to reduce the size of the field by introducing into the eye piece of the microscope a disc of paper with a hole in it. At least 1000 red cells should be counted, and the number of reticulocytes among them is expressed per 100 red cells, the normal figure being less than 2 per cent. The percentage should be interpreted in conjunction with an absolute red cell count, haematocrit or haemoglobin value.

Reticulocytosis is an indication of increased marrow activity and is encountered in the recovery phase from haemorrhage, in the response of anaemia to specific haematinic therapy (sometimes a useful diagnostic observation) and in haemolytic disease. The last should always be suspected when there is persistent unexplained reticulocytosis.

**The Platelet Count.** On Romanowsky stained films, platelets appear as blue granular bodies and if some can be easily seen without an extensive search it can be assumed that the platelet count is in excess of $50 \times 10^9$ l of blood.

A platelet count may be carried out using a 1 in 200 dilution of blood in 3·8 per cent (w/v) sterile sodium citrate solution. The mixture is placed in a Neubauer counting chamber. Platelets can then be seen as small refractile bodies among the red cells and counted in a manner similar to that described for leucocytes. Calculation of the result differs only in respect of the greater dilution. The normal range is $100 - 400 \times 10^9/l$.

## Measurements of the Red Blood Cells

**Packed Cell Volume (PCV).** The PCV expresses the percentage volume of red corpuscles in uncoagulated whole blood. Being potentially an accurate determination it is useful as a screening test for anaemia. The PCV is essential to the calculation of the 'absolute values' such as the mean corpuscular haemoglobin concentration.

The PCV is usually measured in a special microhaematocrit capillary tube or Wintrobe's haematocrit tube. The latter is a thick walled glass tube approximately 11 cm long with an internal diameter of 3 mm and graduated up to 100 mm. It holds about 1 ml of blood which is added after careful mixing from a Pasteur pipette.

The amount of packing of the red cells depends on the centrifugal force which is a function of the speed of rotation and the radius of the circle described by the centre of the packed cell mass. The corpuscles will not be packed to constant volume unless the blood is rotated for at least 30 minutes at 3000 r.p.m. in a centrifuge intended for haematocrit determinations (i.e. with a radius of at least 15 cm). Unless these conditions can be ensured the PCV may be seriously inaccurate. When completely packed the red cell layer becomes translucent to transmitted light. If it appears opaque packing is not complete and the result will be misleading. It should be remembered that the 'buffy coat', which may be of considerable depth in patients with leukaemia, is above the red cell layer and is not included in the PCV.

The normal range of the PCV in men is 40 to 54 per cent and in women 36 to 47 per cent.

**Mean Corpuscular Haemoglobin Concentration (MCHC).** The mean corpuscular haemoglobin concentration refers to the haemoglobin content in grams decilitre of blood and not to the haemoglobin content of individual red cells. The MCHC depends on the PCV and haemoglobin level of the blood.

The MCHC in g Hb per decilitre of red cells is obtained as follows:

$$\frac{\text{Haemoglobin in grams per decilitre of blood}}{\text{Volume of packed red cells in ml per decilitre of blood}} \times 100$$

i.e. $\dfrac{\text{Hb in g}}{\text{PCV}} \times 100.$

The normal range for the MCHC is 32 to 38 g/decilitre and when the MCHC is less than 30 it can be taken that red cells contain less than the normal complement of haemoglobin.

## Tests in Haemorrhagic Diseases

The great majority of disorders of coagulation require specialised laboratory investigations. The blood clotting time is an insensitive measure and is abnormally prolonged only when the coagulation factors are seriously deficient or if they are antagonised by the administration of heparin.

### Fibrinogen

Special problems from massive haemorrhage may sometimes arise in relation to childbirth, after incompatible blood transfusion, in carcinomatosis and as a result of prostatic operations or surgical procedures using an extracorporeal circulation. These are usually due to pathological fibrinolysins in the patient's circulation or to the development of acute fibrinogen deficiency. With pathological fibrinolysins, coagulation time may be normal but lysis of the clot will be seen to take place soon afterwards; if dissolution of the clot has not occurred after one hour it can be taken that fibrinolysis of clinical significance is not present. On the other hand, when fibrinogen deficiency is the cause of serious bleeding, the coagulation time is markedly prolonged and the clot formed will be small; further emergency investigation should be by the Fibrindex test.

**'Fibrindex' qualitative test.** This is a useful rapid qualitative test for fibrinogen as follows:

Place in a small (10 × 75 mm) test tube 0·5 ml plasma from citrated or oxalated normal blood to serve as a control. Place in a second similar test tube 0·5 ml plasma from the blood to be tested. Add 0·2 ml reconstituted Fibrindex (human thrombin diagnostic reagent) solution to each test tube. Fibrindex is supplied in 1 ml ampoules as lyophilised standardised human thrombin and is reconstituted by dissolving the contents of 1 ampoule in 1 ml of normal saline. Start stopwatch immediately. Mix by shaking very gently for 2 seconds or less. Then tilt test tubes slowly backwards and forwards.

If the fibrinogen concentration in the plasma sample is normal visible fibrin formation will be seen after 5 to 12 seconds. After 60 seconds there should be a firm, stable clot, extruding no serum and sticking to the test tube wall. If fibrinogen concentration is subnormal there will be delay in initial fibrin formation beyond the control plasma time. If no fibrin forms in the test plasma within 30 seconds a severe defect probably exists. If the normal control plasma forms no fibrin within 5 to 12 seconds, the test should be repeated with fresh materials.

The following points must be closely observed. Blood must be drawn without allowing clot formation to take place. Only citrate or oxalate should be used; excess anticoagulant (i.e. more than a few crystals of oxalate or more than 1 part in 5 of 3·8 per cent sodium citrate solution) may inhibit fibrin formation, giving unreliable results. Use only dry, clean glassware and tubes of standard size. Remaining Fibrindex solution may be used for further tests if performed within six hours; thereafter it should be discarded.

### Bleeding Time

Ivy's method is recommended. A sphygmomanometer cuff is placed round the patient's upper arm and inflated to a pressure of 40 mm Hg. With a disposable blood lancet three punctures are made in the flexor aspect of the forearm to the depth of the lancet hilt, avoiding veins and scars. A stop-watch is started as the stabs are made and the exuded blood absorbed with the edge of a filter paper, without spreading it or touching the skin, until all bleeding ceases. The longest of the times taken for the bleeding to stop from the three puncture wounds is the 'bleeding time'. The normal value is 2 to 8 minutes. It is prolonged in thrombocytopenia and in capillary defects.

### Cleaning and Decontamination of Glassware

Much time can be wasted and many results will be worthless if dirty apparatus is used. All glassware that has been in contact with blood and is not disposable should be immersed first in a detergent solution such as Diversol and then in a solution of hypochlorite (e.g. 10 per cent Chloros) and left overnight. Thereafter it should be washed in running water and dried in a hot air oven at 140°C.

## EXAMINATION OF VOMIT AND FAECES

### Vomit

**Quantity.** The quantity of vomit produced at any one time varies considerably and is naturally influenced by the amount and the time of the last meal. In the presence of pyloric obstruction the quantity vomited may be very large and amount to several litres in the course of the day. An approximate estimate of the volume and of the duration of the vomiting is necessary in judging fluid replacement therapy.

**Content.** The presence of food in a vomit before breakfast indicates delayed gastric emptying. This may be due to pylorospasm from a gastric irritant such as alcohol. In the absence of a history of alcoholic excess, obstruction at or near the pylorus should be sought by radiological examination. A yellow colour to the vomit indicates the presence of bile and means that there has been regurgitation of duodenal contents into the stomach. This has no serious significance, but the patient usually experiences an intensely bitter taste in the mouth. A dark red vomit, sometimes in company with large red clots of blood, often described by the patient as looking like liver, is due to profuse bleeding such as may occur from a peptic ulcer or oesophageal varices. Severe and possibly recurrent bleeding of this type is hardly ever due to gastric carcinoma. In haematemesis the vomit is very often blackish or dark brown and contains a sediment like coffee grounds. This is due to the conversion of haemoglobin to acid haematin by the hydrochloric acid in the gastric juice. Pink vomit sometimes indicates the sinister combination of a gastric lesion causing oozing of blood and anacidity; this occurs in gastric carcinoma in its later stages. In cases of poisoning, residues of drugs may be seen and it is important to keep vomit for analysis when poisoning is suspected. When acute dilatation of the stomach is present or in paralytic ileus watery black fluid may well out of the mouth without actual vomiting.

**Odour.** Vomit usually smells sour and the patient is aware of an acid or bitter taste. Sometimes the vomit contains food which does not taste or smell unpleasantly; this arises either in regurgitation from an obstructed oesophagus or from an oesophageal pouch, or in vomiting of gastric contents in the presence of achlorhydria. Vomit with a sulphurous smell like rotten eggs suggests the possiblity of an ulcerating carcinoma of the stomach or of pyloric obstruction. Faecal vomiting may occur in intestinal obstruction.

**Acidity.** An opportunity should be taken to test vomit for the presence of hydrochloric acid if there is any suspicion of pernicious anaemia. If the pH of the vomit is below 4·0 units pernicious anaemia can be excluded and the patient may then be spared the need for a pentagastrin test.

## Faeces

**Inspection.** The colour, consistency and bulk of the stool should be noted. A liquid stool of uniform consistency occurs with small intestinal diarrhoea, while in diarrhoea of colonic origin the loose stool usually contains numerous small pieces of faeces. Abnormalities such as the presence of blood, pus, mucus, worms or undigested food may be recognised. The absence of stercobilin gives rise to the characteristic clay-coloured stool in obstructive jaundice, while in steatorrhoea the pallor is mainly due to chemical reduction of pigment by intestinal organisms. On exposure to air the surface of the stool from a patient with steatorrhoea frequently darkens in colour. A pale, bulky, soft, frothy, smelly and fatty looking stool is characteristic of steatorrhoea from various causes; patients also sometimes notice that these fatty stools float and say that it may be necessary to flush the pan two or three times after defaecation. Black and often loose stools (melaena) occur following haemorrhage into the upper gut. The presence of blood must be confirmed chemically since medicinal preparations of iron and bismuth also produce black stools. Bright red blood suggests bleeding from the lower alimentary tract. In addition, threadworms, roundworms and segments of tapeworms may be recognised.

**Microscopic Examination.** A film is prepared by emulsifying a small portion of faeces with a drop of isotonic saline on a microscope slide and applying a cover-slip. Most information is obtained from an examination with the low-power objective of the microscope, and under illumination suitably reduced by lowering the sub-stage condenser.

The principal value of this examination is in the detection of pus cells, red blood cells and macrophages, all of which are usually found in large numbers in ulcerative diseases of the large intestine, and in the finding of parasitic protozoa and metazoal ova. The presence of meat fibres, fat globules and starch granules signifies food which has escaped the action of the digestive juices and the bacteria of the bowel. This may arise from acute conditions with intestinal hurry but more frequently indicates disease of the pancreas or small intestine.

**Occult Blood in the Faeces.** The chemical detection of occult blood in the stools is frequently of key importance in the investigation of gastro-intestinal and haematological problems. Since decisions regarding the further investigation and management of the patient often depend on the results obtained, an assessment should be made on at least three examinations. When difficulty is encountered in obtaining specimens sufficient material for testing can usually be obtained on the gloved finger at rectal examination. In patients with haemorrhoids it may be necessary to obtain the stool specimens through a proctoscope above the pile-bearing area if bleeding from the upper gastro-intestinal tract is suspected. Stool specimens from out-patients are conveniently collected in small waxed carboard containers. Methods for the chemical detection of occult blood in the faeces depend on the oxidation of one of a number of colourless compounds into a coloured salt. The reaction occurs when a solution of the compound is mixed with an oxidising agent (usually a peroxide of hydrogen, strontium or barium) and comes in contact with haemoglobin. Haemoglobin and its derivatives function as carriers of oxygen from the peroxide. Medicinal iron does not interfere with the reaction and in the tests described a moderate meat intake can be allowed. Liver and 'black' or 'blood' puddings should be avoided for one week before the test.

Orthotolidine is the most useful reagent for this purpose for it is rapidly converted into an intensely blue coloured salt on oxidation. The possibility that it may be carcinogenic in man has lead to its withdrawal from use in Britain though it continues to be used in almost every other country in the world in the form of Hematest. For this reason it is described here.

HEMATEST TABLETS. These tablets contain o-tolidine, strontium peroxide and buffers. A thin smear of faeces (undiluted with water) is made on the test paper provided. The test tablet is placed in the centre of the faecal smear and two drops of tap water are placed on the tablet. The results are recorded according to the time taken for the first occurrence of a blue colour on the paper around the tablet and range from strongly positive (within 15 seconds) to negative (after 2 minutes); no attention is paid to colour appearing after two minutes or to colour appearing in the tablet itself.

While it is hoped that the withdrawal of *o*-tolidine in Britain will prove temporary, a number of alternatives have been sought and some of these have become available commercially, among which the Hemoccult slide test, using guiac and hydrogen peroxide and the Scotland Yard Test are recommended.

SCOTLAND YARD TEST. This test is based on the use of the following reagent: *o*-ammo-phthalic-cyclic-hydrazide, $1 \cdot 5$ g; anhydrous $Na_2CO_3$, $30$ g; 10 per cent (w/v) NaOH, $37 \cdot 5$ ml; $H_2O$, to 600 ml. One ml of the solution, prepared in a laboratory, is added to a previously boiled suspension of faeces and shaken. To this is then added $0 \cdot 5$ ml solution of $H_2O_2$. When viewed in a darkened room a positive result is a striking violet fluorescence.

# EXAMINATION OF THE CEREBROSPINAL FLUID

**Appearance.** Cerebrospinal fluid should be inspected in a test-tube in good daylight or against an X-ray viewing box, using a control test-tube containing a similar quantity of water. Normal CSF is clear and colourless. Abnormalities which may be noted are turbidity, blood-staining and xanthochromia.

Turbidity indicates the presence of excessive cells or organisms. Marked turbidity indicates pyogenic meningitis. Blood-staining may be due either to traumatic contamination or to subarachnoid haemorrhage. In the former the degree of staining is much more marked in the initial specimen. In subarachnoid haemorrhage the staining is uniform in all tubes. Further information may be obtained by centrifuging. In traumatic contamination the supernatant fluid is colourless, whereas in subarachnoid haemorrhage a yellowish tinge (xanthochromia) persists in the supernatant fluid if the bleeding has occurred more than twelve hours previously. Xanthrochromia, in the absence of blood staining, may occur when there is a very high protein content in the cerebrospinal fluid as a result of a block in flow due to a spinal compressive lesion (Froin's syndrome).

**Cell Count.** This must be done as soon as possible after the CSF has been collected. Counts done some hours later, especially if clot formation has taken place, give very inaccurate results. A 1 in 10 dilution of CSF is used with 1 per cent methylene blue.

The count is best done in a Fuchs-Rosenthal counting chamber, in which the depth is $0 \cdot 2$ mm (Fig. 125B). The entire ruled area of 16 mm$^2$ is counted. The total volume of CSF examined is approximately 3 mm$^3$. The count in cells per mm$^3$ is therefore obtained by dividing the total count by 3. Red blood cells and polymorphs can readily be distinguished from each other and from other cells in this preparation.

**Gram Stain of Centrifuged Deposit.** This is of value mainly in suspected meningitis, especially when the CSF is obviously turbid. A specimen of fluid is centrifuged and films made from the deposit. Gram's stain will serve to identify provisionally many of the common bacteria, thus enabling appropriate treatment to be instituted without delay. The proportion of polymorphs and lymphocytes can also be confirmed with this technique.

**Culture.** While culture of the CSF should normally be in the hands of the bacteriologist, it may occasionally be desirable, as an emergency measure, to set up a culture with turbid CSF from a patient with suspected meningitis. The reason for this is that some organisms may fail to grow on culture if inoculation is delayed. A chocolate agar slope is inoculated with a drop of the turbid fluid using a heat sterilised wire-loop. The slope must then be placed in an incubator.

# BACTERIOLOGICAL EXAMINATIONS

Occasionally it is advisable to make a rapid bacteriological diagnosis and the doctor finds it necessary to examine sputum or CSF for tubercle bacilli or for other organisms. These should not replace expert examination by a bacteriologist as soon as possible, but in a few circumstances the correct treatment requires to be given urgently and sufficient information may be obtained by using the Gram or Ziehl-Neelsen staining methods.

## Gram's Staining Method

This method serves to identify many common bacteria present in sputum, pus or CSF and is carried out as follows:

1. Stain the smear of pus, after fixation, with methyl violet solution for one to two minutes; pour off the stain.

2. Wash off the methyl violet with iodine solution; allow the iodine solution to act for one to two minutes.

3. Drain off excess iodine.

4. Decolourise by flooding the slide with acetone, several changes being used until further stain ceases to be removed.

5. Wash quickly in water. The smear should be examined at this stage under the low power of the microscope; the nuclei of the pus cells should be a pale violet colour. (*Note*—Thick parts of the film will not decolourise and are in any case unsuitable for examination.)

6. Counter-stain with dilute basic fuchsin till the film is pink (not dark red)—10 to 25 seconds; wash, dry. As an alternative a neutral red counterstain is often preferred for intracellular gram-negative organisms.

## Ziehl-Neelsen Staining Method

This method is used to detect tubercle bacilli in smears for example, of sputum, which are spread on glass slides. For this purpose opaque or purulent portions of the sputum should be selected. Using a sterile platinum loop, the material is spread on a clean slide so as to make thick and thinner parts. The loop should be resterilised in a flame. The smear should be allowed to dry by gentle heat above a flame. The film should then be heated in the flame for a few seconds, allowed to cool, and then be stained by the Ziehl-Neelsen method as follows:

1. Cover the fixed smear with concentrated carbol-fuchsin and heat gently above the Bunsen flame till steam rises (avoid boiling); repeat the heating three or four times in the course of five minutes. The film must on no account become dry; add fresh stain, if necessary, to prevent this.

2. Wash in running water for one minute.

3. Decolourise with 20 per cent sulphuric acid solution in water (several minutes).

4. Wash in running water for one minute. At this stage the smear should be colourless or of a faint pink colour; if it is definitely red, repeat stage (3) and then wash again.

5. Pour on methylated spirit and allow this to act for one minute; wash off with water.

6. Counter-stain with 1 per cent aqueous methylene blue for half a minute or longer.

7. Wash in water; dry.

# NOTES ON INTERNATIONAL SYSTEM OF UNITS (SI UNITS)

## Units of Volume and Concentration

*Volume.* The basic SI unit of volume is the cubic metre (1,000 litre). Because of its convenience the litre is used as the unit of volume in laboratory work.

*Amount of Substance ('Molar') Concentration* (e.g., $mol/l$, $\mu mol/l$) is used for substances of defined chemical composition. It replaces equivalent concentration $(mEq/l)$ which is not part of the SI system—for reporting measurements of sodium, potassium, chloride and bicarbonate. The numerical value of these measurements is unchanged.

*Mass Concentration* (e.g., $g/l$, $\mu g/l$) is used for all protein measurements, for substances which do not have a sufficiently well defined composition and for plasma vitamin $B_{12}$ and folate measurements. The numerical value in SI units will change by a factor of 10 in those instances previously expressed in terms of 100 ml.

Haemoglobin is an exception. It is agreed internationally that meantime haemoglobin should continue to be expressed in terms of $g/dl$ ($g/100\,ml$).

Non-SI units are employed for enzymes and immunoglobulins.

# Appendix

'There is no authority except facts. These are obtained by accurate observation. Deductions are to be made only from facts.'

Hippocrates, 5th century B.C.

Details are given, in this Appendix, of stages in the development of infants and children, average weights and heights for boys and girls (Table 4), average crown-rump lengths and sitting heights (Table 5), average head circumference (Table 6) and average times of eruption of teeth (Table 7). These are followed by charts for recording growth.

Desirable weights for men and women are presented in Table 8.

Nomograms in Table 9 give the metric equivalent for measurements, in other systems, of volume, weight, length and temperature.

A method of case recording is presented on page 466.

## Stages in Development

Illingworth, R. S. (1972). *The Development of the Infant and Young Child*, 5th ed. Edinburgh and London: Churchill Livingstone.

### 4 weeks

Prone position—pelvis high, knees under abdomen.
Almost complete head lag on pulling into sitting position.
Grasp reflex present.

### 6 weeks

Head held momentarily in same place as rest of body on ventral suspension.
Prone—pelvis high, knees no longer under abdomen.
Considerable, but not complete head lag on pulling into sitting position.
Grasp reflex may be lost.
Smiles at mother.
Follows objects with eyes.

### 3 months

Head held beyond plane of rest of body on ventral suspension.
Prone—pelvis flat on couch.
Only slight head lag on pulling to sit.
Momentary grasping when object placed in hand.
Squeals of pleasure.
'Hand regard' evident, i.e. visual study of his own hands.
Turns head to sound.

### 6 months

Sits supported by his own hands.
Supine—spontaneously lifts head off couch.
Bounces when held standing.
Feeds self with biscuit.

Transfers object from one hand to other.
Responds to name.

### 9 months
Crawls by pulling forward with hands.
Can pull himself into sitting position.
Sits steadily without overbalancing.
Can stand holding on to furniture.
Can release grasped objects.
Waves 'bye-bye'.

### 1 year
Walks supported by one hand.
Beginning to throw objects to floor.
May understand simple phrases.
Uses two or three words with meaning.

### 18 months
Walks up stairs with support.
Seats self on chair.
Builds 3 to 4 cubes on top of each other.
Takes off socks, gloves.
Scribbles with pencil.
Points to parts of body.

### 2 years
Goes up and down stairs.
Runs.
Turns door knob.
Kicks ball.
Puts on socks, etc.
Turns pages of book singly.
Asks for things.

### 3 years
Jumps off a step.
Rides tricycle.
Dresses and undresses.
Copies circle with pencil.
Knows nursery rhymes.
Can count, e.g. up to 10.

### 5 years
Skips on both feet.
Ties shoelaces.
Gives age when asked.
Can name four colours.

TABLE 4. AVERAGE HEIGHTS AND WEIGHTS OF BOYS AND GIRLS

| Age | BOYS | | GIRLS | |
|---|---|---|---|---|
| | Height cm | Weight kg | Height cm | Weight kg |
| Birth | 50·7 | 3·4 | 49·8 | 3·3 |
| 2 weeks | 51·7 | 3·4 | 51·0 | 3·3 |
| 3 months | 60·2 | 5·8 | 58·8 | 5·4 |
| 6 months | 66·6 | 7·9 | 64·9 | 7·4 |
| 9 months | 71·2 | 9·2 | 69·6 | 8·7 |
| 1 year | 75·1 | 10·3 | 73·9 | 9·8 |
| 1½ years | 80·6 | 11·4 | 79·1 | 10·9 |
| 2 years | 86·2 | 12·6 | 84·3 | 11·9 |
| 2½ years | 90·5 | 13·6 | 89·1 | 13·0 |
| 3 years | 94·7 | 14·6 | 93·2 | 14·1 |
| 3½ years | 98·7 | 15·7 | 97·4 | 15·1 |
| 4 years | 102·0 | 16·7 | 100·9 | 16·2 |
| 4½ years | 105·5 | 17·7 | 104·2 | 17·1 |
| 5 years | 108·6 | 18·6 | 107·6 · | 18·0 |
| 5½ years | 110·4 | 19·0 | 110·4 | 18·9 |
| 6 years | 112·4 | 20·0 | 113·0 | 19·8 |
| 7 years | 118·8 | 22·4 | 118·4 | 22·0 |
| 8 years | 123·7 | 24·5 | 123·3 | 24·0 |
| 9 years | 127·9 | 26·4 | 127·8 | 26·3 |
| 10 years | 133·3 | 28·9 | 132·8 | 28·7 |
| 11 years | 138·7 | 31·8 | 138·4 | 31·7 |
| 12 years | 144·7 | 35·2 | 144·9 | 36·3 |
| 13 years | 150·3 | 39·5 | 151·8 | 41·8 |
| 14 years | 156·0 | 44·0 | 156·1 | 46·4 |
| 15 years | 163·3 | 50·3 | 159·6 | 50·5 |

NOTES. (i) *Height* can be measured as standing height from the age of 18 months onwards, the child standing barefooted with heels and back against a vertical surface or rule. The head should be held upright with the line of sight parallel to the floor. A right-angled block held against the vertical surface or a sliding bar at right angles to the rule should then be moved down until it touched the child's head. One standard deviation from above means would be approximately ± 4 per cent. (ii) Weight should be measured in the nude or with child wearing thin pants. One standard deviation from above means would be approximately ± 12½ per cent. (iii) These tables are derived from the data of Thomson J. (1954), *Hlth Bull.* **12,** 25; Acheson R. M., Kemp, F. H. & Parfit, J. (1955), *Lancet,* **1,** 691; Provis, H. S. & Ellis, R. W. B. (1955), *Archs Dis. Childh.* **30,** 328.

TABLE 5. AVERAGE CROWN-RUMP LENGTHS AND SITTING HEIGHTS

| AGE | BOYS | | GIRLS | |
|---|---|---|---|---|
| | Crown-Rump Lengths | | | |
| | in | cm | in | cm |
| Birth | 13·5 | 34·3 | 13·2 | 33·6 |
| 2 weeks | 13·7 | 34·8 | 13·5 | 34·2 |
| 3 months | 15·6 | 39·5 | 15·4 | 39·0 |
| 6 months | 17·4 | 44·2 | 16·9 | 42·9 |
| 9 months | 18·3 | 46·5 | 17·8 | 45·2 |
| 1 year | 19·1 | 48·4 | 18·5 | 47·0 |
| 1½ years | 20·4 | 51·8 | 19·8 | 50·2 |
| 2 years | 21·5 | 54·5 | 20·8 | 52·9 |
| 3 years | 23·0 | 58·4 | 22·5 | 57·2 |
| | Sitting Heights | | | |
| 3 years | 22·4 | 57·1 | 21·8 | 55·3 |
| 4 years | 23·6 | 59·9 | 22·7 | 57·7 |
| 5 years | 24·4 | 61·9 | 23·9 | 60·6 |
| 6 years | 25·1 | 63·7 | 24·8 | 63·0 |
| 7 years | 25·9 | 65·8 | 25·9 | 65·7 |
| 8 years | 26·6 | 67·6 | 26·7 | 67·9 |
| 9 years | 27·4 | 69·7 | 27·4 | 69·6 |
| 10 years | 28·3 | 71·8 | 28·1 | 71·5 |
| 11 years | 29·0 | 73·8 | 29·2 | 74·1 |
| 12 years | 29·9 | 76·0 | 30·5 | 77·4 |
| 13 years | 31·0 | 78·6 | 32·0 | 81·3 |
| 14 years | 32·1 | 81·6 | 33·1 | 84·0 |
| 15 years | 33·6 | 85·5 | 33·9 | 86·2 |

TABLE 6. AVERAGE HEAD CIRCUMFERENCE

| Age | Inches | Cm | Age | Inches | Cm |
|---|---|---|---|---|---|
| Birth | 13·8 | 35·0 | 6 years | 20·2 | 51·2 |
| 3 months | 15·9 | 40·4 | 7 years | 20·3 | 51·7 |
| 6 months | 17·1 | 43·4 | 8 years | 20·4 | 52·0 |
| 9 months | 17·8 | 45·2 | 9 years | 20·6 | 52·2 |
| 1 year | 18·3 | 46·4 | 10 years | 20·7 | 52·5 |
| 1½ years | 18·8 | 47·7 | 11 years | 20·8 | 52·9 |
| 2 years | 19·3 | 49·0 | 12 years | 21·0 | 53·4 |
| 3 years | 19·5 | 49·6 | 13 years | 21·2 | 53·8 |
| 4 years | 19·7 | 50·0 | 14 years | 21·3 | 54·1 |
| 5 years | 20·0 | 50·7 | 15 years | 21·6 | 54·8 |

One standard deviation from these means is approximately $\pm 2\frac{1}{2}$ per cent.
(Data derived from Provis, H. S. & Ellis, R. W. B. (1955). *Archs Dis. Childh.* **30,** 328; Thomson, J. (1956). *Br. J. prev. soc. Med.* **10,** 128; Nelson, W: E. (1959). *Textbook of Pediatrics,* 7th ed., Philadelphia: Saunders.)

TABLE 7. AVERAGE TIMES OF ERUPTION OF TEETH IN PRIMARY AND SECONDARY DENTITIONS

| Deciduous teeth | Date of eruption | Permanent dentition | Date of eruption |
|---|---|---|---|
| Central incisors | 8th month | First molars | 6th– 7th year |
| Lateral incisors | 10th month | Central incisors | 6th– 7th year |
| First molars | 12th month | Lateral incisors | 7th– 9th year |
| Canines | 18th month | First premolars | 10th–11th year |
| Second molars | 24th month | Canines | 10th–12th year |
| | | Second premolars | 10th–12th year |
| | | Second molars | 12th year |
| | | Third molars | 17th–25th year |

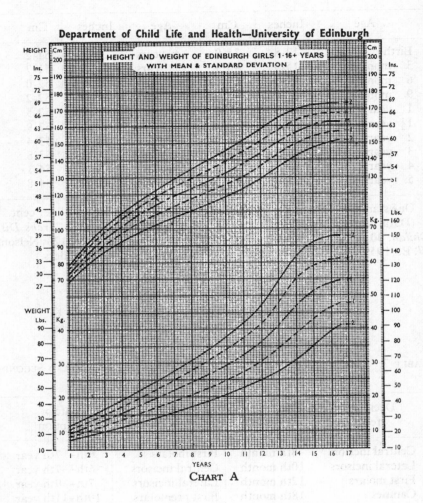

CHART A

Charts A and B can be used in a variety of ways, for instance (i) to compare a single observation of height or weight with the normal means and ranges for children of similar weight in the community; in interpreting such observations the height, but to a much lesser extent the weight, of the parents should be taken into account—thus a normal height for a child whose parents' heights

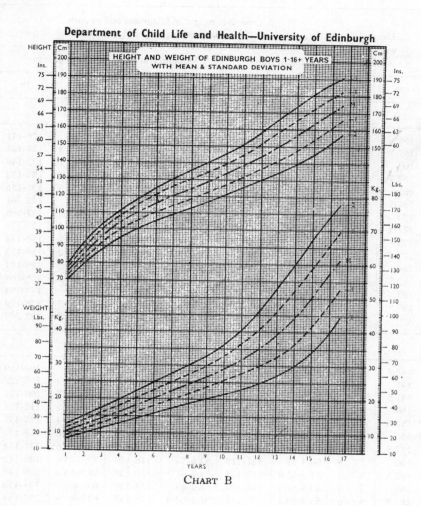

Department of Child Life and Health—University of Edinburgh

HEIGHT AND WEIGHT OF EDINBURGH BOYS 1-16+ YEARS
WITH MEAN & STANDARD DEVIATION

CHART B

were below average would be below the mean on the chart; (ii) to plot serial observations with a view to detecting any trend; (iii) to make a comparison between height and weight in respect of their relationship to community values, e.g. dissociation between height and weight on the graphs would indicate that a child was light for height or overweight for height.

## TABLE 8. DESIRABLE WEIGHTS OF ADULTS
### According to height and frame.

| Height without shoes | | | Desirable weight in kilograms and pounds (in indoor clothing), ages 25 and over | | | | | |
|---|---|---|---|---|---|---|---|---|
| | | | Small frame | | Medium frame | | Large frame | |
| cm | ft | in | kg | lb | kg | lb | kg | lb |
| | | | | Men | | | | |
| 155 | 5 | 1 | 50·8-54·4 | 112-120 | 53·5-58·5 | 118-129 | 57·2-64 | 126-141 |
| 157·5 | 5 | 2 | 52·2-55·8 | 115-123 | 54·9-60·3 | 121-133 | 58·5-65·3 | 129-144 |
| 160 | 5 | 3 | 53·5-57·2 | 118-126 | 56·2-61·7 | 124-136 | 59·9-67·1 | 132-148 |
| 162·5 | 5 | 4 | 54·9-58·5 | 121-129 | 57·6-63 | 127-139 | 61·2-68·9 | 135-152 |
| 165 | 5 | 5 | 56·2-60·3 | 124-133 | 59 -64·9 | 130-143 | 62·6-70·8 | 138-156 |
| 167·5 | 5 | 6 | 58·1-62·1 | 128-137 | 60·8-66·7 | 134-147 | 64·4-73 | 142-161 |
| 170 | 5 | 7 | 59·9-64 | 132-141 | 62·6-68·9 | 138-152 | 66·7-75·3 | 147-166 |
| 172·5 | 5 | 8 | 61·7-65·8 | 136-145 | 64·4-70·8 | 142-156 | 68·5-77·1 | 151-170 |
| 175 | 5 | 9 | 63·5-68 | 140-150 | 66·2-72·6 | 146-160 | 70·3-78·9 | 155-174 |
| 177·5 | 5 | 10 | 65·3-69·9 | 144-154 | 68 -74·8 | 150-165 | 72·1-81·2 | 159-179 |
| 180 | 5 | 11 | 67·1-71·7 | 148-158 | 69·9-77·1 | 154-170 | 74·4-83·5 | 164-184 |
| 182·5 | 6 | 0 | 68·9-73·5 | 152-162 | 71·7-79·4 | 158-175 | 76·2-85·7 | 168-189 |
| 185 | 6 | 1 | 70·8-75·7 | 156-167 | 73·5-81·6 | 162-180 | 78·5-88 | 173-194 |
| 187·5 | 6 | 2 | 72·6-77·6 | 160-171 | 75·7-83·5 | 167-185 | 80·7-90·3 | 178-199 |
| 190 | 6 | 3 | 74·4-79·4 | 164-175 | 78·1-86·2 | 172-190 | 82·7-92·5 | 182-204 |
| | | | | Women | | | | |
| 142·5 | 4 | 8 | 41·7-44·5 | 92-98 | 43·5-48·5 | 96-107 | 47·2-54 | 104-119 |
| 145 | 4 | 9 | 42·6-45·8 | 94-101 | 44·5-49·9 | 98-110 | 48·1-55·3 | 106-122 |
| 147·5 | 4 | 10 | 43·5-47·2 | 96-104 | 45·8-51·3 | 101-113 | 49·4-56·7 | 109-125 |
| 150 | 4 | 11 | 44·9-48·5 | 99-107 | 47·2-52·6 | 104-116 | 50·8-58·1 | 112-128 |
| 152·5 | 5 | 0 | 46·3-49·9 | 102-110 | 48·5-54 | 107-119 | 52·2-59·4 | 115-131 |
| 155 | 5 | 1 | 47·6-51·3 | 105-113 | 49·9-55·3 | 110-122 | 53·5-60·8 | 118-134 |
| 157·5 | 5 | 2 | 49 -52·6 | 108-116 | 51·3-57·2 | 113-126 | 54·9-62·6 | 121-138 |
| 160 | 5 | 3 | 50·3-54 | 111-119 | 52·6-59 | 116-130 | 56·7-64·4 | 125-142 |
| 162·5 | 5 | 4 | 51·7-55·8 | 114-123 | 54·4-61·2 | 120-135 | 58·5-66·2 | 129-146 |
| 165 | 5 | 5 | 53·5-57·6 | 118-127 | 56·2-63 | 124-139 | 60·3-68 | 133-150 |
| 167·5 | 5 | 6 | 55·3-59·4 | 122-131 | 58·1-64·9 | 128-143 | 62·1-69·9 | 137-154 |
| 170 | 5 | 7 | 57·2-61·2 | 126-135 | 59·9-66·7 | 132-147 | 64 -71·7 | 141-158 |
| 172·5 | 5 | 8 | 59 -63·5 | 130-140 | 61·7-68·5 | 136-151 | 65·8-73·9 | 145-163 |
| 175 | 5 | 9 | 60·8-65·3 | 134-144 | 63·5-70·3 | 140-155 | 67·6-76·2 | 149-168 |
| 177·5 | 5 | 10 | 62·6-67·1 | 138-148 | 65·3-72·1 | 144-159 | 69·4-78·5 | 153-173 |

Based on weights of insured persons in the United States associated with lowest mortality (*Statist. bull. Metrop. Life Insur. Co.*, 40, Nov.-Dec. 1959).

## TABLE 9

| VOLUME | WEIGHT | TEMPERATURE |
|---|---|---|
| 28·4ml | 1kg = 2·2lbs | To convert °F to |
| (30ml approx.) | | °C, subtract 32 |
| =1fl oz | | then multiply |
| | | by ⅝ |

**VOLUME**

| ml | fl oz |
|---|---|
| 1,000 (1 litre) | 35 |
| 900 | 30 |
| 800 | |
| 700 | |
| 600 | 20 (1 pint) |
| 500 | |
| 400 | |
| 300 | 10 |
| 200 | |
| 100 | |
| 0 | 0 |
| ml | fl oz |

**WEIGHT**

| kg | lb |
|---|---|
| | 14 (1 stone) |
| 6 | 13 |
| | 12 |
| 5 | 11 |
| | 10 |
| 4 | 9 |
| | 8 |
| | 7 |
| 3 | 6 |
| | 5 |
| 2 | 4 |
| | 3 |
| 1 | 2 |
| | 1 |
| 0 | 0 |
| kg | lb |

**TEMPERATURE**

| °C | °F |
|---|---|
| 40 | 104 |
| | 103 |
| 39 | 102 |
| | 101 |
| 38 | 100 |
| | 99 |
| 37 | 98 |
| 36 | 97 |
| | 96 |
| 35 | 95 |
| | 94 |
| 34 | 93 |
| | 92 |
| 33 | 91 |
| | 90 |
| 32 | 89 |
| | 88 |
| 31 | 87 |
| 30 | 86 |
| °C | °F |

## LENGTH

2·54cm = 1in , 30·48cm = 1ft

cm
0   1   2   3   4   5   6   7   8   9   10   cm

0   1   2   3   4
in                                         in

# A SYSTEM OF CASE RECORDING

Name:      Age:      Sex:      Marital status:

Address:      Telephone No.:

Occupation: In the case of a married woman give that of her husband and her own if she also works. In the case of a child give the parents' occupation.

Family doctor:

Date of admission to hospital:

Date of examination:

## History

**Present Illness.** Begin by naming the presenting or principal symptoms and the duration of each. Proceed with a chronological account of the mode of onset and course of the patient's illness. *Systemic enquiry:* record any symptoms such as cough, breathlessness, digestive or urinary troubles, pain, insomnia or change in weight. Note any *drugs* taken and any *allergy*.

**Previous Health.** Illness, operations, accidents, and their dates. Note any travel abroad. Date and result of any previous medical examination (e.g. for life insurance) and of chest or other radiological examination. History of birth in the case of infants and children.

**Family History.** Note age, health, or cause of death of parents, siblings, spouse and children (Fig. 1, p. 6).

**Social and Personal History.** Record the relevant information about occupation, housing, and personal habits regarding recreation, physical exercise, alcohol and tobacco, and in the case of children, about school and family relationships.

## Physical Examination

**General Assessment.** In an introductory statement comment on the patient's *demeanour* and *general condition*, i.e. physique, nutrition, state of hydration, gait, posture, personality and mental state. Record height and weight. Note any abnormality not recorded under a systemic heading, e.g.:

*Hands and Arms.* Note any information of diagnostic value obtained from inspection of hands and nails. Epitrochlear and axillary lymph nodes.

*Head, Face and Neck.* Describe in detail any abnormality such as goitre or enlarged lymph nodes.

*Skin.* Colour; pallor, cyanosis, pigmentation, jaundice, etc. Specific lesions.

*Subcutaneous Tissues.* Nodules; vascular abnormalities; oedema.

*Breasts.*

### Cardiovascular System

**Arterial Pulse and Pressure.** Rate, rhythm, wave form and volume of radial pulse. Blood pressure.

**Jugular Venous Pulse and Pressure.** Note form of the jugular pulse wave and height of the jugular venous pressure.

**Heart.**

*Inspection.* Pulsations and deformity of anterior chest wall.

*Palpation.* Position and character of apex beat and other pulsations; thrills.

*Auscultation.* First and second heart sounds; added sounds; murmurs.

**Peripheral Circulation.**

*Arterial.* Pulsation of limb arteries; skin temperature and colour; local nutrition; bruits.

*Venous.* Abnormal vessels; signs of inflammation or occlusion.

## Respiratory System

Note cough, character and quantity of sputum, wheeze or other respiratory difficulty.

**Upper Respiratory Tract.** Nose; tonsils; pharynx; position of trachea.

**Chest.**

*Inspection.* Shape and lesions of chest wall; respiration rate and depth; chest expansion; mode of breathing.

*Palpation.* Range of movement; vocal fremitus.

*Percussion.* Anterior, lateral and posterior chest wall; hepatic dullness.

*Auscultation.* Breath sounds, vocal resonance and added sounds.

## Alimentary and Genito-Urinary Systems

**Mouth.** Lips, tongue, teeth, gums. Character of any vomitus.

**Abdomen.**

*Inspection.* Scars; veins; hair. Abdominal wall: shape, general and local changes, e.g. hernias and movement of respiratory, peristaltic, vascular or foetal origin.

*Palpation.* Tenderness; guarding; individual organs and abnormal masses; hernial orifices; inguinal lymph nodes.

*Percussion.* Fluid, gas, and individual organs.

*Auscultation.* Frequency and character of bowel sounds; vascular bruits.

**Rectum.** Inspection of the anus and examination of rectum if indicated; inspection of and testing of faeces for occult blood, if indicated.

**Genitalia.** *Inspection.*

*Palpation.* Vaginal examination in special circumstances only.

**Urine.** Volume, colour, opacity, odour, reaction, specific gravity; microscopy; chemical tests for protein, glucose and other substances as indicated.

## Nervous System

**Intellectual function.** See Psychiatric State (p. 468).

**Speech.** Language function, articulation, phonation.

**Cranial nerves.**

*First.* Sense of smell.

*Second.* Ophthalmoscopic examination; visual acuity; visual fields.

*Third, Fourth and Sixth.* Eyelids, ptosis, palpebral fissures; pupils, size, shape, symmetry and reflexes; eye movements, diplopia and nystagmus.

*Fifth.* Facial sensation; muscles of mastication, corneal reflex and jaw jerk.

*Seventh*. Movements of facial muscles; taste on the anterior two thirds of the tongue.

*Eighth*. Auriscopic examination; estimation of auditory acuity; tuning fork tests; positional nystagmus.

*Ninth*. Sensation of pharynx and of the posterior third of the tongue; palatal and pharyngeal reflexes.

*Tenth*. Phonation; movements of palate and posterior pharyngeal wall; gag reflex.

*Eleventh*. Sternomastoid and trapezius muscles.

*Twelfth*. Inspection of tongue and its movements.

**Motor System.** Inspection of musculature; involuntary movements including fasciculation; tone; clonus; power; co-ordination; fine movements; dyspraxia.

**Sensory System.** Touch and pain sensation; temperature; position and vibration sense; cortical sensory function, e.g. two point discrimination, stereognosis.

**Reflexes.** Tendon reflexes; abdominal and plantar responses.

**Supplementary Tests.** Bruits audible in the neck of skull. Meningeal or nerve root irritation. Tetany.

## Locomotor System

**Spine.** Movements.

**Joints of Limbs.** Movements, deformity, swelling, tenderness, temperature.

**Muscles.** Atrophy, contractures, swelling, tenderness.

**Bones.** Deformity, tenderness.

## Psychiatric State

**The Mental State.**

1. *General appearance and behaviour.*
2. *Thought processes. Sample of talk.*
3. *Mood.*
4. *Delusions.*
5. *Hallucinations.*
6. *Obsessions.*
7. *Evidence of intellectual defect.*
    *(i)   Orientation.*
    *(ii)  Memory.*
    *(iii) Attention and concentration.*
    *(iv  General information.*
    *(v)   Intelligence.*
8. *Insight and judgement.*

**Personality Diagnosis.**

## Clinical Diagnosis

Record the differential diagnosis in order of probability.

## Further Investigations

It is helpful to outline a plan of any further investigations considered necessary at this stage.

## Treatment and Progress Notes

These should be entered from day to day.

## Final Diagnosis

## Summary

It is advisable to conclude the case recording with a brief summary incorporating the principal symptoms, the main abnormalities on physical examination, the significant findings on further investigation, the diagnosis, the therapeutic measures employed and the decisions regarding further management. Alternatively the summary can take the form of a 'problem list' as described below.

## PROBLEM-ORIENTATED MEDICAL RECORDS

The traditional method of case recording is now being adapted in many centres to incorporate the problem-orientated medical record developed by Weed and his colleagues (1968). Basic information is collected by the methods described in this book but its recording is orientated around the patient's problems. Weed's system is structured into four main components, the data base, the problem list, the initial plan and the progress notes.

**1. Data base.** This consists of:

(a) the principal complaint.

(b) relevant social data and the 'profile'; the latter is a description of how the patient spends an average day. Therapeutic goals can be related to this profile.

(c) the history.

(d) the physical examination.

(e) laboratory and other basic investigations. such as haemoglobin, urea and electrolytes and chest radiography.

**2. Problem List.** All the patient's problems. physical, psychological and social, present and past. are numbered and named on a list displayed prominently on the front of the patient's notes. Problems are then classified as either active or resolved. The former category includes not only those which have been diagnosed but also all unexplained or ambiguous findings.

In the case of hospital patients the problem list is best prepared about 24 hours after admission. It is open ended and is modified as the situation is clarified. New problems are added as they are recognised. The problem list serves also as a guide to the case notes and provides a summary which helps not only the medical staff but also nurses, physiotherapists, social workers and others to assess the position 'at a glance'. An example of a problem list is given in Fig. 126.

---

**Problem List**   (1.5.74)
Mrs. A.B.C.   (Date of birth 1.5.34)

|  . **Active** | **Inactive** |
|---|---|
| 1.  Acute abdominal pain<br>   acute cholecystitis (2.5.74)<br>   cholecystectomy (10.5.74) | |
| 2.  Obesity | |
| 3.  Varicose veins | |
| 4.  Hysterical psychoneurosis | |
| 5.  Psoriasis | |
| 6.  Left facial pain<br>   secondary to 4 (4.5.74) | |
| 7.  Social deprivation<br>   (divorced; 4 children;<br>   2 rooms) | |
| | 8.  Duodenal ulcer (1970) |
| | 9.  Penicillin allergy (1968) |
| 10.  Pulmonary embolism<br>   (16.5.74) | |

---

FIG. 126   An example of the basic features of a Problem List. A glance at this gives an overall view of the current situation in the context of the patient's total medical needs. *Note*. Problems 1 and 6 were redefined when their aetiology became clear on the dates shown. Problem 8 signalled the need for particular care in the use of anticoagulants for problem 10. Problem 9 warned the clinician that ampicillin was contraindicated in the treatment of problem 1. The patient required realistic advice about problem 2 in relation to problem 7, which itself received attention from social workers. Further treatment was planned for problems 3 and 5.

**3. Initial Plan.** For each active problem an initial plan is organised from three aspects:
(a)  the collection of further data to establish the diagnosis.
(b)  therapy.
(c)  education of the patient in active participation in the management of his disease.
**4. Progress Notes.** The records are kept up to date by entering all additional relevant information, as it is obtained, under the named and

numbered title of the problem to which it pertains. The notes are further structured by sub-headings:

   (a) subjective data; prominence is given first to the patient's reactions.

   (b) objective data.

   (c) interpretation; this includes both decisions and impressions.

   (d) therapy; this includes education of the patient.

   (e) immediate plans.

These notes are supplemented by '*flow sheets*' when dealing with fast moving situations such as diabetic ketoacidosis, peripheral circulatory failure or acute ventilatory failure. Then the inter-relationships of data and therapy are crucial; time, serial measurements, therapy and comment are recorded side by side and repeated as frequently as the situation demands.

Finally a *discharge report* is prepared summarising each numbered problem on the list; particular attention is paid to any problems which may not have been fully elucidated or which may recur.

## Conclusion

Weed's original work must be consulted for further information about problem-orientated medical records, including illustrations of these methods in practice and the philosophy on which they are based.

The system presents data in structured dynamic ways readily amenable to assessment. The methods, however, are time consuming and this has been a barrier to acceptance in their entirety. Many clinicians have particularly welcomed the problem list as a flexible, intelligible and up-to-date summary which allows an immediate grasp of the medical and social situation and reduces errors of omission and commission in treatment. Weed's methodology also reminds us that the quality and scope of medical care is reflected in its recording.

*References*

Weed, L. L. (1968) Medical records that guide and teach. *New Eng. J. Med.*, **278**, 593 and 652.

Weed, L. L. (1970) *Medical Records, Medical Education and Patient Care— The Problem-orientated Record as a Basic Tool.* Cleveland, Ohio: Press of Case, Western Reserve University.

# Index

## A